Discovery of Magnetic Health

A Health Care Alternative

D0441860

GEORGE J. WASHNIS
AND
RICHARD Z. HRICAK

NOVA Publishing Company
Rockville, Maryland, U.S.A.

This book is published by

TM

NOVA Publishing Company
11607 Nebel Street
Rockville, MD 20852
1-800-637-0067 or 301-231-8229
Fax 301-816-0816

ISBN 0-9639560-1-9

Library of Congress Cataloging-in-Publication Data

Discovery of Magnetic Health; Magnetic Therapy;
Alternative Medicine; Effects of Magnetic Fields;
George Washnis and Richard Hricak; includes index

This book is offered for information purposes and to present
research opportunities for government agencies and private
foundations. It is based on the best biomedical data, clinical and
controlled tests by leading physicians and other experts that have
been made available at this time. Any advice or information
offered here if acted on is intended to be adjunctive to the advice
and care of a physician or other trusted health professional.
Information on proprietary products in connection with illnesses
or procedures does not represent the opinion of the providers of
these products.

To all
those people sincerely interested in
improving their health and all those
already using this medicine who
desire more information and all those
dedicated physicians and other
professionals who want to
give all their patients
every possible reliable
and safe alternative
for better health
and happiness.

Table of Contents

List of Exhibits

Page

List of Exhibits (cont'd)

Acknowledgments

A special note of commendation goes to **Richard Z. Hricak** who, after discovering that little was available on the subject of magnetotherapy, inspired this enterprise and encouraged its research and completion, as well as providing study materials. His exposure to and interest in magnetic products brought him closer to the understanding of the therapeutic effects of various magnetic devices and their influence on human stress, sleep, and other problems. He has also experimented with the effects of magnetic fields on plants, auto engines and other processes. The experiments and tests that he has conducted on reducing auto emissions could very possibly be a breakthrough for pollution control. Without his avid interest, this book probably would not have gotten underway. His wife Astrid and daughters Salina and Sandra have waited patiently and supportively while this work has come to fruition. Families must always be given so much credit.

As with most ventures, credit must go to a lot of people. Regina and Jack Snyder saw the value of this very important book for the safety and health of society and gave materially so the work could be carried forth. Their integrity and concern for the general welfare of people are highly commendable.

The series of typists and word processors and helpers has been wonderful. Jack Snyder's daughter Cathy word processed a first draft of the book. Arun Bhatia went through the document for a second draft. Thanks also goes to Neal Farrell for typing a lot of the correspondence and for monitoring communication links.

Devotedly, Vivian Kwok, an initial supporter of the project, brought the camera-ready copy near to completion. This was no easy task as she read through scribbled notes, but still beautifully aligned the paragraphs and chapters in readable order. Her choice of varied styled print, shading of information, creation of graphs, corrections, etc., made it a desirable product to envision and worth all the effort. I'm sure she'll be in demand for more of this quality work from us and others.

A final commendatory note for preparation to get the book to the printer goes to Neha Sharad who made the absolute final page and alignment corrections. Those last minute word changes and print selections were hers to make while she performed with the highest skills and devotion regardless of time constraints and computer idiosyncrasies. And the job got done. Thanks.

So much credit needs to go to all those medical and scientific experts who gave so freely of their advice and talents, but only a small number can be mentioned here. Dr. William H. Philpott, M.D. and Dr. Dean Bonlie, D.D.S. were probably the major expert contributors. This author talked or interviewed these people dozens of times. Dr. John Zimmerman was another meticulous reviewer and provider of information. Both Bonlie and Zimmerman went over almost every paragraph of the book, making valuable comments. This subject is so complex, I'm sure more questions would have been raised without their insistence of unique points-of-view and scientific analysis. And Robert R. Barefoot, a chemist and holder of several international patents, was a must in explaining the human biological process, as we conversed dozens of times over the phone, passing materials back and forth. Much thanks also goes to Dr. William Pawluk who reviewed and commented on the manuscript extensively. Dr. Harry Park, M.D. and Duwayne Loberg and many others were simply marvelous in their candor and expertise and for passing on valuable research materials.

Of course, Dr. Philpott, founder of the Orthomolecular Psychiatric Association and author or co-author of a number of books, including **Brain Allergies**, **Victory over Diabetes**, **New Hope for Physical and Emotional Illnesses**, etc., was very much fundamental to many of the book's concepts. He is a physician who has treated more than 100,000 patients and, most recently over the past decade, has treated thousands of patients with magnetotherapy. His clinical experience and precise record keeping have provided an invaluable source of documentation of exciting cases. His recommended research, prescribed in the appendix, if supported by the Congress and undertaken by the NIH and private groups could mean a vast improvement in our health system and the medical profession.

For me, this has been the most interesting project that I have worked on. I chose not to lay it aside for anything, although there were some trying times when I was financially strapped. I apologize especially to my two lovely daughters Zoe and Serena who may have wondered at times when it was all going to end. Their patience has been miraculous.

I hope this book makes a worthwhile contribution to the medical world and all those people who use magnetic therapy and all those whom it may help. For me it is more important to make an honest and important contribution to society than to find gold at the end of the rainbow. But perhaps the pieces will fit and we will all be better off.

George J. Washnis

Preface

Any material that deals with the basic mysteries of life by its very nature is complex and controversial. Experts on both sides of the question claim to know the efficacy or function of magnetic fields on the human body. Some controlled and anecdotal case studies are presented here that verify degrees of effectiveness, yet much more research needs to be done.

Symptom relief and stages of healing take place from the application of magnets with the negative (north) or positive (south) polarity or bipolar use. Nevertheless, different effects are demonstrated from various combinations of polarities. Some American and Canadian doctors and researchers believe that the negative fields provide the best of long-term healing and in the safest fashion. Many other nations, including Japan, China, India, and European agree that there are polarity differences but also that most combinations are safe and effective when used at appropriate gauss strength. Some companies with millions of satisfied users space magnets in their mattresses and pads sufficiently distanced so that they are actually getting a bipolar effect and a safe gauss strength. Traditional viewpoints should be respected and, of course, new evidence and case histories equally evaluated.

Those using age old, successful methodologies should be encouraged to utilize what has proved safe. But new thought must also be explored concerning effects of magnets from different polarities, field power, weight, frequency, size, and duration of use, among other factors discussed in the following pages from hundreds of sources. This information should benefit all providers, physicians, patients, and the medical community in general, making this therapy even safer and more effective. Some of the marvels expressed here for improving sleep, eliminating pain and stress, attacking chronic fatigue syndrome, replacing electro-shock treatments with more benign procedures, and helping to resolve epilepsy, psychosis, drug and alcohol addiction, and much more may be too hard to believe but not too hard to research further from existing credible data. It is a matter of convincing unwilling minds to redirect their thoughts. We cannot let the naysayers hold progress back to the detriment of society. Over 50 million people use this therapy, hundreds of thousands in the U.S. alone. They deserve answers. Advanced knowledge should allow us to improve on this natural technology, increase the percentage of patient cures, gain acceptance from the conventional community, and help to improve the health system here and worldwide.

March 25, 1994

EXPLANATORY NOTICE

Some distributors and users of magnetic health products have been concerned about the efficacy and safety of various polarities and gauss strengths of magnets. Hopefully, the following explanation will clarify those questions.

Magnets of different gauss strength and polarity are used for different therapeutic purposes. Higher strength magnets of about 3500 gauss and up have been found useful for more serious or complex ailments. In this range polarity and duration of use are more important. In the case of lower strength magnetic beds and other magnetic devices of 850 gauss or less, for use on the human body, application is considered safe regardless of polarity but with certain limitations associated with adaptation.

Most practitioners and long-time observers, such as Dr. William H. Philpott, M.D. agree that low gauss magnets of either polarity do not cause cell damage and are safe in other respects with the stipulation that a brief rest period may be necessary after two or three months of continued use, in order to rebalance the body's energies due to the reflexology response that leads to adaptation. Use can be resumed immediately thereafter and this same procedure followed as many times as necessary, perfectly safe to the human body and desirable from the standpoint of rebalancing.

Importantly, Dr. Philpott defends the right of distributors and health providers to use magnetic beds and magnetic devices of varying polarities and liniments, acupuncture needles, massage and other methodologies that create the counter-irritant effect which draws essential magnetic fields to areas of the body where most needed. He also accepts the validity of testimonials that report the success of these methods.

Health ministries worldwide and the U.S. Food and Drug Administration also declare these therapies, that harness the body's energies, as medically safe and valid. Interestingly, the FDA does not recognize any medical difference between polarities and has declared magnetics in human diagnosis and therapy, within certain limits, as "not essentially harmful," allowing further study and medical use for additional toxicity evaluation. With the above information in mind, users should feel comfortable and safe, particularly when applying low gauss magnetic products.

William H. Philpott, M.D.

Introduction

We might ask how there can possibly be a health problem when life span has increased and we experience less disease today than ever in history. Impressively, life span took its big jump early in the century, increasing about ten to fifteen years; but there is little evidence that it will advance significantly beyond an average of eighty years unless we begin to engage in preventive techniques and health building. The emphasis now is too strongly on drug therapy and surgery, which do little to increase life span or general health. For a number of reasons, including lifestyles, pollution, a new crop of carcinogens, and the lack of preventive methods, cancers have increased.

Dr. Samuel Epstein of the University of Chicago Medical Center states that over the past decade, lymphoma, myeloma, and melanoma have increased 100 percent, breast cancer 31 percent, testicular cancer 97 percent, cancer of the pancreas 20 percent, cancer of the kidneys 142 percent, and colon cancer 63 percent. Drugs have helped us cut infectious diseases dramatically, but we have accomplished little in the area of cancer and heart disease, our biggest killers. We keep searching for miraculous, "magic-bullet" drug cures and advanced surgery suited for a small percentage of the populace, with little success for improving general health.

It is curious that magnetotherapy has been around for centuries, yet so many people are unable to appreciate its value. Only during the last few decades have we really begun to study scientifically its effects. Now there are controlled studies we can point to for efficacy, clusters of healing, and predictable results that an increasing percentage of physicians are willing to accept. A lot more documentation is needed, but at least we have enough to forge ahead. Importantly, we must keep the charlatans at bay and the fast-buck entrepreneurs under control, or all will be lost again. Society cannot afford to let that happen. This medicine is too important, for it can dramatically improve our health. And with its acceptance, the medical profession can be further guided into the realm of prevention.

The U.S. is the most technologically advanced nation in the world, able to provide the best possible medical care for a large segment of society. But this mostly occurs after disease erupts. We have largely forgotten that medicine is an art—not pure technology. We need the old

1

family doctor technique back again, where the patient finds love and understanding, long-term care and prevention, truth about effectiveness and less greed on the part of providers. Technology has raised the cost of medical care while promises of golden health and extended life have turned empty. The degenerative diseases of heart attack, arteriosclerosis, cancer, stroke, arthritis, hypertension, and ulcers have replaced infectious diseases as our major enemies. We have to stop looking only for a "cookbook" of one shot cures and begin to treat the whole body and its immune system in a preventive fashion by means of proper lifestyle and nutrition, exercise, mental conditioning, and natural therapies of little or no risk.

Self-help can benefit individuals and the nation's health status immensely. People need to begin to take greater charge of their own health. Surely see a doctor for any serious ailment and weigh that advice. If it's a serious matter, a second opinion ought to be sought and the patient (you) ought to ask about alternative cures and preventive techniques. If the doctor doesn't give any alternatives, one must question whether he has done his job. The doctor should communicate with you, educate and promote proper lifestyle, and not be in a rush. Speed is equivalent to productivity improvement, not effectiveness.

The nation has lost much of the preventive health character that our parents and grandparents taught us—much of it wiser than the dangerous drugs recommended to us today. A good preventive maintenance program in our daily lives including alternatives can improve chemical balance, the immune system, pain reduction, and mental well-being. Back problems alone, as just one example, affect eight out of ten people, and the direct and indirect costs run as high as $100 billion a year. Certainly a new approach is needed to get the nation back in shape. We must take the time to understand what is happening to our bodies. We must take control of our own lives. Magnetotherapy is just one of the alternatives that can lead in that direction.

Many people approach the use of magnetic devices as a simple matter. After all, if Queen Cleopatra and others throughout history wore magnetic bracelets and necklaces, why can't we simply do the same and if we heal—fine? Why all the fuss? Well, it's true. A magnetic necklace or wrist or ankle band may help some people. However, if you want to achieve a high degree of success, one must use the proper magnetic strength, magnetic size, polarity, and length of exposure. Simply wearing something, any place, won't do very much for your health. A magnet needs to be placed where the ailment is located for specific periods of time and of sufficient strength to cure a special problem. Bone fusions may require ten or twenty times the strength and depth of penetration as may be necessary for applications on outer tissues and minor bruises and aches and pains.

A magnet placed in a limited location won't do much for the whole body or immune system. Magnetic beds with magnets that provide magnetic fields to every part of the body are necessary for full body treatment, much as the Earth emits a magnetic force evenly over our entire bodies. A magnet in one location will primarily affect that spot without the ability to reach much farther unless at a central nerve center. An 800-gauss, lightweight magnet, for example, may penetrate effectively only a few millimeters into the body. From there, the magnetic fields dissipate rapidly.

Importantly, we must be able to differentiate between the polarities and avoid semantic confusion. The New Encyclopedia Britannica clarifies the difference as it is used here. We are not interested in direction of north and south but rather the biological effect of negative (north) and positive (south) as used throughout this book. Evidence is available that the negative polarity predominates for long-term healing and whenever the need exists for high gauss strength; while, it is shown that the positive fields are especially suited for stimulative functions and special disease characteristics. Both polarities used simultaneously provide what some believe is similar to a pulsing effect that gives quick acting symptom relief. This is perfectly safe if of the proper gauss strength and used for the appropriate duration of time, depending on the human condition at hand and the ailment. Others insist that there is no pulsing at all, rather a biofeedback effect that acts quickly on the painful site since the bipolar magnet influences a minimal amount of surface tissue, as explained in the chapters ahead.

A most common question raised by physicians and others is whether the alternative healing business is all in the mind. The psychosomatic role is significant in healing but scientifically becomes a rather predictable figure according to a number of studies, regardless of the type of therapy. The Johns Hopkins Treatment Pain Center tested the use of magnetic devices with a control group and found that only 13 percent were influenced by the placebo (sham) effect. In a variety of tests by a number of institutions over the years, it has been shown that only about 11 to 13 percent of subjects respond to the placebo effect. The Food and Drug Administration (FDA) concurred in a series of rather elaborate tests by the Japanese that about 17 percent is a consistently reliable figure of psychosomatic response or placebo effect for most types of therapy. Success rates higher than this in most cases show actual physical or therapeutic effect. Magnetotherapy has shown success rates of 70 percent and higher, depending on the ailment. Of course, animals are cured with magnetotherapy at about the same rate as humans. And very infrequently is mind manipulation a factor with animals other than that involving love and respect of the master.

On the other hand, positive mental attitudes, in contrast to unfounded placebo beliefs, improve chances of healing. Visualization of curing and good mental imagery are known to assist in striking away cancers and other diseases for at least a small number of people who have the conviction to do this. It's better to think soundly than not to, but in almost all cases it's still going to take a good treatment or physical regimen to wipe away illness.

Little question exists that we need to know more about magnetic field therapy. The benefits of magnets have been known for thousands of years, yet we are still searching for answers. Most of the medical profession, government agencies, and pharmaceutical companies appear to prefer to wait rather than to find the answers. Over 50 million people use magnetotherapy worldwide so we cannot afford to wait any longer. It is not fair to them or to the rest of the population who possibly could realize healthier lives through proper use of magnetic fields. Furthermore, we are being hurt by magnetic frequencies of the wrong type on our bodies. We need to proceed to take the safest steps for we cannot simply wait and assume that we will be able to find the ultimate mysteries of life. The health industry isn't waiting to experiment with drugs or new technology on our poor bodies. In this respect, we have an obligation to further examine alternatives already deemed safe.

Assuredly, more clinical and double-blind controlled studies are needed. But much of the basic data already exists. Most of the answers could emerge in one or two years of in-depth research. Meanwhile, if there is no hope from conventional medicine for a particular ailment, the patient has the right to try an alternative therapy that shows efficacy. Since magnetotherapy is many times safer than almost all drugs and has demonstrated effectiveness, proper application is warranted. Magnetic field therapy to ailing bodies can relieve pain, improve sleep and quality of life, and can make all the difference in the world for many people. For some, it may do little or nothing, yet it has been shown to have effect in about 70 percent or more of cases. Only the user can judge for himself. Many therapists report that the predictability of success with magnetotherapy is higher than any other treatment.

A single-blind, controlled study simply means that the same procedures and methodology are used on an approximately equal number of subjects receiving treatment and a second group not receiving treatment, called a control, in a test to determine effect. The control group is not administered the key therapy under experimentation, such as a particular drug or magnetic device. Of sixty subjects, for example, thirty would be actually treated with magnetic devices and thirty would not. No individual would be told in advance if he or she were actually being administered the real device. The other control, called double-blind, is when those administering the therapy also do not know which devices have real magnets and which did not, in order to eliminate any bias on the part of the providers. The control subjects are actually the placebo group. A triple-blind is when those measuring outcomes also do not know who was being treated or not treated.

Clinical testing may involve strict observation by doctors or other professionals, of subjects as a group or individually, accumulating results over time under actual treatment conditions. A control or placebo group may or may not be part of this process. A placebo does not necessarily make a double-blind, controlled study any more valid than clinical testing with proper recording, although a good deal of the scientific community considers control trials more acceptable. Nevertheless, if a high number, such as 100 or 1000 patients, are cured by a particular methodology, the fact that some other group was not administered the same therapy as a placebo group does not mean any smaller number of people were cured or the effect is any less. A control group may let us assume greater validity but not necessarily greater effectiveness. Since studies show that the placebo effect occurs in only about 12 to 17 percent of subjects, this phenomenon does not overwhelmingly detract from the success of trials that do not use control groups. The most reliable indicator of efficacy is how often a particular therapy is effective and to what extent. The placebo can help make that judgment yet not invalidate all other clinical tests.

Many doctors and institutions refuse to use control groups in the belief that all patients should be given the best available care without some being fooled. Dr. David Kessler, head of the FDA, believes that there is a valid risk/benefit scenario which postulates that if the risk is low and benefit high, especially for serious illnesses, experimental therapies may be worth it. After all, most of FDA drug validation involves double-blind controlled tests of as little as six weeks of observation without long-term assessment of effect, relying on the anecdotal histories from the drug companies themselves. The FDA is now moving to strengthen this process.

Anecdotal cases (personal descriptions of cures before and after) if of sufficient number and validated with a sense of truthfulness (possibly detailed affidavits) can demonstrate effectiveness. Taking into consideration the usual psychosomatic response, hundreds or thousands of people can't all be fooling us. And for what purpose? Many doctors in the studies reported here keep well recorded results of their patients from beginning to end of treatment, with observation for months, sometimes years later for follow-up. The placebo effect, of course, is used not only to determine psychosomatic response but also to show whether the control group heals just as well without the medication on trial. Most colds, for example, go away just about as quickly without any medicine.

It is important for us to remember that certain kinds of magnetic fields are considered harmful. Perhaps the most controversial, but with ever-increasing evidence, are the adverse effects from high pulsating magnetic pollution all around us—high-power transmission lines, computers, TVs and radios, microwave and other electric appliances, electric blankets, shavers, hair dryers, and possibly even the phones you and I use every day. The ordinary 60 cycle household A.C. electricity and also other higher frequency currents can cause memory loss, headaches, changes in heartbeat and blood chemistry, and general malaise. Significantly, exposure is cumulative, contributing further to human sluggishness and digestive problems and other ailments. Death and cancer rates have been found almost four times as high in areas near high current overhead wires. This "electric smog" can block out the brain's electromagnetic signals to the cells, diluting the body's disease-fighting ability. And unfortunately, with the multi-millions of dollars spent on trying to determine the adverse effects of electromagnetism in regard to cancer and leukemia, we have failed to consider seriously other possible adverse effects and what we might be able to do about them therapeutically. We often keep scientists in business looking at the wrong things, or certainly not all of the right things.

Now even the pharmaceutical companies are coming around to the understanding that there may be tests that better relate to quality of life and cost effectiveness than the disparate clinical evidence of the classical FDA placebo—based trials. Companies are engaging in scientific marketing in more combative head-to-head comparisons of products directly against each other. No longer is it enough to prove that a new drug is effective, it also must be better in price and performance. It appears the percentage of

6

the research budget for this will grow from 10 percent to a third or more over the next few years.

Certain Genentech Inc.'s drugs have been tested against Hoechst and Merck Company products, demonstrating greater effectiveness under specific circumstances. SmithKline Beecham PLC has done direct comparisons of its non-steroid, anti-inflammatory drug Relafen to show that it has a better "side-effects profile" than its competitors.

Upon this type of realistic recognition of direct comparison testing and documented clinical trials that show efficacy and safety, the FDA ought to proceed to the next step of requiring comparison of these products to alternative medicines that claim similar results and fewer side effects. Pills that put people to sleep ought to be directly compared to magnetic beds or magnetic head boards that make similar claims. Over 100 million Americans have sleep problems and many experts say that sleeping pills may do more damage than good. To be fair and honest to society, drugs for pain, inflammation, chronic fatigue syndrome, and various other ailments ought to be compared to alternative methodologies, including inexpensive and safe magnetic products.

The drug companies might not like "comprehensive comparison," yet doctors might and our health system ought to endorse it if comparisons have any merit at all. As much as 80 percent of doctors' treatments are for pain (10 percent for chronic pain) of about $23 billion for doctor services and many times that of total remuneration. This excludes drug costs. Can one imagine what the appropriate magnet could do for the health care system? For example, using just the one alternative of acupuncture, which unquestionably cuts pain for most causes, better results and higher quality of life could be attained for masses of ailing people. Some drugs and herbs might do a better job at healing than acupuncture for certain ailments. Astonishingly, magnetotherapy could supplement or even exceed the efficacy of acupuncture and some other alternative therapies, allowing the average physician to use this less complex technique for both pain relief and healing. Although acupuncture may heal, this benefit occurs with magnetotherapy to a much greater extent. If these statements are valid, it would be pure negligence on the part of the government and medical community not to use this medicine. Let's prove that it works or doesn't work and let's see if the NIH and other federal agencies have enough courage "to come out of the closet."

Unfortunately, some improperly designed electromagnets that are used for therapy may also pose some of the adverse consequences found in appliances and devices that operate in the 60 cycle range. The electromagnet (essentially an iron bar inside a solenoid through which an electric current passes) can be controlled in strength by the amount of voltage and current used. Power is typically generated from an alternating current (A.C.) 60 cycle electric source. On the other hand, the permanent magnet (also called steady or solid state, natural, premier, static, D.C.) does not generate a frequency from an external power force and is considered a safe instrument.

Magnetism can be defined simply as the alignment of dipoles in a ferrous or other material so that the molecules face in a uniform direction. The molecules form a natural balance between the positive and negative fields. The more molecules aligned, the greater the magnetic intensity.

All electric currents generate magnetic fields and the rate of current flow through a coil determines magnetic strength. In the permanent magnet, strength is determined by the transfer of power from another stronger magnet or the alignment of molecules from an external power source. The electromagnet can be made quite safe by using a D.C. source that processes frequencies within the human body's frequency range of 2 to 20 cycles per second. Many electromagnets are now designed to emit 14 cycles per second. As a consequence, they have been found to be considerably more effective in securing healing and symptom relief and, of course, safer than the higher frequencies, especially the 60 cycle range that can disturb normal body resonance.

Use of a constant frequency, even that compatible to human tissue and organs, can create an adaptation response over time which may mean one has to rest the body for a period in order to balance energy forces. The negative fields of the permanent magnet do not appear to create such an adaptation condition.

Different effects are obtained from different modes of the permanent magnet. The possible ill effects from using permanent magnets of incorrect polarity or gauss strength over an extended period of time must be considered. Short periods of use over weeks, even a few months, does not appear to be a problem when using positive (south) or bipolar (north/south) oriented magnets of low strength in the range of 200 or less gauss against the body. This translates to about 10 or 20 gauss to the body tissue when placed further away, as in a mattress or pad. But even at this gauss strength, when using the positive (south) pole, therapists advise resting the body a few weeks by staying off the positive oriented pad after continual use for two or three months or when bodily stress develops. Similar adaptation stress symptoms do not appear to occur when using the negative magnetic fields even after extended or continuous use.

A number of experts believe that it is the negative polarity that encourages deep restorative sleep, fights infection, supports biological healing, normalizes pH acid-base balance, brings more oxygen into the cells, and relieves pain. On the other hand, positive energy stimulates wakefulness and can jump-start immobile muscles, but is considered less effective on long-term biological healing.

Most human illnesses are positive oriented, such as intestinal disorders, seizures, infections, and toxic and acidic states. The positive fields have been shown to eat away at tumors at least temporarily, yet may also spread infectious bacteria and cancerous virus, while the negative fields have been shown to arrest cancerous growth and reduce tumors, as evidenced in a number of studies and case histories. What is important is that positive and bipolar magnetic fields attract the negative polarity to the injury site by biofeedback and other mechanisms in order to heal. And this is accomplished as long as the gauss strength from positive or bipolar magnets is sufficiently low.

Several companies space the magnets in mattresses, pads and seats several inches apart, which allows the opposite pole to rise and mix with the polarity facing the body, creating a bipolar effect. The beds of Nikken and Japan Life, for example, have been tested to show negative (north), positive (south), or bipolar fields facing the body, depending on where the measurements are taken. If a compass indicator is held directly over the magnet, the reading will be different in attraction than when held between magnets. The Ameriflex company uses a bipolar concentric pattern. Magnetic X Corporation and MagnetiCo, Inc., use negative-oriented magnets toward the body, spread one inch apart and in larger numbers to render a predominantly "extra strength" negative field, more beneficial for specific purposes. But all of the different configurations of beds have demonstrated healing or symptom relief for millions of people.

Differences between the two magnetic poles are still argumentative for many. Nevertheless, the two poles are diametrically opposite. The force of each field is exerted around the magnet in opposite directions. Also both clinical and laboratory trials show a definite difference between the negative and positive polarities.

We also need to place considerable attention on resonance as it is a key factor in healing. Since body tissue vibrates at about 7.5 cycles per second (CPS), the heart and central nervous system at 14 CPS, and the brain from 2 to 22 CPS, one can visualize that if the pulse repetition of an external frequency is tuned to match exactly the beat of the heart, for instance, cardiac rhythm could go into sympathetic resonance and the heart's amplitude would be increased. Out-of-step beats and extra systoles (contractions) can occur, causing stroke or other forms of cardiac disturbances, very much exemplified during solar storms. The body accepts these varying frequencies at the expense of cell efficiency since body tissues are thrown out of molecular resonance.

We can liken body performance to a radio receiver, able to modulate almost any level of frequency into the human acceptance range. No matter whether from the extremely high frequencies of light waves or satellite or radio emissions, or the lower frequencies of household current or high-power transmission lines, evidence indicates that the body is capable of accepting these frequencies. Dispute exists concerning the body's ability to accept the very large wave forms that may range from the size of football fields to miles in length, yet a number of consequences have been recorded. As for smaller waves, you have probably experienced placing your hand on a radio and TV set, for example, where your body acted like an antenna attracting those frequencies. Scientific studies show the human body can assimilate frequencies as low as .00005 (cps) and, of course, be significantly damaged by the higher frequency microwaves that cause ionization of cells.

Both the electromagnet and the permanent magnet emit magnetic fields that are essentially the same when frequency and wave form are discounted. Differences lie in gauss (unit of measurement) strength, polarity orientation, duration of use, frequency and the shape of waves emitted, although the latter is more controversial and short of necessary evidence. The size and the weight of the permanent magnet are also important. Weight is very much related to depth of penetration as is strength or intensity. Size is extremely important because the more area covered, the greater the volume of tissue influenced and the more effective the results. Too often it is forgotten that the amount of tissue affected is directly related to the rate of healing.

Thousands of scientific studies, including clinical trials and various double-blind placebo controlled tests exist to demonstrate the usefulness of electromagnetic therapy. The FDA approved electromagnetic devices in 1978, primarily for bone fusions and relief of body pain, edema, and similar ailments. Their attitude at first was that these instruments were harmless, perhaps useless, so the idea would most likely fade away. But that didn't happen as hundreds of thousands of individuals in the U.S. alone were cured or relieved of symptoms using these procedures. Dozens of instruments are on the market and used successfully today. Over 100,000 surgical procedures are performed annually with electromagnets, many by orthopedic surgeons with incomes of $400,000 or greater earned with the help of this technology.

Remarkably, success rates for bone fusions, pain relief, and healing of many types of ailments range 70 percent or higher when procedures are properly applied. A pioneer in electromagnetic therapy, orthopedic surgeon, Dr. Andrew Bassett has demonstrated success rates of 80 percent in healing non-union bone fractures. Dr. John F. Connolly, M.D., using electromagnetic devices, recorded success in almost all cases involving 100 consecutive fractures, as described in the chapters ahead.

We know electromagnetic therapy works but, one might ask, how can a simple, little permanent magnet do the same thing and possibly heal many other types of diseases as well. Simply trying it may be the best answer. After all it is safer than drugs, and just about everybody is on drugs. Under most circumstances, if it holds true for electromagnets it holds true for permanent magnets with the differences already enumerated. A permanent magnet of the correct size and strength utilized for the proper duration of time has proven to be as effective in most cases. And for healing of the whole body and immune system, the long-term application of the permanent magnet appears to be the most appropriate, especially for self-help treatment such as with a magnetic pad.

Skepticism abounds in the professional medical community about the healthful effects of magnetic fields. This idea is derived mainly from magnetotherapy's competitive nature to conventional medicine and the lack of education in this field, as well as very little being published in the peer-review medical journals. Yet the average person can prove a point to himself by trying this therapy without fear or danger. Importantly, for any serious ailment or for periodic checkups, one should see his or her physician. But if after many visits of ineffectiveness from conventional therapy, one should be able to determine for himself the effectiveness of a safe magnetic device—perhaps a clearer barometer of efficacy than a mixture of conflicting scientific voices.

Anecdotal cases are never sufficient proof of predictable effectiveness but do reflect the personal experiences of thousands of individuals whose claims cannot be entirely discounted. The wife of a close friend sprained her upper thigh in a horse accident. When she applied a simple, 550 gauss strength, bipolar permanent magnet to her swollen leg, the pain went away immediately. Swelling receded more rapidly than she had ever experienced in previous injuries. When she took the magnet off, the pain came back instantly. Whenever she applied the magnet the pain disappeared.

Many people with whom I personally visited have witnessed pain relief from such things as tennis elbow, back problems, gout in the foot and hands, shoulder spasm, among a variety of ailments. Relief from gout occurred in minutes and arthritic fingers have moved in short order where they were stiff before. In one case of a close friend, gout in his feet disappeared in minutes after applying a bipolar magnet of 550 gauss. He was able to move his toes for the first time in years.

A female custodial worker, with whom I have spoken over the past year, and a male carpenter carry a concentric, bipolar magnet to place on sore spots whenever they feel the need during the work day. I relieved a toothache of mine in about 15 minutes and observed the infection disappear in a couple of days. Back pain from strenuous tennis exercise is relieved when I sleep on a magnetic pad, and has usually remained when I loaned the pad out to my teen-age daughter to determine her experience. She says that after studying hard, she needs less hours of sleep than usual to feel fully energized after sleeping on the pad. I have noticed that I require less hours of sleep as well. Of course, endless anecdotal cases can be cited, but also at least some double-blind, controlled studies are available and a few cited within these pages.

Professional observation may add some credence to efficacy. In 1992, Dr. Dean Bonlie, D.D.S. Calgary, Canada, was requested by an ophthalmologist to see a patient who had lost vision in her left eye. Her history revealed pain heart surgery that caused massive infection in the area of the brachial plexus, resulting in permanent nerve damage that appeared to set up a chain reaction of tetanic contraction in the muscles of the neck, scalp and finally the eye. Prescription pain killers had been the only relief for ten years, although 108 different physicians and health-care providers had treated her.

She was treated for one hour and 15 minutes using a ceramic magnet 4"×6"×2" with the negative side placed against these muscle groups. As each area was treated, the muscles relaxed and the pain relieved, vision was regained, and finally she was free of pain as tears of joy filled her eyes and she thanked her providers over and over. She now successfully treats herself.

A U.S.A. Nikken distributor of wellness products states his lady friend would not be able to walk or function if it were not for a series of bipolar magnets that she wears on her body at all times to provide balance and muscular movement. Treatments over the years from a number of doctors failed to alleviate this serious problem. The magnets have created a new life for her and is probably one of the reasons the distributor remains in the business.

Something unique is happening here. I try to explain as fairly as possible the different sides of the arguments, but opinions are sufficiently diverse that analysis is not an easy task. Yet, after looking at this from many sides, some commonality arises that can lead in the direction of strategies for further controlled tests and additional documentation. Various types of research are suggested here that would be desirable.

We know that this therapy is not successful on everybody for a variety of reasons. The successful anecdotal cases are marvelous but what about the failures? Some answers are presented. A success rate approaching 70 percent is not to be scoffed at. Few drugs can claim such a high rate, perhaps aspirin alone and we don't really know how that functions. For magnetic therapy, we have a reasonable theory of a biofeedback effect where the brain causes increased negative magnetic energy to rush to the site of pain, energized by the injury itself or the irritant effect of a positive magnetic field, heat pad, homeopathic remedy, acupuncture, mustard plaster or other medication, including aspirin. In any case, it works to various degrees in the majority of circumstances. Other reasons for the healing powers of magnetotherapy are also enumerated, including cell changes, increased blood flow and improved oxygen intake.

In the therapeutic application of magnetic fields, both positive pole and bipolar magnets of about 500 gauss strength or less are effective and safe for symptom relief for many ailments. It is believed by some that dual polarity magnets create a pulsing type effect that treats more rapidly than single polarity magnets of similar gauss strength. Some believe that there is no pulsing in reality. The quick response to the bipolar magnet is believed to be a more rapid reaction of a biofeedback effect in its desire to counteract the irritant effect of the positive polarity. A higher gauss, negative poled magnet might be required to create a similar response The negative polarity is the more effective long-term healer because it adds negative energy rather than taking it from other body sources.

Health authorities from nations around the world vary in their idea of what gauss strength is most appropriate or which may cause human adaptation response where effectiveness no longer takes place and stress might develop. The Japanese Health and Welfare Ministry will not approve magnetic therapy devices unless they approach the 500 internal gauss strength level, believing anything less may not demonstrate effectiveness. But there is wide disagreement as to what level may cause human adaptation, assuming this may be in the range of 100 to 200 gauss against the body.

Adaptation can occur from many treatments including drugs or almost any medication that elicits a reaction from the brain to provide additional energy for healing or relief. Dr. William H. Philpott, M.D., and certain other practitioners believe that this adaptation response does not occur when using negative magnetic fields because this polarity provides the healing negative energy directly to the injury. They believe that positive and alternating (negative and positive) poles stimulate the brain in the biofeedback process that passes negative magnetic fields to the site of injury, while the negative polarity alone simply places it directly on the site. Over the long-run, the negative fields would essentially be healing the entire human body and not draining negative energy from other body sources. Attracting negative magnetic energy from other parts of the body in order to heal an injured site may gradually deplete this vital energy from elsewhere. And for some ill patients substantially depleted of internal electromagnetic energy from the start, instead of experiencing symptom relief from the counterirritant reflex response, symptoms may actually increase even from low-level positive or bipolar magnetic fields.

Some have assumed that the adrenal gland function may decrease with extensive use of the negative fields. However, Dr. Dean Bonlie observes that although adrenalin levels may drop, it is not due to suppression but rather because the body no longer is in an emergency state where it needs additional adrenalin. He confirms this with athletes whose performance improved under competition when using negative magnetic pads.

Another use for positive magnetic energy is to apply it directly over the sternum to stimulate the thymus gland. Theoretically, this increases the production of the T-cells and therefore aids the immune deficiency system, but Dr. Philpott, for one, recommends that the treatment should be limited to three minutes of application three times daily, followed by negative energy treatment for as many hours as possible. The positive polarity has been used to reduce tumor size; but again, evidence seems to indicate that the negative fields should be applied afterwards.

Magnetotherapy is probably the least complex of treatments, perhaps the reason some doctors choose not to use it because it takes the mystery out of much of the world of complex medicine. For most ailments, 550 or 850 gauss strength magnets are all that is needed, applied for periods of ten, twenty, or thirty minutes several times daily until the ache or pain or swelling recedes. More serious problems require professional help and further instruction and may take a 2000 or 3000 gauss magnet. Some problems may require a 12,000 gauss magnet for serious diseases. These high-strength applications should only be done under the direction and advice of a licensed professional. The high gauss fields should not be used directly in the head area or the central nervous system without full knowledge of what one is trying to accomplish.

Pregnant women should avoid being exposed to magnetic fields in order to be on the safe side; however, there are no reports of adverse effects from use of the proper polarity for women or children. But magnetic devices should be kept away from anyone using a pacemaker or any health device that can be affected by magnetic force.

Effect also depends on how magnets are placed in mattresses and seats and other devices. Check the diagrams, construction sheets, and make your own personal observations as to how many magnets are in a bed pad including their size, strength, and spacing to meet your purposes. For most ailments, the magnetic devices and beds on the market will serve people well. If you are receiving satisfactory results, fine. But if your ailment persists or you are searching for peak performance, you may require extra strength magnets. For example, a twin-size magnetic bed would need 665 magnets of ¾ inch diameter and 850 gauss to give a two gauss field to the center of the body. It takes 218 miniblock magnets ¾"×1¾"×(3/8)" of 1100 gauss to render four gauss to the center of the body. Remember some people experience stress over the first few nights even from weaker magnetic pads because their bodies are throwing off toxins or meridians, associated with acupuncture, that are being stimulated. Others feel little difference even from the stronger strength pads, noticing a difference only over a period of weeks or months as the body's energy level improves and physical performance is tested higher. The desirable magnetic strength of the pad depends very much on what you are seeking and your body condition.

Once you are accustomed to sleeping on a magnetic bed, it will be habit forming for life. An important issue in improving the nation's health is changing behavior patterns. For example, surveys show that fully half the men told by their doctors to take aspirin regularly—to reduce their risk of heart attack and stroke—do not do it. According to research by the National Council on Patient Information and Education, noncompliance involving prescription medicine ranges from 30 percent to 50 percent. "Programmable pill boxes" that beep and whistle when its time to take medicine may be the order of the day, they say. On the other hand, people never forget to sleep on a magnetic bed because it's always there. Is that why 10 million Japanese sleep on magnetic beds?

The elimination of pain, better sleep, and greater energy are just some of the uses of magnetic fields. The chapters ahead will not only demonstrate the usefulness of permanent magnets for these purposes but also the astounding effect magnetic treatment can have on such serious illnesses as epilepsy, schizophrenia, chronic fatigue syndrome, depression, diabetes, premenstrual syndrome, and many other complications as it strengthens the immune system and balances the electrical signals of the brain. Drug and alcohol abusers are helped from their addictions by minimizing withdrawal symptoms. Many drug treatment centers in the U.S. now use acupuncture with a high degree of success. Can one imagine how much more effective our drug treatment programs could be through the use of magnetotherapy, which can largely override acupuncture and be administered by a larger pool of trained providers and counselors? It could make the nation's anti-drug and anti-crime programs a real success. And controversial electric-shock treatments can turn to more benign permanent magnetic therapy, minimizing the dangers from these 100,000 plus treatments per year. A whole list of diseases can be attacked. Rising health costs could be cut.

If just one-fourth or even one-tenth of disease was helped by magnetotherapy, it could be the most important discovery or awakening of the century. And to think for all these years, we have tinkered uninformed about gauss strength, polarity, and treatment protocol. It is time the Congress, National Institutes of Health, medical professions, and private foundations took this matter seriously regardless of competitive opposition, and conducted the necessary studies, laid out the answers once and for all, and moved courageously forward for the benefit of the nation's health and world health.

Chapter 1

Meeting the Health Challenge

Magnetic Energy is Fundamental to our Health

The healing of our bodies should not be left to chance alone. Simply to let nature take its course in this adverse environment is contrary to sound judgment. It might have made some sense centuries ago; unfortunately, our internal metabolic energy system will not always produce the necessary healing energies we need to deal with modern life. The healing process, whether in a cut, burn, blood clot, allergic reaction, addictive or toxic state, infection, emotional and mental reaction and other metabolic disorders, responds to magnetic energy—something which many therapists have known for years but which most of the medical profession has been unwilling to take seriously. Cells are alive, constantly forming and renewing themselves in a process called cell division, activated by a number of forces, one of which is magnetic energy that can assist in healing specific organs or the whole body (Becker and Tarcher; Davis and Rawls; Evans).[*]

Scientific experiments demonstrate that the interaction of all organs and systems is dependent on the constant influence of magnetic energy. Of equal significance is the body's natural vibration frequencies that produce biological responses from the energy of positive and negative magnetic fields (Gerber). Tests show that the positive energy increases frequencies, while the negative energy decreases them. Albert R. Davis and Walter C. Rawls, Jr. in **Magnetism and Its Effects on the Living System**, describe this process. We are reminded that most human organs have a unique functional vibrating rate of approximately 7.96 cycles per second (CPS). The heart and liver have higher vibration rates at 15 cycles, which is also

---

[*] See full references and readings chapter by chapter at the end of the book.

the natural pulsing frequency of the Earth. From these normally low frequencies, we can visualize how 60 cycle A.C. electric currents and high frequency radio and TV waves, for example, might disturb our system by interrupting natural body vibration rates (Gerber; Savitz; Blackman).

Importance of the Body's Magnetic Energies

Many of our disorders and diseases are the result of electrochemical breakdown. When a magnetic or oxygen deficiency occurs in an organ or system, symptoms of illness arise and normal cell division is adversely affected, resulting in a high risk of cell mutation. An effective treatment, a growing cadre of doctors and researchers believe, is application of negative magnetic fields that causes the oxygenation of tissues by creating a field of high energy and an increased number of electrons (Philpott and Bonlie). Dr. William H. Philpott, M.D., has successfully used magnetotherapy on thousands of patients over the past decade. He, among a variety of researchers and practitioners, believes that negative magnetic energy is the primary healer and induces melatonin production which is anti-aging, anti-stress, and controls free radical cell formation that causes many of our known diseases. Melatonin, as the master hormone of the energy system, controls the immune, hormone, and oxidation systems. Both positive and negative magnetic fields, plus a variety of other treatments are believed to increase negative magnetic energy to injured sites and to the body as a whole. We know that states of excitation cannot be maintained for extended periods of time without undue stress and fatigue. Organ functions and metabolic processes can become over-worked and prematurely wear out. We know that to stimulate our system with caffeine or amphetamines can be unhealthy and risky, whereas the proper method of restoring energy is rest and sleep. Upon awakening from restorative sleep, negative energies are rejuvenated, allowing appropriate physical and emotional responses to be initiated so that adverse environmental or other influences can be counteracted.

We absorb energy directly from the Earth's magnetic fields and also from inhaling oxygen that carries the Earth's magnetic fields into our cells. Oxygen is para-magnetic, meaning that it takes on the magnetic field that influences it. The higher the surrounding magnetic fields, it is believed the higher the human level of energy (Philpott).

Sharks and insects, as observed by the Smithsonian Institute, obtain as much as 90 percent of their energy from the Earth's magnetic fields rather than from food. Our nauseating pest, the cockroach can live six months or linger without any food. Both sharks and insects are highly resistant to viral infectious diseases, including cancer, even though insects do not have an immune system. Can this simple idea of magnetic force be a chief answer to health and well being? Dr. Philpott believes magnetic energy is our first line of defense and that it can solve a lot of human ailments without even involving the immune system, which may be described as our second line of defense.

The laws of physics state that a conducting fluid flowing through a magnetic field produces an electro-motive force. The water flow over the Niagara Falls, for example, creates electromagnetic energy and voltages that can be measured by meters as it passes through the Earth's magnetic field. It is reasonably assumed that blood flowing through the body, which is also in the Earth's magnetic field, produces an internal source of magnetic field energy. Also, a certain amount of electromagnetic energy is generated from bone stress during exercise called the piezoelectric phenomenon, encouraging us to just say "yes" to exercise. The sophisticated instrument called the SQUID measures electrical currents of the brain and other organs. When death occurs the SQUID no longer registers magnetic energy in the body. At this stage, the magnetic energy that produces physical and mental functions no longer exists. It is understood that electrons or the atoms of the body are in constant movement through the geomagnetic and electromagnetic fields of the body. Moving a charged particle through a magnetic field will increase its energy as it does in a generator and other devices.

For example, the process of how non-ionizing magnetic fields interact with lung and other human systems to cause alteration in cells is still somewhat of a mystery, even after 30 years of research. A model was presented in 1984 by Abraham Liboff during a NATO Advance Research Workshop in Euce, Italy, that suggested ion cyclotron resonance could occur in the membrane of individual cells and generate increased transport of ions such as calcium, magnesium, potassium, and other ions. Since that time, researchers have written countless papers, both experimental and theoretical, supporting ion cyclotron resonance for specific ions. It is rather easily explained for charged particles moving in free space in presence of static magnetic fields. Also, it is well *demonstrated that frequencies can be changed from the resonance frequency to either add or subtract energy. **

Where Energies Come From

A multiple of energies function within our bodies and around us for which we are constantly searching to improve our well-being and vitality. The principal energy fitted for our biological system is called the Krebs Cycle (named after the German Chemist Hans Krebs) used for processing nutrients. But biologists believe it is capable of providing no more than 70 percent of the energy necessary to promote human metabolism (Daniels and Martin; Davis and Rawls). No matter how much we apply ourselves to eat the best foods and consume quantities of recommended vitamins and minerals, still another 30 percent of non-nutritional energy is needed to function at the peak of good health. Athletes may reach for the top while the average person simply seeks a healthy, well-balanced mind and body. In any case, we must extend our interest beyond nutrition, beyond simply the right foods, diet, mega-vitamins or herbal supplements. It seems clear that our system needs more.

Science tells us that it is the 30 percent, non-nutritional energy that may give one human being the advantage over another in health, performance, and life span. Dr. Philpott insists that it is this energy that gives humans the benefit over pathological microorganisms, as well as the ability to maintain an alkaline pH balance and an important way to build plentiful amount of intracellular oxygen. It can also assist the human system in fighting and developing mastery over environmental hazards such as chemical and electromagnetic contamination. A plentiful supply of cellular oxygen acts as a defense against microorganism invasion, since these organisms have less tolerance for oxygen than human cells. In addition, much of our energy is supplied by the exitonic process that is also experienced in the photosynthesis of plants. This is one reason our veins are close to the surface of the skin (Barefoot and Reich).

Evidence shows that it is magnetic negative energy rather than magnetic positive that maintains proper blood and tissue alkaline pH, the medium in which oxygen can survive and fight off unwanted organisms.

---

* The italicized text refers to more complex information.

The pH measures the relative acidity or alkalinity of human blood with 7.4 being about right. It seems evident that non-nutritional energy must be magnetic negative poled, Dr. Philpott says, otherwise we would die of inflammation, microorganism infection, cancer, and other illnesses. Robert Barefoot explains that exitonics also create a negative field (Barefoot and Reich). It is recognized by an increasing number of researchers and practitioners that the way to correct negative magnetic deficiency states of stress is to provide consistent and frequent exposure to an artificial source of negative magnetic energy. Properly constructed magnetic beds and seats and other devices can alleviate magnetic energy deficiency.

Importantly, it has been shown that the most dreadful cancers can be attacked by magnetic fields if used properly. Negative fields raise the body fluid pH to the alkaline state which kills cancers quickly. The medical establishment admits that cancer rates are increasing rapidly, striking one in three people. The cause is not only from smoking and dietary fat but also from carcinogens in our environment, from smoke-filled and smoke-free work places, from pesticides, from electromagnetic pollution and such things as annual mammography radiation tests on highly sensitive female breasts. Science journalists, says professor Samuel S. Epstein, University of Illinois Medical Center in Chicago, base their cheer leading for cancer cures on initial reduction in tumor size rather than on prolonged survival. Certain forms of electromagnetic fields, radiation, and chemotherapy can spread cancer to normal cells and may do more damage than good. It 's like trying "to make a rabbit out of rabbit stew."

The Magnetic Earth and Our Health

The Earth has two magnetic poles—north and south—but is also influenced by a positive charge below the crust of the Earth and a negative charge at the Earth's surface under the positive oriented upper atmosphere which emanates from the sun's rays. This gives us, happily and propitiously, a negative magnetic field on the surface where we live, otherwise we would be terribly sick animals if we continuously lived in a positive magnetic field. Not surprisingly, many of us are ill not only from a weakened field force but also from extensive man-made electromagnetic pollution. As a matter of fact, in some areas where unusual cracks exist in the Earth's crust from quakes and volcanoes—or where the molten mass beneath the Earth's plates is closer to the surface—greater amounts of positive magnetic fields enter the Earth's surface, causing serious medical problems and disorders with both human and animal population. Unusual eddy currents are also noticed in these areas.

On the other hand, there are areas where greater negative magnetic fields prevail. Some believe that certain health resorts, such as Sedona, Arizona and Lourdes, France are such places. Lourdes is a city of only 18,000 people but gets 5,000,000 visitors every year during a six month period who come to replenish their stock of water, bathe in the water and dab it on their eyes, making emergency trips when necessary. All seem to feel better, as pain and stress are relieved, while over 2,000 inexplicable cures (with 65 so-called miracles) have been recognized by the authorities. But psychiatrist Armond-Lareche says many of the ills of people return and he is surprised that more people do not get sick from drinking the bath water which is changed only twice daily. He sees no medical value, yet people are healed.

Can the science behind this and similar circumstances be our old friend negative magnetic fields, where negative means beneficial and healthful? It appears, at least with this one term, that we must change our understanding of what it connotes—negative is healthy and it is good. But it is also helpful if we think positively about magnetic fields as we try to understand this fundamental mystery of life.

If we picture the Earth as a bed we sleep on, we would want to rest on negative magnetic fields. Luckily the Earth's surface is predominantly electrically negative oriented. Yet unfortunately, the Earth is rapidly losing its magnetic strength. So if we sleep on a bed that had negative magnets pointing toward us, this could be good for our health.

The Earth's magnetic strength is relatively mild, only ½ gauss (.5), compared to 10 times that centuries ago and many more times higher a million years back, verified by atomic lysterises dating from core drilling of volcanoes. All of the Earth's surface is negative except at the south magnetic pole and over eddy currents at various locations.

You may have noticed when a storm first brews, the body is stimulated. It is a period when animals stir and jump, horses kick their stalls, institutionalized and other mental patients are noticed to react excitedly, and we all are affected if we take the time to notice. In one study that observed 28,000 patients in psychiatric hospitals involving 67 magnetic storms, serious alterations occurred in a large percentage of these subjects. This is a time when positive ions from storms predominate (similar to those evoked by solar flares), the same positive ions that have been observed to precipitate human illness and microorganism replication. As the storm subsides, the negative magnetic fields take over and we begin to feel relaxed and comfortable, animals stop stirring, and we experience a feeling of pleasantness and ease. This negative charge is the technical name for "fresh." The magnetic fields are caused by the electrostatification of the air and water which creates a negative charge differentiated on the ground.

We are fortunate that the Earth is oriented to the negative field, but yet not so lucky that the Earth's magnetic fields are decreasing in strength year-by-year. Sleep helps us to recharge the trillions of tired body cells after a busy day, like so many microscopic batteries that need a boost or electric car batteries that need to be recharged after a day of use. The Earth's natural negative magnetic field is intended to do this but has been greatly reduced in strength over centuries and now even these limited fields are shielded from us by our urban environment of concrete and steel, the encased auto, and other barriers intertwined with many complex and counteracting, man-made electrical fields. Since a five percent loss of the Earth's magnetic strength has occurred in the last 100 years alone, we must ask the question how long it will take for yet another, even a small amount of gauss strength to deteriorate to the extent that it will affect future generations of life. We are experiencing lower levels of magnetic energy compared to past generations and we are encountering an unusual amount of electromagnetic pollution from a variety of sources which distort our bodies' chemical and immune balances. These immense quantities of electrical and magnetic energies which enter our bodies are mixed positive and negative magnetic fields of varying frequencies and with overpowering positive fields that twist and distort our immune system and level of magnetic energy. Some evidence indicates that these mixed forces may very well be the reason for much of our stress, cancers, weakness, immune system imparities, and a host of disorders.

Electromagnetic Pollution

We have heard that there are electromagnetic sources of pollution all around us. The White House, the Congress, and most industrial and utility companies are still unwilling to admit to any serious problem, yet even Vice President Al Gore's office tested for an unusually high degree of adverse electromagnetic pollution. We are slowly coming around, but it may be too late for some people already infected with maladies.

The U.S. Department of Energy (DOE) funds millions of dollars every year in studies associated with extremely low frequency (ELF) electric and magnetic fields and related matters, but still they don't have the answers they want. Therefore, some local governments are taking the matter into their own hands. Seven states have regulations limiting the intensity of magnetic fields from transmission lines, while multimillion dollar suits are pending in several other states against polluting utilities. One of the risks is that we may focus too much on cancer as the major health effect and ignore such things as depression and chronic fatigue syndrome and other diseases. A strong reluctance is evident against admitting that any correlation exists between ELF fields and disease, but the battle goes on and the association to cancer and leukemia appears stronger than ever. The DOE concludes, "in our view, the emerging evidence no longer allows one to categorically assert that there are no risks." The latest federal reports are being held off for another year pending further analysis, although a good deal of the data are in as described more fully in Chapter 4.

Some academic experts and medical practitioners believe that the problem may be at least partially alleviated by the proper and sensible application of negative magnetic fields to our bodily systems to raise appropriate magnetic energy levels and ward off some of the effects of adverse frequencies.

How Magnetic Fields Work on the Body

Studies of athletes using negative polarity magnetic beds show an immediate increase in the body's ability to pick up and use oxygen from the air we breathe. Dr. Dean Bonlie of MagnetiCo, Inc. of Calgary, Canada,

Information Brief

Magnetic Water Treatment

Controversy exists over the effectiveness of magnetic water treatment for industrial purposes, such as that used to keep scale from building up in water heaters and boilers. A well-financed water-softening industry that funds many of the water quality studies attacks the use of magnets as fraudulent. One reason may be that magnets are relatively inexpensive, last almost forever, and would save industry and commerce and residential users billions of dollars annually but cut profits for the chemical industry.

The Department of Energy in 1986 stated "Magnetic water conditioners...are operating extensively throughout the world today with tremendous economic effect. Marked reduction in scale formation in steam boilers has been verified in practice and confirmed in laboratories." Cost-conscious and maintenance--plagued building managers are among the satisfied customers. The technology is used at the medical school building of the University of California at San Diego and San Antonio's Victoria Towers. Magnetic water treatment has been used successfully for over 30 years in Europe. Less scale accumulation on magnetized heating elements was demonstrated by Dr. Kenneth Busch, chemist at Baylor University, in a controlled study using magnets on some stills and others without magnets. Dozens of companies in Norway alone use magnet water treatment and the U.S. Navy has used it since 1903 to prevent scale buildup.

Chief design engineer, Denver Collins of State Industries, one of the largest water heater manufacturers, found that inexpensive magnets mounted on water inlets extended heater life beyond the warranty period when previously these $2000 commercial heaters were failing well before warranty, causing costly problems. Mor-Flo, another heater manufacturer, markets a $30 inexpensive magnetic device for use on heaters.

Field tests by the City University of London, England, found that both descaling and scale prevention occurred when water was magnetized. X-ray diffraction and electron microscopy showed magnetic treatment increased the size of the precipitated crystals. This report in the *New Scientist* magazine also revealed compositional change in hard-water scale from evaporated untreated water in a ratio of 4 to 1 calcite and aragonite (two types of scale) changing to a ratio of 1 to 4 when magnetically treated. They concluded that when surface charge of scale-providing crystals is altered, scale accumulation is reduced. These results were verified at a Bedford automotive plant, where industrial-grade magnets reduced maintenance costs 22,000 pounds in one year.

The opposing view is expressed by Jim Rober, chairman of the National Association of Corrosion Engineers' committee that investigates the nonchemical treatment of water, who believes magnetic water softening is pure fiction. The question arises as to whether both the chemical industry and the pharmaceutical industries are in the same non-progressive climate of protecting their profit levels against more effective and safe procedures. In humans, magnetic energy alters the surface charge and electrical potential of the cell, opening ion channels and raising pH levels. Magnetic fields work in both humans and water pipes. Simple tests have demonstrated this.

Source: Magnetic Water Treatment, Merle Henkenius, *Popular Mechanics*,
June 1992; author.

has conducted such tests and found that sleeping in an enhanced magnetic field speeds recovery from disease, strengthens the immune system, improves muscle function and repair, and increases overall body endurance and mental alertness. Complementary to this, Albert Roy Davis demonstrated how prior (preventative) negative magnetic exposure arrested active intake of infectious cancer and other diseases. Davis showed that both negative and positive fields can relieve pain and symptoms at specific sites, and negative magnetic energy can safely treat the whole body over the long-haul. As already mentioned, the positive fields in low gauss strength will also attract negative magnetic energy wherever the body indicates deficiency but will do this at the expense of taking it away from other parts.

The science behind magnetotherapy, like any biological science, is not simple, many factors are at work. One involves electrical charges within cells. All cells have a positive and negative electrical charge differential between the inside of the cell and the outside of the cell wall. For proper functioning, this differential must be at least 60 millivolts. The greater the electrical charge differential, the greater the exchange of nutrients and water through the cell wall. By increasing the body's negative magnetic fields, a negative electric charge is assumed to take place in the plasma and tissue. As a result, fluid is induced that creates more hydroxyl (OH⁻) ions which combine with other ions to raise the body fluid pH to alkaline. This increase in pH increases the oxygen carrying capacity of the blood (Barefoot and Reich).

When hydroxyl ions attach to the glyco-proteins of the outer cell wall, the electric charge differential is increased. When increased substantially, old waste and toxins that have been held in the cell for long periods are drawn out of the cells into the bloodstream and can cause a degree of discomfort. Increased absorption by the red blood cells results in more surface area made available for the exchange of oxygen and carbon dioxide. [*]

However, although oxygen carrying capacity is enhanced by an increased negative charge on the outside of the red blood cells causing cells to repel each other, this is considered a very minimal effect. Both Dr. Dean Bonlie and Dr. William Philpott, among others, indicate that this process is secondary to the increase in the energy level of electrons and other

---

[*]   The italicized text refers to more complex information.

particles and that it is this energy transfer to various parts of the body that magnetic fields and certain other therapies create that are primarily responsible for symptom relief and healing.

Positive or negative magnetic fields alone, as well as bipolar fields plus other types of application, including acupuncture, homeopathy, and various surface medications are able to excite the brain through the biofeedback effect to send increased levels of negative magnetic energy to the site of injury in order to countermand the accumulation of positive magnetic energy which occurs at all injured locations. (The terminology "energy" is used in many instances in place of "fields" because it is more easily understood and less confusing to the average reader, although perhaps technically annoying to the trained physicist, so please excuse.) Negative magnetic field application places negative ions at the site directly to join and assist the brain's output of negative fields. In short, all combinations of polarities work; the question is which functions most efficiently and effectively. If one questions that various combinations work, simply try them and you will prove it to yourself. But take into account the parameters of difference and what is happening.

It is important to underscore that the release of toxins can cause temporary reactions, such as aches or pains, sciatic pain, tingling or itching sensations, or an overall feeling of tiredness. These symptoms will soon subside and the body cells will begin to function at an improved level of effectiveness. A gradual increase in length of time one uses a magnetic system will help reduce annoying symptoms. Also it is significant to note that people on medication may develop symptoms similar to that of excess medication when using an overall body treatment such as a magnetic bed. Drugs become more effective and may have to be reduced or discontinued to match body chemistry changes. As stress and inflammation are reduced, toxins are released, metabolism improves and eventually one feels more comfortable and healthy.

Remember that symptoms can occur when using either the negative or positive polarities. Some people complain about getting up several times during the night to ward off discomfort. This will soon dissipate, while for many healthier systems it may not be experienced at all. Symptoms occur in about 30 percent of cases but soon subside and go away after toxins are released in several days or weeks depending on a person's health. One should not be alarmed at this beneficial effect even though it may be stressful for a while. A growing number of practitioners, such as Dr. Harry Park, M.D., Vancouver, Washington, prefer to use the negative fields, especially for long-term magnetic therapy and use a variety of herbs or liniments to reduce toxin effects.

Scientific Studies of Magnetotherapy

C ase histories and evidence that the application of magnetic fields can cure ailments and relieve pain are both scientific and anecdotal. A reasonable number of controlled studies for electromagnetotherapy are available and are cited in the pages ahead. Fewer studies exist for the application of permanent magnets, but performance of the two therapies demonstrate that results are the same when gauss strength and duration of application are taken in consideration. Over 1000 articles appear in scientific journals on the effects of electromagnets but considerably fewer are available concerning permanent magnets. However, physicians and researchers have documented subjects in detail prior to treatment with permanent magnets and for a reasonable study period afterward to verify lasting results. Cases are cited here so that the reader can gain an understanding as to what has actually occurred under investigative procedures.

Nevertheless, scientific double-blind, controlled studies are needed which could take place over the next several years to answer many remaining questions. It is such an important health question, that government and private foundations ought to provide sufficient research funds as soon as possible. The newly created Office of Alternative Medicine has been allocated $2,000,000 to examine alternative therapies with $600,000 to be used for research, parceled out in maximum $30,000 grants, hardly enough to find the answers to this very important medicine. The study of magnetotherapy may not even receive a grant. Many believe that a minimum of $100 million ought to be allocated for the very important purpose of alternative medicines, particularly when we spend tens of billions of dollars on space exploration and super conducting colliders, and still many unnecessary defense projects. What is the sense of it all and where is the political courage to tackle the nation's real priorities!

Electromagnets versus Permanent Magnets

As pointed out in the introduction, in the U.S. alone, over 100,000 treatments annually are given using electromagnetic devices for such things as bone fusions, inflammation, tennis elbow, sprains, back aches, and most types of pain. In addition, tens of thousands of cases are treated with permanent magnets for similar ailments and also to give people higher energy levels, improve immune systems, or simply to provide the means for better and more restful sleep. It seems the electromagnet is rapidly becoming the therapy of choice for healing bone fusions, for aches and pains, and for a variety of muscle and tissue ailments; while, permanent magnets are recognized more for improving energy levels and immune function and alleviating symptoms from many diseases. The professional appears to prefer the most sophisticated electric devices, perhaps to make the process appear more complex than it is. On the other hand, the layman is more suited for the application of permanent magnets.

Permanent magnets are similar to the magnets hanging on your refrigerator door that have no electrical power source, just the magnetism built into them. The magnetic energy fields that they emit are static or non-pulsed (as opposed to A.C. electromagnetic pulsing of various frequencies) and can be pointed to give off either negative or positive fields from one side or the other. A D.C. current can make a non-pulsed field in an electromagnet as well, which means that a battery operated electromagnet would perform much like a permanent magnet.

The growth of this industry is rapidly expanding. Nearly 100,000 providers of these services operate in the U.S. alone. One Japanese-American company, Nikken, supplies magnetic health products in the United States through over 40,000 distributors, and has many times that number of users. Japan Life and Ameriflex have thousands of distributors also. Japan Life has been operating in the U.S. since the early 1980's and has a half dozen or more distribution outlets that have demonstrated highly successful results. Worldwide, over 50 million people in eight countries are users of magnetic beds and other magnetic devices. If you want case histories, these companies have thousands. Magnetic healing is not going to go away. When people realize results, of course, they continue to use the therapy. It does little good for the medical community or government agencies to hide their heads in the sand as if nothing were happening or, by keeping tight-lipped, believing it might all go away. That will not happen and we may as well face up to it. We need to become educated on the topic, not hide from it.

The use of magnetic devices early in this century expanded quite rapidly, but then suddenly faded away because of entry into the field by quick-buck artists and charlatans, as well as lack of scientific investigation and research. Today, much more scientific information and documented experiences are available. If the subject is approached genuinely, we may witness an innovative health success. The NIH position appears too politically cautious, seriously lacking the necessary innovative spirit that brings new and viable medicine onto the market for the benefit of the health system. Even the new Office of Alternative Medicine had to be mandated by the will of Congress. That seems a sad commentary on the affairs of state. Opposition to organized innovation often comes from the medical community based on traditional practice paranoia or medical school infatuation. Concomitantly, the FDA has taken a conservative stance on the efficacy of magnetic devices for generalized disease therapy until sufficient data are available to demonstrate the risk/benefit tradeoff. Yet these agencies have largely conceded that magnetotherapy is a benign, safe procedure. Something else must be paramount in the decision-making process. The purpose in these pages is to bring forward ever more needed information on this subject to help direct people who use magnetism into the best possible and safest treatment protocols at this time when it is so important to millions of everyday users who could be otherwise hurt or discouraged by improper use. Even doctors are confused, especially since so few have ever been taught anything about magnetotherapy. With an NIH budget of $10 billion it would seen that one percent of that devoted to this question would not be too much.

We might ask why so little information is made available to the public. The competitive nature of the medical business, government fear and ignorance are the main reasons. The FDA remains almost neutral; insurance companies rarely reimburse for this therapy or most preventative measures; and pharmaceutical companies would rather sell drugs at extremely high profit levels. Also, too many doctors want to maintain the mystery of their healing powers learned from narrowly defined and overly complex medical school curricula in order to keep patients bewildered and dependent. Just recently, President William Clinton said that there is a need for Americans to "take responsibility for our own health as much as we can." Alternative therapies would be a good start in that direction. There is no safer self-help methodology.

However, natural methods of healing appear too simple and straight-forward for most of the medical community. Can you imagine of a single basic therapy were able to relieve countless ailments and what this would mean to the medical profession and our national health bill?

After brief instruction, magnetotherapy can be performed at home by any reasonable person. Of course, providers are instructed always to advise every person to consult a physician for diagnosis and periodic examination for any serious illness. Yet for certain ailments and long-term magnetic maintenance therapy, one can do this as a self-help, home procedure with proper instruction. Instruments can be used for many years or decades and may only weaken if exposed to other, stronger magnetic fields. This means that almost anyone can begin to oversee his or her own body. The occasional visit to a doctor will not do it. Except for the most serious sickness or surgery, our parents and grandparents took charge of illness for most of their generation quite successfully and many are still doing it. The last chapter of this book reports an analysis of 7000 people that shows how plain, sensible lifestyles allow 70 year old people to live as healthy a life as 30- to 40-year-olds who do not lead the lifestyle traditionally espoused by most of our parents.

Today, we need to integrate the old and the new. A recent Rand Corporation study indicated that for most middle-class Americans in particular, no matter how we re-structure the health system, it won't change health status one iota unless we engage in preventive medicine. It emphasizes that what we are doing is essentially meaningless. We need greater concentration on effective preventive health measures and for people to understand what best to do for themselves. Family doctors are too rushed and, sad to say, too many not prevention minded. In order to receive preventive care for most of our health system, one usually has to go into full and costly diagnosis and visitations which most people refuse to do or can't afford, and unfortunately for which they are not reimbursed.

Magnetotherapy could add to our health and to the financial success of American companies and the entire medical community, including pharmaceutical companies. American business will certainly find ways of adding new and improved devices and profitable systems. As long as it is beneficial to humankind, we could all support that. In Japan, ten percent of households or over ten million people use magnetic beds and a total of 30 million use a variety of magnetic devices approved by their Ministry of Health and Welfare. It has not damaged the profits of the wellness industry. On the contrary, it has made for a healthier, more productive society that can take advantage of the diversity of comprehensive health services. Even with their notorious and vigorous work ethic, Japan is number one in the world in life expectancy; the United States eleventh. Just one of many companies, the Nikken corporation, which sells magnetic beds and other health products, is the 21st largest corporation in Japan at over one billion dollars annually.

The squeamishness for professional use of the permanent magnet has something to do with methodology. For electromagnetism, the provider operates an electrical device that requires a current and various controls for manipulation, allowing it to appear more sophisticated. When professional and business people get hold of devices or services where they see medical as well as business opportunity, they are more likely to pursue it. In fact, as already pointed out, many of the orthopedic surgeons who use electromagnetism earn incomes of $400,000 or more a year. The same interest has not occurred for using or promoting permanent magnets, yet evidence exists that the permanent magnet can do essentially the same thing as electromagnets and more safely. The differences lie primarily in speed and power, which can be obtained in both kinds of devices to meet various conditions. The electromagnet can achieve a more effective resonance with the body if designed properly. Used together, electro and permanent, may be the most effective methodology.

The Placebo Effect versus Real Treatment

As stated earlier, it would be foolish to discard the benefits of permanent magnetic therapy simply for a lack of certain placebo (without intrinsic therapeutic value), control studies. Of course, more such studies are needed, yet the thousands of case histories and studies that already exist should not be ignored simply because they are not of a particular nature. Observers working with our team have examined or witnessed first-hand a variety of successful cases watched over a long period of time in order to eliminate the possibilities of placebo reaction. These experiences are in addition to thousands of case histories reported from across the United States. Multiply this by the 50 millions of people using magnetotherapy all over the world and one comes up with real success and, importantly, a high percentage of effectiveness.

Several double-blind, control studies are being undertaken by Dr. Zimmerman, Ph.D, president of the Bio-Electro-Magnetics Institute (BEMI), Reno, Nevada. One involves plant life and growth; a second, implanted tumors in mice where the entire body is exposed; and a third, monitoring pain and quality of sleep.

As stated in the introduction, the placebo effect or psychosomatic response to healing is not as important as once assumed. The double-blind placebo study conducted by the Johns Hopkins Pain Treatment Center indicated that at most 11 to 15 percent of subjects experience the placebo effect.

In the case of magnetotherapy on animals, used extensively by veterinarians and other animal keepers, little to no placebo effect on these unsuspecting dogs and cats and horses occurs, except possibly from the loving care of the master. Yet this therapy is effective in the vast majority of cases.

Some of the most prominent thoroughbred stables report continual success and some instant cures on race horses where hope once had been given up. Henry Arsenault of St. Pierre Health Corporation, Taunton, Massachusetts, reports excellent results attained in as little as 15 minutes when magnets are placed on both sides of a horse's shanks. Energy is increased and pain appears to be eliminated. Inflammation subsides much more quickly and bones heal in one-fourth the time. Veterinarians nationwide use magnetotherapy successfully and placebo effect has virtually nothing to do with it.

From these studies, the conclusion can be fairly drawn that for the majority of those who experience symptom relief or healing from magnetotherapy, it is due to the treatment not the mere idea of treatment. For many therapies, only a fraction, some 20 to 30 percent on average find effectiveness. In the case of magnetic fields, figures from providers suggest unusual, overall success rates of 70 percent or higher. This may not necessarily mean a cure, but relief of symptoms and stress, greater mobility or increases in energy levels and, importantly, without side effects when properly used.

Dr. Philpott has found that magnetotherapy has a much higher success rate and predictability of effectiveness than any other treatment method that he has applied over his lifetime. Almost everyone experiences some good and many show remarkable recovery. He has closely monitored and documented his cases as described in some detail in later chapters.

Would instituting controlled studies prove more about the effectiveness of magnetotherapy? It most likely would. All agree that such studies should be undertaken. However, a great many providers refuse to participate in double-blind, controlled studies where one group of people will not be given the treatment, therefore will not be healed. R. Lightwood, Medical Associate of the Department of Surgery at Queen Elizabeth Hospital in Birmingham, U.K., says his staff can not ethically use control groups while others are being healed. He and the hospital staff have administrated hundreds of successful cases with electrotherapy ranging from the ordinary to difficult war wounds, but all patients were treated. Later, in the description of his methodology, we are to be reminded of his insistence that it is time that all of the medical profession accept this therapy for its genuine effectiveness on a variety of illnesses.

Anecdotal cases cited in this book involve real healing and no control group can change that. In this regard, the millions of people being treated and healed by alternatives such as holistic medicine and natural products, homeopathy, acupuncture, reflexology, biofeedback and all the rest, are not about to cease treatment because there are no control groups to prove they have been healed. In fact, it is very difficult to be able to establish a control group of precise physical and mental equivalency as those under treatment that would allow a fair comparison. Sorting out age, sex, and the type of ailment is usually not enough to match differences in life styles, immune systems, genes, emotional well-being or general health that may influence conclusions.

For more complex illnesses, longer periods of time are needed to validate results. Too many of the controlled studies conducted by the FDA, for example, take place over a six-week period. This is notoriously insufficient to determine adverse side-effects, let alone long-term health, making much of drug testing inconclusive or inappropriate. In so-called anecdotal cases, providers of magnetotherapy can cite numerous cases where people have had ailments for 10 or 20 years and were completely relieved of pain and remain so. These people had tried an endless variety of treatments, including many alternative therapies without result. Perhaps the timing was just right or some other circumstance may have entered into the picture, yet the fact is they were healed by magnetic fields where nothing else worked. The point is that we should not be so scientifically pompous that individual cases or massive clinical trials cannot be treated as success simply because a control group was not used. True science cannot call the six week FDA drug tests effective either.

A Mixture of Cases and Polarities

In magnetotherapy, relief may come immediately or may take hours, days or weeks to reduce pain inflammation or influence more serious ailments. It is difficult to believe that some patients begin to move fingers or arms more freely in a matter of minutes from arthritic-type stiffness, tennis elbow and neck or back pain. People carry small 550 gauss magnets that they place on sore points whenever they feel the need. Others tape a magnet to their backs. Strains and inflammation of many sorts are usually healed in less than half the normal time. In almost all of these cases, pain is taken away when magnetic fields are applied and pain comes immediately back when the magnetic fields are removed. This is continually reflected until the final healing process takes place which may take days or weeks. This characteristic surely discounts any placebo effect.

In the past year, a conference attended by over a thousand back and spine specialists took place in Washington, D.C., concluding that the best thing that can be done about back pain is to do nothing. In most cases, they said, the pain will go away on its own anyway. It appears that the medical profession has given up on this one. Yet, these are the very conditions where millions of sufferers can be helped, and many are with magnetotherapy.

The most interesting of cases, however, are those people who have suffered with illness for many years—where nothing has worked—but are healed in a short-time by magnetotherapy. Dr. Dean Bonlie, himself having suffered from arthritis since the age of 21, has verified the complete elimination of symptoms after sleeping on a negative field magnetic bed for two and one-half months.

Another individual who suffered a broken neck and crushed disk for over 20 years from an automobile accident was very skeptical, even sarcastic that anything could help after trying pills, electric shock, biofeedback, hypnosis, acupuncture, and a variety of other therapies. Nevertheless, the application of permanent magnets to the appropriate place on the body plus a magnetic bed made a difference in one day. His doctor could not believe it. The patient is in his second year of living without pain and has had no need to continue his former medications.

A number of exciting cases are described in this book, but it is not the intention to enumerate hundreds of cases to impress skeptics. These are samplings. Impressive cases exist for cancer, PMS, heart disease, epilepsy, a variety of mental disorders, chronic fatigue syndrome, and for most kinds of ailments. If the immune system is strengthened and energy levels raised, most diseases will be attacked. But these are still anecdotal histories, even as doctors and physical therapists heal case after case in their own medical centers and the typical self-help patient does it in his home.

Dr. David A. Kessler, head of the FDA, states that in life threatening cases, controlled studies for a group of sufferers in a placebo environment is not demanded. Risk/benefit is the more important criterion. People who have suffered for a number of years should not be required to suffer any more under placebo conditions, even though acceptable circumstances for controlled testing must be found to satisfy the medical community. Dr. Kessler speaks of the importance of risk/benefit for breast implants and drug treatments and other therapies. All therapies involve risk/benefit. The patient must eventually control his or her own destiny and help make the assessment. Fortunately, in the case of magnetotherapy, a favorable risk/benefit exists when properly administered.

Citing thousands of cases of effectiveness may not be convincing. For some, famous personalities are impressive. Marvin Fernandes, leading wide receiver for the National Football League's Los Angeles Raiders, sleeps on a Nikken magnetic bed. He testifies. "I don't get tired running and running. I stay fresh, so I get and stay open. I run right past the younger guys. I go to sleep faster...and it helps keep me at peak performance. It's non-chemical, non-invasive...I sleep great, I'm totally rested." Some of his teammates are now using magnetic bed pads.

Nikken, Japan Life, Ameriflex and certain other companies manufacture a complete series of magnetic pads and beds of various polarities. Japan Life also has a blanket with magnets so that one can experience magnetic effect from above as well as below. A number of companies and manufacturers around the world still do not recognize a difference in polarity effect or they use an incorrect designation of which is negative (north) and which is positive (south) poled. The method for designating positive and negative orientation is described in the following chapters.

In many instances, athletes, decathlon competitors, weight lifters, and other energy seekers are now using magnetic devices to gain strength and endurance. Thomas Hanley, Mr. Canada and World Championship qualifier of 1990, sleeps on an extra-strength magnetic bed in a negative field orientation. Body pain has been reduced 80 percent after major workouts, heart rate at post exercise did not increase, squat lifts increased by 20 percent, and leg extensions increased 46.4 percent after being on the pad for six weeks. It is significant that he had not experienced any increase in strength in this exercise in one and one-half years before using the magnetic bed. Also his weight dropped seven pounds while his muscle dimensions remained the same, which is a better definition for a body builder. (See Exhibit 1, Extra Strength Magnetic Bed Pad related to the negative oriented pads used by both Magnet-X Corp. and MagnetiCo Inc., Calgary, Canada.)

The significance about the above two methodologies is that people are healed or their performance improved by using either the negative or positive magnetic fields. Also, some providers make magnetic beds with simultaneous positive and negative orientation. Over the years, it appears all sorts of combinations have been tried. Certain specialists, such as the late Richard Broeringmeyer, N.D., D.C. Ph.D; Albert Muller, M.D.; and Ted Zablotsky, M.D. believe that the simultaneous positive and negative orientation is perfectly acceptable, particularly for localized application. Certain researchers, Coesta Wollen, Ph.D and Erik Enby, M.D., report important clinical success in treating cancer with the positive pole alone placed over or near the heart, but this essentially promotes the stimulation of the immune system which the positive polarity will do at least temporarily. Nevertheless, positive fields might also eventually accelerate cancer cell growth as shown by Dr. Robert O. Becker.

Other scientists, Elizabeth Rauscher, Ph.D and William Van Bise, E-E., believe magnetic fields in general are dangerous because of the deleterious effects evidenced from electromagnetic pollution, but this has much to do with frequency rates not applicable to permanent magnets (discussed in greater detail in Chapter 3). And finally, researchers and practitioners Albert Roy Davis (deceased), Harry Park, M.D., William Philpott, M.D., Tom Nellessen, Dean Bonlie, John Zimmerman, Robert Barefoot and a vast number of others agree that biomagnetic north (negative) is the polarity that should be used for treating almost all illnesses and is the safest, particularly for long-term or accumulative exposure at the higher gauss strength.

The data presented here must be digested fairly on balance, keeping in mind that further research is necessary. Human beings can experience healing and energy increases from either pole or both poles together. Bipolar magnets have been shown to function more quickly than a single pole magnet of equal strength, perhaps because of a quicker biofeedback response. Both poles will produce energy, the positive through stimulation, the negative from rest. After sleeping on a south pole mattress for several weeks or a few months, depending on one's constitution, the user might feel a loss of energy or even a stressful condition. Providers of

Exhibit 1   Extra Strength Magnetic Bed Pad

Subject: Tom Hanley

1. Mr. Alberta Master Light Weight, Mr. Canada, World Championship Qualifier, 1990.

2. He does not use drugs of any type and for the last six months has not taken enzymes or vitamins, nor has he changed his work-out program. He started sleeping on a Magnet-X Extra-Strength Pad, September, 1991.

3. The maximum weight he could lift--in equals of 20 repetitions--was 309 lbs. (this amount had remained the same for the last 1½ years before pad use.) After lifting a series of lesser weights but just before reaching the 309 lbs. and before using the negative magnetic pad, his pre-exercise heart-rate was 84 beats/minute and 150 beats/minute post-exercise. Two-minute post exercise heart-rate was 102 beats/minute. After six weeks of sleeping on the negative magnetic pad, his pre-exercise heart-rate was 72 beats/minute.

4. After 6 weeks sleeping on the negative pad, Tom was able to do 25 repetitions rather than 20 (which is a 20 percent increase), yet both his immediate and two-minute post-exercise heart-rates remained the same.

5. His leg extensions were also tested, which he does at the end of his exercise program. Before using the pad, he was able to lift 6 plates, 28 times. After being on the pad for 6 weeks, his leg extensions were increased to 41 times; a 46.6% increase. It must be noted that he had not experienced any increase in this exercise in 1½ years.

6. Hanley reports that soreness after a major workout, such as described above, has been reduced by 80%. He stated that normally the next two days after a major workout is like "hell" in the mornings, and that now this is no longer the case. During the six week time period of sleeping on the magnetic pad, Hanley's weight dropped seven pounds, yet his muscle dimensions remained the same. This, of course, is very important to the body builder, as it gives better definition to muscles with less fat.

Source: Dr. Dean Bonlie, formerly with Magnet-X Corporation and now with MagnetiCo Inc., Calgary, Alberta, Canada.

Note: MagnetiCo and Magnet-X sleeping pads are of similar construction, gauss strength, and polarity.

positive oriented beds instruct people to halt use temporarily—for a few weeks—if stress develops, in order to allow the body to rebalance itself from what they believe is a state of adaptation, then resume use of the magnetic bed. However, it is important to point out that after continued use, even with a rest period, reports Dr. Philpott and Dean Bonlie, this can result in a persistent level of stress, although one may not feel it directly in pain or immediate symptoms.

As serious as stress symptoms are, a strong positive pole has other problems. The positive polarity promotes the growth of all living things. Davis and Becker and others have demonstrated that the positive fields accelerate the growth of bacteria, virus, fungus, and cancer. A similar conclusion was reported in the (September 1990) Journal of the National Medical Association in reference to cultures that were exposed to both negative and positive poles. These tests showed that an increase of cancer cell proliferation occurred at the positive fields in just a few days; biomagnetic negative exhibited a markedly reduced growth compared to biomagnetic south and a control group.

Assessment of these differences may be the most controversial in the understanding of magnetotherapy. In his research, Robert Becker describes the positive field as the polarity of injury which results in the release of chemicals to the damaged site and correspondingly elicits negative pulsed magnetic energy from the brain to that area. This is believed to be largely a biofeedback response. Importantly, overuse of the positive field makes it less effective because other areas of the body also regularly call for negative magnetic energy from the brain; therefore, there are limitations on its use.

Positive magnetic fields redirect energy but do not produce new energy as do the negative fields, according to both Philpott and Bonlie. The magnetic energy from the brain is distributed to the body by D.C. currents flowing through the Schwann cells that surround the nerves in the periphery of the body outside the central nervous system. Some believe that dual polarity magnets (concentric, checkerboard, magnetic foil and other configurations) will not penetrate body tissue as deeply as single poled positive magnets of the same gauss strength, because one polarity is offsetting the other to some extent. If this is true, it would be easier for the body to accommodate long-term use of alternating polarities. Still, the body must have sufficient vital forces (D.C. current) to do so.

In the treatment of severe muscle spasm, for instance, Dr. Bonlie first uses the positive field for 10 minutes to stimulate the process; then, he uses the calming negative field for 15 minutes or longer until the muscle is completely relaxed. Clinical evidence supports his theory that positive exposure stimulates the biofeedback response, increasing the pulsed D.C. current to the area of injury. The pulsed D.C. current and its accompanying magnetic field interact with the negative magnetic field when it is next applied. The interaction of these two enhanced fields increases magnetic resonance in the tissue being treated. The resulting increased orbital energy of the affected electrons causes enhanced chemical activity and diffusion of gases in the tissues, speeding recovery. The use of the positive field alone to increase the biofeedback response is not as effective or as fast as the use of the two fields in the above sequence, reports Dr. Bonlie.

Meeting the Challenge

Much of our health and treatment philosophies are affected by magnetic energy forces that we really don't understand. We know more about how to build atomic bombs and get to Mars than we do about the basic mysteries of life. Many alternative therapies function largely from magnetic effect. Suppose this medicine does cure many diseases or at least arrests or relieves ailments and prevents the onslaught of disease through preventative therapy—then we truly have found a marvel of life. For some, it has been that very thing. Why don't we unravel the blindness of this centuries' old medicine and undertake whatever experimentation is necessary to open or close the doors? For the benefit of society and world health, the unwillingness to percolate resources for research and development of this alternative medicine must be overcome in a free society against the odds of all opposition. We must ask and answer these questions as to whether we are dealing with real science or something else.

It seems that there is common interest here for government, the medical community, providers, and patient users to be concerned and earnestly willing to find answers. Since millions of people are already making use of magnetotherapy, it is paramount that they be guided in the proper direction. Let us at least begin seriously to take up the challenge.

Chapter 2

How Magnetism Relates to Human Life, Planets, and Alternative Therapies

Man is an Electromagnetic Creature

Magnetism is a force all around us and within us. It is universal in nature, in the planets and stars, the sun and moon—all of which replicate giant magnets that extend their magnetic fields for thousands, even millions of miles. Each influences the other, depending on the extent of its power and location. The Earth is particularly influenced by the sun and moon and other heavenly bodies. It emanates its own magnetic field from several sources—electric current within itself, from atmospheric electricity, and likely its own rotation. Human bodies and even the smallest atom within us are forms of magnets. Each cell has a north and south polarity in our DNA that affects our lives and health in many different ways (Semm; Bradford). Surely, we would want to know how it influences us.

Over our long history, it is unfortunate that some have manipulated magnetotherapy and certain other natural therapies for their selfish motives of profit or personal fortune. Electrotherapy was applied over-enthusiastically to claim cures for almost any disease without the studies to defend it. This approach has largely driven the subject from medical classrooms and clinics. Only in the last couple of decades has renewed interest come about. Yet, much of the medical profession tends to shy away from any treatment that cannot demonstrate successful double-blind, placebo controlled studies, or does not provide physicians a regimen in which they can feel comfortable in prescribing a very definite amount of something—usually a drug for a precise disease.

Most doctors can't seem to find the time to get close to patients any more, in order to get to know them, to understand their condition fully, or to comfort and work with them like the traditional family doctor used to do. It doesn't seem to pay so we continue to lose family doctors. Push is too great to rush patients through the office and to identify a magic bullet that will cure a specific condition after one gets sick rather than before. Prevention seems not to be in the realm of the physician's work any more. Good nutrition, exercise, positive thinking, and a variety of therapies seem all too conditional and require too much time and effort on the part of the doctor to encourage or guide his client. For too many physicians, it appears easier to prescribe a drug, a test or an operation.

Drugged Nation

It would seem enough that doctors over-prescribe drugs for their patients, but we are also bombarded by the drug companies with endless advertising to buy more drugs and constantly flooded or betrayed by the over-the-counter pills we take. A good example of deception is enumerated in the Public Citizen Health Research Group's book, **Over-the-Counter Pills that Don't Work**, that asks the question "...what is the only safe and effective ingredient for treating pain contained in the following products: Alka Seltzer pain reliever, Antacid, Anacin, Maximum Strength Anacin, Bayer Aspirin, Bayer Time-Release Aspirin, Bufferin, Arthritis Strength Bufferin and Cope?" The answer is aspirin alone. The rest of the ingredients lack evidence of safety or effectiveness.

Most drugs are essentially the same. The drug companies spend more of their resources on developing competing drugs that are basically the same than on new drugs that may offer true cures, simply to increase profits. And the costs of drugs have gone up three to four times the rate of inflation. The drug industry as a whole spends more on advertising than they do on research. Now there's got to be something wrong with that. If drugs were so effective, advertising would hardly be necessary.

The nation is buying over 300,000 different over-the-counter drugs concocted out of a mere 1,000 ingredients—two-thirds of which have not been proved safe or effective. Furthermore, most diseases for which typical self-medication is appropriate are self-limiting, like a cold which usually gets better no matter what you do. Nevertheless, over $1 billion a year of anti-histamines are pushed on us for colds when, according to a congressional study, they have no effect. The FDA, according to Ralph Nader's Public Citizen, is violating the drug laws by allowing these untested ingredients to be marketed, but pressure from the drug companies and the medical profession keeps them on our shelves to the tune of $10 to $15 billion a year. We can double this figure for prescribed drugs, knowing that emphasis on pharmacology permeates the training of our physicians. Furthermore, one-third of prescription drugs are illegal drugs. We are a drugged-out society that needs safe, non-drug approaches to problems that affect us every day of our lives, problems such as sleeping difficulties, excess weight, coughs and colds, constipation, depression, chronic pain syndrome and many other ailments.

Looking back, you may recall how penicillin made medicine almost exclusively drug oriented. We are still looking for more like that. No matter how clinically effective a therapy is, most of the medical community seems to believe that to work it must work chemically or not work at all. We assume that the cure for cancer will be a chemical that kills malignant cells without harming healthy ones. Promises of a technological fix and golden health and extended life have turned out to be empty, points out Dr. Robert O. Becker, nominated several times for the Nobel Prize. The degenerative diseases—heart attack, arteriosclerosis, cancer, stroke, arthritis, hypertension, ulcers—have replaced infectious diseases as the major enemies of life. Failure of technology medicine, Becker says, paradoxically is due to its success, sweeping away all aspects of medicine as an art. Doctors seem unable to learn from patients, only from their professors, he says. We know a great deal, yet we are no closer to the truth. We know virtually nothing about basic life functions of pain, sleep, control of cell differentiation, and growth and healing. We remain almost totally ignorant of nearly every aspect of consciousness, instinct, choice, memory, learning, individuality, and creativity. And we know little about how the human organism regulates its metabolic activity in cycles to the fluctuations of the Earth, moon and sun. Becker flatly states that the chemical-mechanistic model has failed.

Most Important Discovery

Only recently are technicians reexamining and applying therapeutic technology previously discarded as "unscientific" by the academic and medical world. Orthodox treatments are not healing the masses. For example, patients are becoming increasingly dissatisfied with their care. Over 25 percent of hospital deaths are the cause of the hospital visit itself. Many enter with a minor illness and come out with a major complication. We know that people heal faster at home. The old adage of "the doctor knows best" many times means the doctor is wrong or can make you sicker.

Most medical professionals are saying that the doctor should make sure his patient knows all there is to know about illness and the therapeutic possibilities, both orthodox and unorthodox. Most progressives say that a maximum level of control by the patient over his treatment will reduce stress and improve the outcome. The doctor must let the patient help make decisions. We must begin to understand that the ill person cannot safely delegate responsibility to any one else.

Magnetotherapy is just one alternative treatment that requires trial and error, demonstrates some uncertainty like most therapies, and works best under extensive personal and continual observation of the patient. It also includes choice by the patient. Doctors complain that this type of treatment takes time and time is money. Unfortunately, most physicians don't seem to want to learn alternative therapies. These treatments appear too fundamental to be real. How many doctors are willing to stand up and dare to say that your life is in any sense electrical or magnetic and your health is dependent on it? Dr. Becker sums it up by stressing the importance of including the Earth's normal geomagnetic field as an environmental variable when we deal with basic bodily functions: "In my opinion, this knowledge is probably the most important discovery of the century."

History of Magnetism

Some of you may recall how your mother walked across the dewy grass early in the morning encouraging you to come along as you danced and felt so good—fatigue and dullness leaving the body. The soles of our feet are a network of nerves that stimulate the entire body. We never knew why it felt so good, only that it did. We know more clearly now that a magnetic energy force passes liberally through our bodies from many sources, including more centered areas like the feet and hands.

Some therapists insist that sleeping with the head to the north and feet to the south facilitates the flow of the Earth's magnetism and assists in restful sleep. Dr. H. L. Bansal, in his book **Magnetic Cure for Common Diseases**, points out the age-long Hindu custom of placing a person near death with his head to the north and feet to the south to reduce agony. Dr. William H. Philpott, psychiatrist and practitioner expert in the field of electromagnetic therapy, has designed a head board where negative (north polarity) magnetism is set up to flow through the crown of the head, with amazing therapeutic effects. He emphasizes the importance of the negative (north) magnetic field as the healing polarity.

The geophysical magnetic lines of the Earth essentially run straight up into the sky and then toward the magnetic poles. Robert O. Becker conducted an experiment in which he aligned a magnetic field parallel to the Earth's magnetic field and another at right angles. When cancer cells in culture were exposed to the field at right angles, they showed several abnormalities and did not replicate; when exposed in the parallel position, no alteration occurred in the cells. This embodies the principle of the Hall Effect which states that magnetic fields influence a substance when its force is at right angles to it.

Human beings have used the beneficial powers of magnetism for thousands of years even with little knowledge of its scientific reasoning, knowing only that it works. More than 100,000 years ago magnetite was ground up to be used in potions and foods and topical applications. Our knowledge of this can be traced to African bloodstone mines. In fact, most of the ancient civilizations used magnets for healing, including the Hebrews, Arabs, Indians, Egyptians, and Chinese. Aristotle was the first in recorded history to speak of the therapeutic properties of natural magnets on the body. About 200 B.C., the Greek physician Galan found that pain could be relieved for many illnesses with natural magnets. A Persian physician documented the use of magnets in 1,000 A.D. to relieve disorders, such as gout and muscle spasms.

In 1991, one of my close associates, suffering from gout since childhood was instantly relieved of pain in a matter of minutes with the application of a permanent magnet on his big toe. He now sleeps and sits on a magnetic pad with excellent results. Dozens of cases of relief from pain or lack of muscular movement from gout, arthritis, backache, tennis elbow, sprains, inflammation, and a variety of other conditions have been personally witnessed. Hundreds of thousands of cases are reported worldwide. It is fascinating, from B.C. until now, the same simple magnets have been used to cure or bring relief.

In the 17th century, English physicians wrote of the positive effects of magnetism. Also the first in-depth study of the history of magnetic treatment of diseases was undertaken by the Royal Society of Medicine in France. Numerous other studies have continued through the years, some confirming effectiveness, some not. There is never a 100 percent cure factor or even close to it with any medicine. Controlled, double-blind studies are considered effective if there is simply a marked improvement in a reasonable percentage of the patient population.

The Egyptians, builders of the pyramids, were well acquainted with the properties of magnetic force, utilizing it for the preservation of mummies to delay the decay of lifeless bodies. The legendary beauty Queen Cleopatra of Egypt (69 - 30 B.C.) wore a magnet on her forehead to preserve her figure. Ancients believed that the magnet had magical healing powers. It was not until the 16th Century that a Swiss alchemist and physician, P. A. Paracelsus, researched and observed that the magnet could cure inflammations, influxes, ulcerations, and diseases of the bowels and uterus. And Dr. Mesmer (1734 - 1815) of Mesmerism fame succeeded in curing serious and complicated disorders, although he went overboard with claims and lost his credibility. Also, Dr. Samuel Hahnemann (1755 - 1843), the father of homeopathy, was fully convinced of the powers of the magnet and recommended its use. Today, some therapists believe that magnetotherapy can largely supplant homeopathy and acupuncture because it essentially does the same thing. Unfortunately, the mystery and doubt about the effectiveness of magnetotherapy prevail in the medical world and in the training of doctors generally.

Our Amazing Magnetic Earth and Planets

The Sun

The whole idea of geomagnetic fields and their respective effects is absolutely fascinating. The spinning molten iron, miles beneath the surface of the Earth, creates a dipole magnetic field similar to a bar magnet.

The sun's energy distorts and converts this field to a magnetofield from the solar wind crashing into the outer layers of the Earth's magnetic field, compressing it until energy matches that of the solar wind. On the other side, away from the sun, the Earth's magnetic field is drawn into a long magnetotail which stretches far out into Space. From this, high energy particles are trapped in the Van Allen belts and bounce back and forth between the north and south ends of our planet.

Besides solar wind, the sun emits deadly ionizing radiation (X-Rays) and other high energy particles, largely blocked out by our own magnetosphere, without which we could not survive. Space flights beyond these boundaries must be of short duration and timed for a tight solar cycle, otherwise astronauts would perish. Recent experiments by NASA confirm this. We must be grateful for the magnetosphere that protects our small island from a very hostile universe filled with enormous forces.

Over hundreds of millions of years, the Earth's magnetic poles reportedly have changed places a number of times and its fields have declined substantially. A collapse or partial collapse of the magnetosphere could occur again, exposing the Earth to the full force of solar winds and ionizing radiation that would kill organisms, you and me, the dog and plants.

Outer space bombardment creates enormous electric currents to the tune of billions of watts and ionizing radiation of electromagnetic waves in the range of extra-low frequencies (ELF) between 100 and 1,000 cycles. A rather "quiet field" can result from an inactive sun. The aurora borealis is caused by solar storms that enter the Earth's magnetic field at the polar regions into the atmosphere and interact with gas molecules to produce unusual and beautiful lights. Many magnetic dust particles enter the atmosphere and drop to the ocean floor like a layer cake of magnetite deposits, along with a vast number of radiolarians or skeletons of minute single celled sea creatures. Our system is composed of a rather complex array of magnetic forces.

The sun's magnetic field is more than 100 times greater than the Earth's. We depend on the sun for life, light and shade, day and night, seasons, vegetation, fire, heat, and magnetism. Without the sun there would be no life, just a dark, barren Earth. The sun's solar and magnetic storms affect all living creatures here on Earth. Since our cells are small magnets, they are sensitive to the daily cyclic patterns of the Earth's magnetic field. Sun spots can cause restlessness and other adverse effects.

Studies show that mental patients become aggravated and highly disturbed during these periods. Animals stir wildly, horses kick their stalls and a general excitement whips the air. You and I feel it too.

Information Brief

Earth in the Balance

Man-made pollution created right here on Earth is damaging us. The ozone hole that opens up each winter over the Antarctica, and now spreading elsewhere, threatens much of North America, London, Brussels, Berlin, and Moscow, exposing us to even higher doses of dangerous, ultraviolet radiation, according to NASA scientists in a report released in February 1992. Vice President Albert Gore, in his book **Earth in the Balance: Ecology and the Human Spirit**, says it is clear that increased levels of ultraviolet radiation suppress the immune system and increase our vulnerability to disease, raising rates of melanoma and cataracts. He has proposed a Strategic Environment Initiative (SEI) that would phase out older technologies worldwide for a new and better generation of environmentally benign substitutes. Proposals would move up the phase out of chlorofluorocarbons (CFCs) from the year 2000 to 1995 or 1997. If nothing is done, reports the United Nations, new cases of skin cancer will increase by 300,000 (26 percent) and cataracts by 1.6 million (8 percent) per year by the turn of the century. Increases will also occur in cancer of the lip and salivary gland and in infectious diseases, including AIDs. (See Appendix III for latest research on reducing auto emissions; this demonstration by the Eco-Mag™ could possibly mean a breakthrough for pollution control.)

The varying effects come from the positive and negative polarities of the magnetic fields. The positive field and its ions excite us, while the negative calms us down. When a thunder storm first brews up, positive ions are dominant, which stir our senses and excite our bodies. As the storm recedes, negative ions predominate and we begin to feel at ease, even wonderful. Surely, you have noticed this. Next time watch for it. It is the reason why we, as well as animals, begin to stir and become excited at the beginning of the storm during the positive polarity and suddenly relax as the storm recedes and the negative ions flourish.

The moon affects us too; it is not merely some silly superstition. Many of us are skeptics by nature and it has to be proved to us. But we know that calendars are set in reference to the moon and menstrual periods of women are directly linked to the lunar calendar. It is believed that body fluids flow better on full moon days. Some studies show that certain ailments, especially mental conditions are adversely affected during the full moon. A greater degree of magnetism flows to the Earth from the sun during full moon exposure, as the sun's magnetic fields cover a wider

SCIENTIFIC DIGEST

Sunspots, Electromagnetic Fields, and Life Span

Sunspots and life span may be interrelated and may give astrology its best scientific basis, at least as to how it is influenced by one planet—the sun. A study in the peer review journal *Radiation Research* (March 1993) conducted by Barnett Rosenberg, Michigan State University biophysicist, and David A. Juckett, Professor of chemistry, indicates that people born to mothers who were born in sunspot minimum activity periods live several years longer than those born to mothers born in high sunspot activity cycles. Rosenberg previously led development of two of the world's leading anticancer drugs—eisplatin and carboplatin.

Rosenberg and Juckett chose a sampling of groups that had a sizable population for which there are reliable records of birth and death rates over a long period of time. The first group, totaling 7,552, was of U.S. House of Representative members and two other groups were members of the British House of Commons and alumni of the University of Cambridge. The same 9 - 12 year cycles of sunspot activity emerged with similar life-span results.

The importance of the mother's birth is that a woman's ova—or "eggs" that she will release one at a time in each menstrual cycle is formed by the time she is born. During this highly radiation sensitive period, much of the genetic fate of her children is sealed. A gene altering effect could come from this extra dose of radiation that puts out both electromagnetic waves (ultraviolet, X-rays, gamma rays) and charged particles such as protons and electrons which vary with the number of sunspots, the more sunspots, the more radiation.

Another indicator, described elsewhere, is that sunspots throw out very high levels of positive magnetic fields shown to cause mental anxiety and distortion in both humans and animals. Also positive magnetic fields, as experienced in animal studies, shorten life-span as compared to the negative magnetic fields that tend to extend longevity. The Rosenberg study may be a good reason to study further the effects of polarity differences on life-span and health.

Source: *Radiation Research*, March, 1993; *Washington Post*, May 24, 1993, H3, Boyce Rensberger; author.

surface of the moon in relationship to particular sectors of the Earth. Importantly, during this period the positive ions predominate.

SCIENTIFIC DIGEST

Ionization Machines

Ionization machines resemble the calm of storms. They were approved over a decade ago by the FDA as medical devices for allergies, hay fever, and common respiratory disorders. Professor A. P. Kreuger, University of California, says the negative ions kill off bacteria. In a trial of 3,000 patients at a Cologne clinic, 80 percent of those under age 20 experienced complete relief by using the ion machine, while 50 percent of the older group benefited. In heated buildings, the production of positive ions and the loss of negative ions from smoke, dust and fumes take place. Negative ionization helps to clear up the environment in buildings and elsewhere. Executives use them in their offices; thoroughbred horse trainers use them in stalls.

Source: A. P. Kreuger, University of California, 1992; FDA; author.

We have already pointed out that the human body is engulfed in its own magnetic field. Dr. Bansal reminds us that the occultists call it the Astral Body. In any case, the effects influence our inner nature and physical and mental health. The mere touch or laying-on-of-hands by prophets, ministers or ordained persons has resulted in cures, if not permanent, at least relief of symptoms. This is not magic or necessarily spiritual. Dr. John Zimmerman of BEMI, who has studied this phenomenon rather extensively, states that it involves the stronger magnetic force of the "healer" or purveyor to the sick or magnetically underbalanced, undernourished person. This may answer some of the questions as to how an Oral Roberts or other spiritualists heal people before our eyes. Actually, most healers are just ordinary people with plain jobs who heal in their spare time and don't have the slightest idea of how it works. In Poland, for instance, these healers are accepted as valid medical therapists subject to licensing by their government. Sometimes the effect may only take a minute or so to work.

In a significant number of these cases, a hypnotic or psychosomatic effect may also take place where the person being cured is mentally overwhelmed   by a strong belief in a higher power or a powerfully influential individual.   Studies show that the psychological effect may be present only in a small percentage of the cases.   For the rest, something physical is happening or it may be a combination of both.   Zimmerman's experiments demonstrate that it can very well be the transfer of magnetic energy.

The Earth's Decreasing Magnetic Field

The Earth's magnetic field is in constant flux, influenced by solar winds, shifts in the Earth's core, and the presence of ferromagnetic substances in the Earth's crust.   The field varies its intensity periodically and reverses itself about every one-half to one million years.   Scientists report that the most recent reversal was about 700,000 years ago.   What happens is that the strength of the field gradually grows weaker, reaches a minimum or disappears entirely and then builds up again in the opposite direction, resulting in reversal of the north and south magnetic poles.

Robert Barefoot states that the Earth's poles have changed positions many times, as evidenced from geological measurements of iron in volcanic rock.   At one time, the north pole was a few hundred miles north of Hawaii; at another time near Tuscon, Arizona.   This polar shifting is really the Earth's shell or mantle wandering about the fixed magnetic poles, he believes.   Not only do the continents drift apart, they also slide past the poles.   Relative to the Earth's mantle, its molten metallic core is massive.   But its relation is not affected to any degree by the sliding crust.

The laws of physics state that when unlike substances are rubbed together, electrons are stripped from one and passed to the other.   The electrical current generated creates the associated magnetic field, setting up both north and south poles.   As this spin differential is reduced to zero, electric current is no longer generated and poles disappear.   Spin differential is caused by celestial activity and positioning of the solar system, which can cause the reversal of the flow of electrons and of polarity (north pole becoming the south pole and vice versa), according to Barefoot.   Others believe that the evidence of pole reversal is weak. However, there is strong indication that the Earth's magnetic field has collapsed nine different times, resulting in positive fields on the Earth for short periods.

Questions abound about evolution and extinction. Several theories suggest that the extinction of animal life on Earth can be laid to the disappearance of magnetic forces at various periods. It appears that there were many periods of extinction occurring at the end of the geological eras of Devonian, Permian, Triassic, and Cretaceous. During the last period, dinosaurs became extinct. Each period represented a change in the direction of evolution. Humans have never yet experienced it. However, many scientists believe that the creation of our own heavily implanted electric and magnetic energy that is polluting our atmosphere may hasten our demise. Dr. Becker indicates that over the past 50 years we have more than duplicated changes in frequencies and strength of micropulsations that may have been associated with past specie die-outs.

Physicists have documented that the Earth's magnetic field may have degraded 50 percent over the past 500 to 1,000 years, with a full 5 percent decline recorded in the last 100 years. Some believe a sufficient magnetic field to support life within 1,500 years may not exist if this degradation continues at its present rate. Dr. Bansal reminds us that certain locales on Earth have inexplicably retained the strength of their magnetic fields. As already noted, these include areas near Sedona, Arizona, and Lourdes, France, where countless persons travel annually to experience feelings of well-being and to seek healing.

The daily rise and fall of the Earth's magnetic fields cause our biological rhythms. The Earth as a whole measures at a strength of one-half gauss (0.5) today but some researchers believe it was about four (4) gauss centuries ago. The Earth's daily fluctuation of magnetism is about

0.1 gauss. Compare this to the magnet on your refrigerator door of over 200 gauss. And remember, although the Earth's magnetic strength is small, it is constant and is everywhere, therefore highly effective. However, reinforced concrete buildings, elevators and automobiles decrease our exposure 20 percent or more from the Earth's magnetic fields our bodies need. Such distortions also make the use of a compass for directional purposes almost useless. The magnetic force in automobiles and trucks is 50 percent less than that found outside in river beds, for example. Our modern age promotes an unhealthy condition for at least half of our population. You may wonder why we need to worry about the loss of the Earth's magnetism if it is so small. If there were no magnetism, we would not be alive. If this last statement is true, then there should not be a question that the manipulation of magnetic fields can either improve or distort our bodily functions.

Magnetism Defined

The natural magnet has many names. The Greek's call it—Magnetis or Magnesetos; the English—lodestone; the French—Aiment (loving stone); the Indians—Chumbak (kissing stone); the Arabs—Maqnatees; and the Chinese—Chu She. They have all used magnets to make health products.

We manufacture magnets because not enough natural magnets of the proper shape or strength exist. Magnetic materials can be made by rubbing magnets on a substance in a unidirectional fashion or by exposing material to an electromagnet or with a device called a magnetizer which charges the material instantaneously to the desired gauss.

The molecular theory of magnetism can simply be explained by the transformation that takes place. Molecules are tiny magnets misaligned in non-magnetized material, which means similar poles do not point in the same direction—the north neutralizing the south and vice versa. The process of magnetization changes the existing positions to align them properly, the strength determined by the percentage aligned. Also, a magnet can attract a non-magnet because some molecules of the non-magnet will be aligned to the magnet.

Information Brief

Recent Scientific Studies about Geomagnetic Effects

Dr. E. G. Stoupel, cardiologist and Ph.D on the faculty at the Toor Heart Institute, Bellinson Medical Center in Petah-Tiqva, Israel, has conducted a series of studies that show changes in geomagnetic activity that affect cardiovascular health. For instance, there is higher hospital cardiovascular and cerebrovascular accident mortality on active and stormy days of the geomagnetic atmosphere (GMA), higher deaths from acute myocardial infarction (heart attack), higher diastolic blood pressure in healthy blood donors and hypertensive patients, greater human blood plasm viscosity, more severe migraine headaches, higher levels of human prolactin and 17-ketosteroid levels, and higher levels of human growth hormone, among a number of findings. He is continuing to conduct studies in the cosmobiology field and effects on the human body.

Permanent magnets are made from iron or more often from the alloy Alnico—composed of aluminum, nickel, iron and cobalt. Some are made from a synthetic material prepared from oxides of ferric and barium and are called ceramic, ferrite or graphite magnets.

Every magnet has two poles called north (negative) and south (positive). Even the tiniest molecules are magnets. If a magnet is broken in two or into many small pieces, each becomes a magnet with two poles. The poles are simply a concentration of magnetism at the two ends, the most powerful magnetic points. Single poles are primarily used in therapy because greater strength lies with one pole where the opposite pole cannot offset the other. It should be noted that cylindrical shaped magnets have the broadest magnetized surface. It is common understanding that the north and south poles are directly attracted to each other by swinging their fields back to the ends of the magnet (as in a bar magnet). Rawls and Davis stated that these forces converged at the center of the magnet where strength (repelling fields) was the weakest. Evidence seems to be clear that a meridian occurs at the center of the magnet yet lines of force travel all around the magnet to its ends, varied in effect by length and gauss strength. The fields weaken with distance.

It is common knowledge that opposite poles attract each other and that the same poles repel each other. This is important in magnetotherapy as there is a different effect from opposite poles. In homeopathy, for example, medicines are prepared from each pole. Furthermore, the strength of the magnetic field is subject to the strength of the magnet; yet, regardless of strength, the magnetic field is always infinite, much like the circles of sound waves that get bigger and bigger in space but go on forever. The field weakens with distance but never ends as it circles the Earth. However, it cannot reach out into the universe because it is canceled by the magnetosphere.

Frequencies in Magnetic Fields

Let us briefly look at the technical functioning of electric currents in a magnetic field. An electric current flowing through a wire produces a magnetic field around the wire. The strength of the magnetic field is related to the amount of current flow. If the current is D.C., the field is steady like a permanent magnet.   If the electric current in the wire is fluctuating, the magnetic field will have the same fluctuation as the current and be characterized by the rate of frequencies or fluctuations per second. We call this hertz (Hz), rather than cycles per second, after Heinrich Hertz.

The field is called electromagnetic because it has both an electric field and a magnetic field. It also has a wave motion. Its speed is that of light (186,000 miles per second). The wave length depends on frequency. A one Hz frequency has a wave length thousands of miles long; a one million Hz frequency (MHz) has a wave length of several hundred feet; and a one hundred million Hz frequency (100 MHz) has a wave length of about six feet.   About one percent of the frequency spectrum is light. Sunlight and the light from electric lights have the same characteristics as radio waves and X-rays.   Light is electromagnetic radiation.   An individual quantum of electromagnetic radiation equals one photon (Y). We can see light because we have developed our eyes as anatomical detectors, but we cannot see magnetic fields. Magnetic fields have both waves and photon particles but have no mass. In quantum theory, photons carry the entity—the higher the frequency the greater the energy. Any frequency greater than 20,000 cycles per second, as in ultrasound, is beyond human hearing range. Ultrasound therapy, for instance, converts high frequency electric current into vibrating sonic waves from an *oscillating quartz crystal (piezoelectric) substance whose basic science is magnetic energy.**

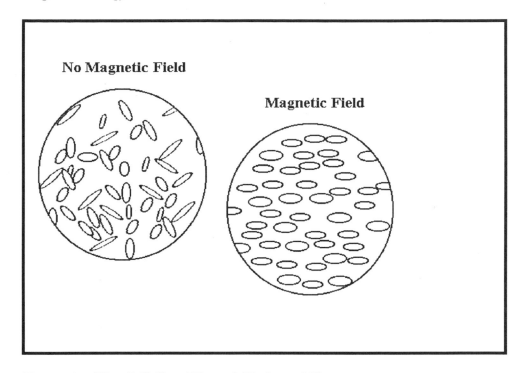

Figure 1   Blood Cell as Viewed Under a Microscope

Frequency, power level, and duration of exposure all have some effect on the human organism. Frequency seems to be the least understood. A very low frequency of 10 hertz has a wave length thousands of miles long so would appear to bypass a six-foot human, while shorter wavelengths (higher frequencies) that approach the size of man may be more easily absorbed. In any case, research shows that all wave lengths produce biological effects. Studies show effect or non-effect from different hertz magnetic fields. Longer time exposure might very well show effect for all wavelengths. This is exemplified by human exposure to high power electric lines (discussed more fully in another chapter) that may not show immediate effect but that can be detrimental. And most importantly, permanent (steady state) magnets without frequency, produce equally fascinating results which lead us to speculate that wavelength is not the

---

* The italicized text refers to more complex information.

controlling factor. It appears that the body can easily modulate frequencies (like a radio receiver), enabling it to absorb most frequencies.

Magnetism and Living Organisms

As far back as the early 1960s, Dr. Robert O. Becker stated that the D.C. current in the brain produces a magnetic field that can be observed at a distance outside the head if we had a magnetometer of sufficient sensitivity to measure it. At the time, this declaration brought considerable laughter from scientists who said such a device could never be made and even if such a magnetic field could be measured, its strength would be so small that it would be of no physiological consequence whatsoever. Of course, we now are familiar with the SQUID (Superconducting Quantum Interference Device) that measures the MEG (magnetoencephalogram) fields from the brain to inform us what is happening inside. Science is now mapping every section of the brain and we may expect remarkable discoveries in the near future. We know now that the electromagnetic fields all about us, considerably weaker than the Earth's 0.5 gauss force, influence our health and the cyclic behavior of living organisms. We know these scientific facts, yet have done little with them.

Scientists, as well as the average person, always knew we had intrinsic cycles of sleep and wakefulness and other regularized activities, but the science mechanics simply explained this as a chemical oscillator or clock timer in the brain. Yet, says Becker, all the cycles had rates of change almost identical to the cycles of the geophysical environment. Long-range effects in human activity have been shown to have a relationship to the 22-year cycle of the solar magnetic field.

Some in science still believe that the physical field, other than light, has no influence on life. But scientists such as Professor Frank Brown of the Woods Hole Marine Biological Laboratory, Woods Hole, Massachusetts, in experiments in the 1960s and the 1970s, established beyond doubt that the cycles of simple organisms could be changed dramatically by exposing them to magnetic fields from a small permanent magnet of the same strength as that of the Earth, but pointing in a different direction. And Professor Richard Blackman, of the same laboratory in 1975, with the eye of an electron microscope, found that bacterium contain a chain of tiny magnets of the mineral magnetite, the original lodestone of preliterate peoples. Bacteria do not know north is the way to swim, they just naturally follow it.

Have you ever marveled at how homing pigeons find their way back home? Experiments have demonstrated that pigeons have several senses to determine direction: polarized light from the sun, remembered visual representations of the ground, and also a magnetic sense. Dr. William Keeton of Cornell University, in 1971, fitted pigeons with translucent contact lenses that permitted light to enter, with the exception of polarized light and any source from visual images. He released these pigeons about 100 miles from their homing grounds. Those with the lenses found their way just as those without lenses, except that those fitted with lenses made a detour far west until they crossed the geographical line of the Earth's magnetic field that told them to fly in another direction. He verified his findings by gluing a small permanent magnet of 0.5 gauss, oriented in the opposite direction of the Earth's magnetic field, on the back of the head of each pigeon with the contact lenses. These fitted birds flew in disarray in all directions, not returning until the contacts fell off. Their magnetic sense had been cancelled by an abnormal magnetic field applied to the head. Now there was no question that their directional control was aided by the Earth's magnetic field.

We can try to explain the mystery of pets, dogs and cats, for example, able to return to their original homes after being lost thousands of miles away. The Duke University Parapsychology Laboratory has authenticated over 50 cases of this kind, attributing the phenomenon to a function of the body's biomagnetic D.C. system as a locator. Tests showed that the accuracy of 40 professional dowsers (who search for underground water supplies) was diminished by three-quarters when a current (magnetism) carrying wire was attached to their wrists, presumably throwing off their ability to detect magnetic lines of force. Metal bending is also attributed to a willed biomagnetic action from the human system interacting with the electromagnetic structure of inanimate matter, which may also explain why certain statues, pictures and other objects cry (sweat) or exude moisture. The mere presence or the touch of a person who possesses a greater amount of either positive or negative magnetic energies can affect other objects. The palm of a mother's hand on her baby's forehead soothes the child. Berkeley physicist Sharon Carlson makes icons weep from ordinary sea salt and calcium chloride that absorb water out of the air until it liquefies itself.

Positive and negative magnetic fields push and pull ions, whether in the human body, animals, or industrial pipes and a myriad of objects. Thousands of industrial firms and office buildings use magnets to dissolve sediment buildup in pipes so that they don't have to spend costly funds on chemical products to do the same job. In Washington D.C. for instance, the Charles E. Smith Company saves thousands of dollars annually by using magnets on its pipes. Magnetism will loosen and make fluid such elements as plaster, ceramics, clay, porcelain, paint, dirt, and many other materials.

Sharks, skates and rays navigate, using the weak geomagnetic field (about 50 micro Tesla), as related by Mote Marine Laboratory. Almost all of their energy comes from the Earth's magnetic field. These species have long, narrow canals in their heads (called Lorenzini Ampullae) filled with a jelly of electrical conductivity as high as that of sea water. The polarity is dependent on the relative orientation of the line of force of GMF with respect to the body axis of the fish, forming an ultra-sensitive navigating compass. They experience almost total confusion during magnetic storms, even of a few minutes duration. Can we learn something of how to prevent disease from these creatures that rarely get sick even though they do not have immune systems as we do ?

Plants and animals are affected by magnetic fields. Faster growth of animals and plants has been demonstrated in a variety of experiments. Fish in magnetized tanks show faster growth, stouter physiques, and lower mortality rates as opposed to those in unmagnetized tanks with otherwise similar conditions. Plants grow faster under a magnetized environment. The Agricultural faculty of the University of Shizuka, Japan, reports increased harvests for tangerines and other fruit under magnetism. Canada's Ministry of Agriculture states that magnetic fields improve germination and bring in at least a 10 percent better harvest.

People witness substantial increases in growth and vitality of plants in both office and home environments from using magnetic fields. Simple observation can verify how plants in such environments flourish compared to similar plants in the same vicinity without magnetic treatment. Anyone can try this in his or her own garden to verify results at very little cost and with likely fascinating results.

In humans, minute copulates of magnetite are found in the central nervous system and the pineal gland, located in the central area of the brain. Similar organs originated very early in evolution in bacteria, insects, fish, amphibians and mammals. Science pretty much agrees now that all living creatures sense the Earth's magnetic field and derive information from it, a heretical statement just a short time ago, Dr. Becker says. It appears that for over two billion years of evolution, living things have taken advantage of two electromagnetic elements in our environment that could always be depended upon—the geomagnetic field and visible light. We know that life develops specific organs to sense light. But would the other key element be left out ? Of course, it was not. We simply haven't been very good at detecting it nor did our human system have to see it or provide us with any directional sight to obtain its benefits. Nevertheless, in certain animals and fish, magnetism is a form of sight. What we must now learn from magnetism is how to let it improve our health rather than destroy it.

Human Magnetic Body Effects

More and more research is being directed toward the electrical nature of life, in that we now know all living cells are electric in essence. Cells of the nervous system in every living being are based on A.C. current as well as pulsed D.C. energy. Without this energy, life does not exist. Each individual cell possesses an electric charge at its nucleus and on its outer membrane, varying in polarity based on the type of tissue.

Positive-negative polarization allows each cell to function in an orderly and healthy manner. There appears to be little argument that this electromagnetic charge wears down as cells perform their normal bodily functions and that the body attempts to revitalize "tired" cells by sending pulses of electromagnetic energy from the brain through the nervous system in order to recharge the cells and strengthen the polarized field. The Earth's own D.C. and magnetic pulses support our natural biorhythm.

Our bodies are run by electrical impulses. Dr. Bansal reports that the average size adult brain generates about 30 watts of electrical energy through its nerve cells, each a tiny dynamo. The heart, stomach, glands, muscles, and other organs generate electricity in order to function. Our bodies can feel electromagnetic waves at the rate of 80 million cycles per second. We can act as aerials by placing a hand on the antenna jacket. Carbon, oxygen, phosphorous, potassium, sodium, chlorine, calcium and other elements in our bodies are the basis for generating electricity. Whenever this activity drops below sufficiency to deal with physical and

Information Brief

What Role Magnetic Energy?

Does the answer to cancer lie with sharks, skates and rays ? Exposing sharks to potent cancer-causing chemicals does not produce cancer, not even in skates exposed as embryos, says Carl Luer, senior scientist at the Mote Marine Laboratory, who has studied this question for the past 12 years. It is hard to find a sick shark—perhaps why they have managed to survive 450 million years as one of the oldest species on Earth. When a tumor forms in humans, blood vessels grow toward the site and provide nourishment for rapid cell growth; while, on the other hand, sharks possess a skeleton made entirely from cartilage that naturally resists penetration by blood vessels, researchers report. These biochemists speculate that there may be an extractable substance in the cartilage that can be used to fight cancer or they say that perhaps sharks have an efficient mechanism to repair DNA. They believe that sharks have only one, non-specific antibody that constantly circulates in the blood stream, produced without bone marrow or a lymph system. In other animals, we study how cancer forms, says Leur, in sharks we study how cancer does not form.

What is the one non-specific antibody? In sharks, Robert Barefoot says, it may be squalene, which is highly anti-carcinogenic. In embryos, cartilage could not be the answer. Yet we have health food stores selling doses of cartilage as though this were the answer. In July of 1993, Dr. David A. Kessler, head of the FDA, warned makers of dietary supplements, who make claims they cannot backup, not to promote the idea that cartilage, colonic rinses, floral herbal teas and a variety of other unproved substances can cure disease. Common vitamins and minerals pose no regulatory problem, as is the case with magnetotherapy which is considered a safe procedure. The FDA approved the use of electromagnets in 1978 for various ailments. Permanent magnets are considered even more benign. Nevertheless claims must be substantiated.

It is estimated that 90 percent of the shark's energy comes from the Earth's magnetic field which is negatively oriented. Evidence exists that negative magnetic fields arrest the growth of infectious cells and cancer. Can this be the answer ? Certainly it is worth the time to investigate seriously the possibilities of negative magnetic energy as a healer and to test scientifically each claim. Areas of research are recommended in this book.

Source: Mote Marine Laboratory, Carl Luer, 1992; *Washington Post*, July 30, 1993, p.19; author.

mental exertions forced on us by stress or improper diet, or whatever reason, we feel exhausted and ready to collapse.

Our weakest magnetic field is the brain. As we have stated, science can now measure the degree of magnetic fields of individual organs with a super sensitive magnetometer. This allows us to read the heart with a magnetocardiogram and the brain with a magneto-encephalogram. Dr. Bansal explains that the peak value of the magnetic field produced by the heart is 10^{-7} and the brain is 3×10^{-8} gauss. But these appear much too high for most experts. Bonlie believes it is lower. Remember that the gauss strength of the Earth is only 0.5 gauss, minute in comparison. Some muscles when flexed produce a value of 10^{-7} gauss. Diagnosis of many organs based on magnetism is now routine. We must now go the next step toward maintaining the proper level of magnetic energy in our body as an essential key to good health. It is as fundamental as good nutrition, exercise, and proper mental conditioning.

Relationship of Magnetotherapy to Alternative Treatments

Magnetotherapy is closely related to the principles of many therapies, including homeopathy, naturopathy, acupuncture, laying-on-of-hands, light exposure, reflexology, essential nutrition, and other treatment methods. This interrelationship is so significant that for some it may even be revolutionary.

Recently, the Congressional Appropriations Committee stated that it "is not satisfied that the conventional medical community as symbolized by NIH has fully explored the potential that exists in unconventional medical practices. Many routine and effective medical procedures now considered commonplace were once considered unconventional and counter indicated. Cancer radiation therapy is such a procedure that is now commonplace but once was considered quackery."

SCIENTIFIC DIGEST

Magnetite Found in Human Brain

Microscopic magnets have recently been found in the human brain by a unique process. Magnetite had already been identified in non-human organisms, including bacteria, mollusks, homing pigeons, whales, salmon, honey bees, jelly fish, and other species. Why our research has been so poorly oriented in humans not to have found these biological bar magnets ——made of crystals of the iron mineral magnetite——is difficult to understand. "This is really an exciting discovery", says geobiologist Joseph L. Krishvink of the California Institute of Technology, who has identified these strong magnetic crystals that measure one millionth of an inch wide and 10 millionth of an inch long.

Primitive bacteria two billion years ago, Krishvink believes, gained a competitive advantage from internal magnets that allowed them to navigate toward nutrient-filled mud that helped to evolve life into more complex cells and eventually into higher plant and animal life and finally human forms. This new study found that an average human brain contained seven billion microscopic magnets weighing a total of one millionth of an ounce. The team dissected brain samples from autopsies using non-metallic instruments treated in a magnetically shielded, dust-free room to avoid contamination. The tissue was liquefied and a magnet was used to pull out the crystals which could be moved about by magnetic fields only slightly stronger than the Earth's natural field.

The movement of magnetite affects the flow of ions across cell membranes, reports Krishvink. This may be the reason why electromagnetic radiation from power lines and other electrical devices can affect our health and also how magnetotherapy is capable of opening the ion channels of our cells. Here science has demonstrated a plausible mechanism by which electromagnetic fields can affect biological tissue.

Source: *Health Journal, Washington Post,* Robin Herman, May 12, 1992; *Washington Times,* May 12 1992; Joseph L. Krishvink, California Institute of Technology, 1992; author.

As a consequence of a Congressional mandate, $2,000,000 was appropriated in 1992 for the Office of Alternative Medicine under NIH. Most of the funds in the first year have been allocated for staff and administration, while some $600,000 is to be used for twenty, $30,000 grants to explore a variety of alternative procedures.

Homeopathy

First, let us look at homeopathy. Many believe that homeopathic remedies are essentially pure electromagnetic energies, derived from various crude substances used to jump-start the healing process. They function as any counter-irritant would, such as a mustard plaster, for example. After a number of steps, the form, smell, and color of the original substances are lost in the final product. In the end, products cannot be differentiated from one another. The final substance, which replicates ingredients of the original ailment is so diluted that it heals rather than creates symptoms, by either manufacturing a negative magnetic field or attracting negative energy to that locale. All drugs are removed, only the memory of the energy remains. Even the founder of homeopathy, Samuel Hahnemann, recognized magnetic energy as a principle of homeopathic effectiveness.

From the review of dozens of national magazines and health books on homeopathy, not one publication ventured into how it works. Dana Ullman, in her book **Discovering Homeopathy** (*North Atlantic Books*, 1991), says "we don't understand how it works...but that doesn't mean we should ignore it." The AMA takes no formal position on it. The FDA says it is not harmful so leaves it alone. Queen Elizabeth II has homeopaths on her medical staff and the British National Health Service covers it in their health services. The *British Medical Journal* (February 1991) assessed 107 homeopathic studies and found 81 that showed positive results, but also some failures. Importantly failure can many times be attributed to incorrect application. In magnetotherapy, failure may be related to such things as polarity, insufficient reactive strength, or too little exposure time, all of which can be corrected if one understands the science.

What is extremely fascinating about homeopathy and magnetotherapy is that they both rely to a large extent on magnetic energy. Millions of people use the healing power of homeopathy, never realizing that it very likely employs the principle of attracting negative magnetic energy to the injury. Medical doctors and many other specialists have never understood how a homeopath could take a substance and dilute it to such an extent that there is no measurement of ingredients left, yet healing or relief takes place. Dr. William Philpott, who has healed thousands of individuals using homeopathic methods for a period of years, believes that what is taking place is a reversal of the magnetic field in the substance from a positive polarity to a negative polarity or the attraction of the negative field to the area by the homeopathic substance. In fact, Philpott says that he has stopped using the rather complex assortment of homeopathic substances designed for specific diseases and ailments. He simply applies magnetotherapy with equally effective results, since these therapies are designed to achieve the same effect but by different procedures.

Information Brief

Unconventional Medicine Users in America

A survey of 1,539 American adults in 1990, conducted by David M. Eisenberg, M.D., and his staff, Beth Israel Hospital, Boston, showed that one-third used "unconventional" therapies, including self-help counseling sessions, nutrition and lifestyle changes. About 10 percent of adult Americans actually sought the help and visited "unconventional" medical practitioners, expending over $10 billion, primarily out of their own pockets rather than insurance reimbursements. There were more visits to "unconventional" therapists than physicians.

Unconventional treatments were used most often for back problems, anxiety, headaches, chronic pain, and cancer. And the prevalence of use was in the age group of 25 to 49, people with some college education and incomes over $35,000. In seven of ten cases, users did not tell their physicians, while 90 percent undertook treatment without the recommendation of a physician. A number of these therapies are now recognized as useful by the conventional medical community, including anesthesiologists who acknowledge the value of acupuncture, for example.

Source: David M. Eisenberg, M.D., Beth Israel Hospital, Boston; *New England Journal of Medicine*, Jan. 1993.

If the similarity between homeopathy and magnetotherapy holds true, this would be a most fascinating discovery, making magnetotherapy all the more relevant for its comparative simplicity and higher degree of predictability. It does not mean that the homeopath should discard his procedure for the more simple magnetotherapy, since each type of therapy has its own intrinsic values. Homeopathy has physical and mental attributes and feelings or beliefs that can be beneficial to particular patients. It does mean, however, that magnetotherapy could very well fit into the regimen of homeopathy and possibly make treatment successful in a higher percentage of cases by a clearer understanding of how it can be applied to achieve specific results, by varying strength and exposure time. Homeopathy may work more quickly in certain circumstances depending on the substance and the extent of dilution. The two methodologies can work hand-in-hand. Most importantly, this observation and understanding can help reduce the skepticism of physicians in order to allow them to consider the use of these therapies.

In short, homeopathy is a function of secussion and dilution, where the secussion or jarring of solutions can create static negative electricity or perform as a positive energy irritant. Symptom producing substances are positive magnetic energy poled that perform very much like any other irritant to stimulate the functioning of the counter-irritant immune system. Each homeopathic remedy carries a very weak magnetic field that relieves a particular symptom by attracting negative ions to the site and allowing the immune system to build resistance to the substance so that the body can better tolerate it. Various levels of dilution give the body time to react with the least stress possible.

On the other hand, many alternative practitioners believe that magnetotherapy involves a strong magnetic field that has a universal value capable of overriding all variables. Magnetotherapy provides immediate relief or extended relief and healing by simply increasing exposure time. Also, magnetotherapy is more predictable and can be used as an antibiotic, providing an anti-cancer effect. It can also produce the hormone mclatonin, when applied to the brain in the area of the pineal gland, and is much easier to use as a self-help medicine—all of these clinically observed by Philpott and other practitioners.

Acupuncture and Yoga

Acupuncture is a Chinese system. Yoga with many similarities has an Indian orientation. They both are influenced by magnetic fields. It is well known that our body has many energy centers or points that control or direct functions of our system. Over 1,000 such centers have been identified.

In acupuncture, usually fine needles are pierced through the flesh at several points associated with the ailment, generally accepted as activating nerves or releasing energy in order to remove stagnation, lethargy or malfunctioning. The saying goes that some doctors can't seem to understand how a needle inserted in the head can cure a pain in the stomach, yet readily accept that a pill in the stomach can cure a pain in the head.

The National Institutes of Health, in the last few years, has funded over 20 studies that have examined acupuncture, finding that at least 25 percent of claimed acupuncture points exist such that they are specific, reproducible, have significant electrical parameters and are found in all subjects. One theory postulates that meridians connect these special points that have electric characteristics (similar to transmission lines), while other areas with non-meridian skin do not have this distinction. Some describe the points as amplifiers, similar to telephone cable boosters. When needles are inserted near the points, they create a current of injury. Since they are metallic, the needles create a tiny galvanic current that boosts the D.C. current flowing in the meridian from acupuncture point to point. The points are capacitors, while the needles "fill" the capacitors. Stoppage of the flow is what presumably causes disease, as explained by Dr. William Pawluk, M.D., a family doctor highly skilled in both acupuncture and magnetotherapy.

The Gate Theory stipulates that stimulation of sensory nerves will so much interfere with the transmission of pain (overloading the sensory traffic in the spinal column) that these signals will be stopped at the gate and not reach the central nervous system or the brain so that pain will not be felt. Dr. Becker states that this theory has been largely discarded because a wide variety of magnetic devices, wave forms, pulses and frequencies can achieve the same results by bypassing the sensory transmission area altogether. However, we have two processes at work. Meridians really are channels. Furthermore, we are dealing with at least two procedures. The first involves short circuiting the nerve tracks that travel at 30 feet per second to immediately cut pain, similar to the idea of the Gate Theory that inhibits circuit flow. But others believe that what is really happening is that the short circuit maintains the flow of electrons to the brain, having been interrupted by the injury. The second process involves the sending or placement of negative magnetic energy to the injured site, which creates cell energy change usually in about 15 or 20 minutes but sometimes much longer, depending on the extent of injury and

Information Brief

The Alternative of Apitherapy

Apitherapy involves injection of bee venom in points of pain, muscle cramp, multiple sclerosis, and other diseases. Basically the same trigger points are used as in acupuncture. The American Apitherapy Society, North Hartland, Vt., monitored by Dr. Brudford Woeks, who records the work of therapist Charles Mraz, states that they have been prompted to use the bee stinging method on such diseases as lupus, asthenia, and inevitably AIDS.

The most intriguing aspect of bee venom is a compound in it called apimin. The symptoms of multiple sclerosis, for example, result from inflammatory degeneration of the nerve sheaths that carry electrical signals to and from the brain. When a sheath degenerates, it doesn't conduct electricity very well, so the nerve impulses get blocked. Apimin doesn't stop degeneration but it improves conductivity. The venom also contains two powerful anti-inflammatory agents, melittin and adolapin.

Bee venom, cobra venom, and certain other natural substances have been touted as promising cures, but no long-term improvement has been shown. A recent national television program showed hundreds of people receiving as many as a dozen bee stings several times weekly as their symptoms disappeared. Even people with severe illnesses walked away feeling better and more mobile. But there is nothing new here. Dr. Dean Bonlie says his mother used bee stings on the family 49 years ago. And you will find thousands of people who have done this in their backyards. Bee stings are not lasting and are painful. On the other hand, magnetotherapy has demonstrated not only an anti-inflammatory capability and improved electrical signal conductivity, but long-term effect from a daily maintenance program or sleeping on a magnetic bed. Negative magnetic energy may even offer some cures as suggested later in this book.

Source: *Washington Post*, June 22, 1993, Ken Ringle; author.

the strength of application. In contrast, magnetotherapy also has direct influence on cells, and negative magnetic fields can change cell composition directly. If a homeopathic substance, for example, is so structured as to place negative magnetic energy directly on the site of pain, the consequences would be similar to the application of magnetotherapy. Here we have at least three of the most important alternative medicines that function essentially by the same human biological processes. Furthermore, many of the hundreds of thousands of drugs on the market (a combination of chemicals and homeopathic type herbs) emulate this process. This understanding could have amazing consequences on our health system.

Each point is actually positive oriented compared to its environment. This means that the opposite pole (negative) may be the most appropriate application. Injecting a needle in an acupuncture site creates a local injury which becomes positive oriented, eliciting more negative magnetic fields to the area. Remember that permanent magnets or electromagnets are able to block pain with almost no skill required in locating acupuncture points, as one can simply lay a magnet near these points. Magnets can locate a greater number of centers with the possibility of accomplishing a more thorough job. In China, practitioners use permanent magnets and also slow pulsing currents of two per second in place of acupuncture. The pulsing current is the delta brain wave frequency of deep sleep.

Yoga and acupuncture also appear to have the same theoretical basis. Yoga concentrates a great deal on spiritual energy in centers called chakras. Postures are designed to create spontaneous pressure on the same centers as acupuncture. This is accomplished by contraction and expansion of nerves and muscles at these points. Specific exercise, reflexology and pressure on various centers, as in acupressure, also elicit a stream of energy by way of the nerve cells. All of these send signals to the central nervous system to concentrate negative magnetic fields at specific organs or tissues for symptom relief and healing. Many acupuncturists worldwide now use either electric currents or permanent magnets at acupuncture points to stimulate energy. When one sleeps or sits on a magnetic pad, he or she does not have to be concerned about precise location of acupuncture points, since the magnet will cover most locations. In other words, as pointed out already, one does not have to be a specialist in acupuncture or point location to apply magnetotherapy to obtain similar results. The same level of knowledge of points is not necessary, although it may help. Also the injection of needles through the skin is unnecessary as a magnet may simply be laid on the skin or muscle. Nevertheless, these therapies function well in conjunction with each other. More and more therapists use both, as they assess the patient's feelings and needs.

Many medical doctors now use acupuncture as an acceptable and reliable therapy. In addition, the State of Washington has cleared magnetotherapy as part and parcel of the license for acupuncture. Many more states will follow this dual licensing. Acupuncture therapy is now approved in over 20 states with over 2,000 licensed practitioners. The Menninger Clinic in Kansas, plus many other clinics and hospitals use acupuncture. If it were as easy to learn and apply as magnetotherapy, many more physicians would use this method of treatment to the advantage of their patients. While acupuncture requires time-consuming involvement by the doctor, magnetotherapy with similar effects allows the doctor simply to apply several permanent magnets on the most vulnerable spots and go about other business as healing takes place without concern for losing time. The physician can also send his patient home with a magnetic device so that it can be used whenever needed. Such practices can certainly help to reduce health costs and improve service.

Dr. Harry Park, M.D., Vancouver, Washington, who has practiced acupuncture for over 20 years, uses acupuncture in conjunction with magnetotherapy, finding much faster results with magnetism. He also prefers not to have to use needles, as most patients don't like them. He says he gets much better results with magnetotherapy and has experienced actual cures for many serious ailments. Contrast this with the simple relief of symptoms as in acupuncture. Importantly, the longer-term application of magnetotherapy that drowns cells in negative magnetic energy can actually heal, not simply bring relief. This may very well be the significant difference between proper magnetic field treatment and other therapies. Dr. Park, for example, has found excellent results using magnetotherapy for patients with multiple scerlosis, breast cancer, arthritis and many other serious diseases. He employs herbal remedies to alleviate the stress of toxin release and he is a strong believer in proper nutrition.

Another facet of acupuncture involves animals. Veterinary acupuncture was approved as an "alternate therapy" in 1988 by the American Veterinary Medical Association which represents 52,000 veterinarians. "It's like a good body massage in a lot of ways," says Wendy Moon, president of the Muirfield East thoroughbred horse farm in Maryland, home of Housebuster, winner of the Eclipse Sprinting Championships in 1990 and 1991. The horse was treated with acupuncture before each race which seemed to relieve muscle and joint softness. "We don't look at it so much for curative type treatment, but as something that treats some of the symptoms of rigorous training," Moon says.

Mereaith Snader, executive director of the International Veterinary Acupuncture Society, treats 100 horses in five states weekly at $75 to $100 each. Small animals cost $50 to $75 per treatment. Harold Alterman, Dale City Animal Hospital, Virginia, uses electrodes to send high-voltage blockage into a dog's spinal cord to undo nerve blockage from a ruptured disc. He treats cats and dogs for kidney failure, acute pancreatitis, arthritis, bad hips, and chronic ear infection. A great deal of success is obtained.

Some animals can't stand needle injection so certain veterinarians use magnets to stimulate to obtain similar effects. And, of course, instead of returning twice monthly for these treatments, the home user can simply take a set of magnets with him and apply it to his animal at anytime. Place a magnetic pad in your pet's bed and watch how other house pets fight for the bed. Owners have found it difficult to get their animals off these pleasurable magnetic pads.

In equine care, magnetotherapy offers a convenient and human approach to injury therapy, especially when compared to blistering or pin-firing. Various types of pads are contoured so that the horse's range of motion is not impaired during usage. Successful treatments for tendonitis, bowed tendons, bucked skins, muscular sprains and strains and other injuries to the musculoskeletal system, plus preventive and post-workout therapy have been documented.

Hall of Fame trainers and Eclipse Award winners recite their success. Jack Van Berg has used Bioflex pads on his two-year olds and three year olds with chronic shins. These pads have also stopped shin bucking. Charlie Whittingham states the strips were very good for his horses' shins and on check ligaments. Trainer Woodford "Woody" Stephens says bipolar magnetic pads have helped with bucking, splints, tendons, and have improved sound horses as well.

For too long, chiropractors and M.D.s have not gotten along. The Chiropractic Association says that the AMA is not the watchdog of our health. Chiropractors say that for many of the drugs prescribed by M.D.s, nobody has the remotest idea of how they work and, assuredly, no one knows the effect of the combination of multi-drug intake. Physicians avoid their own drugs and very seldom find a doctor being admitted to a hospital or accepting care as an outpatient unless he is extremely sick. Chiropractors, on the other hand, say that their approach is normally risk-free, informative, caring and that they take more time with patients.

Arguments persist as to whether physicians should send more patients to chiropractors. Some physicians say, if it is indicated yes; others say, if patients want to go—fine, but they'll find nothing special. If there is no severe underlying structural abnormalities but just generalized complaints of aching back or neck, a physical therapist might make the most sense; and if that doesn't help, physicians say the next step would be to consider a chiropractor. The important thing is what works and what will create a better quality of life for the patient, not a prejudice of one type of therapist over another.

Today, more than ever, the patient must become knowledgeable about which physician or chiropractor to use. He must question whether his doctor is familiar with a variety of alternatives and that he will look beyond drugs and unsafe applications, as well as take the time to get close to the patient.

Chiropractors are one of the first groups to realize the potential of magnetotherapy, since it easily fits into their regimen and may improve their whole field of effectiveness and credibility. Hundreds, perhaps thousands, of chiropractors are using magnetic fields in their practices, with little fanfare as of yet. Magnetism, in conjunction with body manipulations, acupressure, reflexology, yoga, and just plain, good old exercise of the right sort have created a new interest in chiropractic. Also, physical therapists, nurses and home providers carry magnetic devices with them and prescribe home use as well. There should be absolutely no reason why all medical practitioners should not be able to work together as a well oiled machine for the benefit of the nation's health. A shortage of well qualified providers is very evident. Rather than ridicule each other, all ought to be working toward the same sensible goals.

Many chiropractors make extensive use of magnetotherapy along with their regular practice. Dr. Kenneth Bernd was one of these but ended up dropping magnetic field therapy because he felt he was not getting the results he initially expected. He believes it works best on people whose pH is up near the 7.6 healthful range, otherwise it's like beating a dead horse, he states. He strongly favors nutrition in getting the pH up. On the other hand, Dr. Philpott states he gets excellent results whether the pH is up or not. Nutrition is important but need not come first. Robert Barefoot says simply sleep on a magnetic bed and observe the body's pH rise in the morning compared to the night before. "The pH will go up every time," says Barefoot.

The key problem here as with many providers and users is most have never understand how magnetotherapy really works. It should not consist of simply placing some manufacturer's magnets of any gauss strength and polarity on a patient and wishing for results. Bad names will follow magnetotherapy if people don't know how to use it and don't have the proper mix of magnetic tools consisting of various gauss strengths, sizes, and other combinations to tackle a particular problem. And it may not come in one office visit but weeks or months of maintenance therapy. Hopefully, some of the answers come out of this book.

SCIENTIFIC DIGEST

Veterinary Bipolar Magnetic Foil Trials

Over 200 applications of alternating (bipolar) magnetic foil in clinical trials, primarily to the lower limbs of the horse, were conducted by Dr. Leonard P. Blach of Roswell, New Mexico. Complete observations were recorded with highlights presented here. The reactions of these animals certainly dispels the myth that magnetic treatment is largely psychosomatic. It also should be noted that the use of foil emulates the effect of permanent magnets of various construction but that foil has the advantage of adhering to the leg or body more conveniently and lasting when subjected to vigorous movement.

Importantly, much that has proved successful with animals also applies to humans, such as treating ailments of tennis elbow, scar tissue, backache, surgical healing, sinus, bruises, and the list continues. Valuable lessons are also learned so that better results can very well take place by the use of higher gauss strength and heavier magnets as warranted. Dr. Blach, for example, found that his effectiveness was limited (particularly myositis of the back) because the relatively thin foil could not penetrate deeply through the horse's heavy musculature. We know the depth of penetration, in animals and humans, depends on the weight of the magnet and gauss strength. With this knowledge the medical industry can achieve even greater success.

* Bowed Tendon (Tendonitis-Tendovaginitis): Case of three year old quarter horse, Santa Fe Downs Race Track. Both the deep flexor tendon and the superficial flexor tendon, along with both tendon sheaths, were damaged from below the carpus to the top of the sesamoid area. The horse was presented two days after injury. No medication was given except the magnetic foil. Within five days the horse could apply his weight, in 30 days the superficial flexor tendon could be seen and by 60 days the tendonous area appeared normal——no longer bowed. Dr. Blach indicates that this case was as severe as any he ever observed and the results astonishing from his experience around the race track which includes tendon surgery, various other therapies and rest of at least a year for injuries. In 100 days, this horse was healthy enough to sustain training.

* Tearing of Tendon Fibers and Sheaths : Case of two year old thoroughbred. In ten days there was noticeable reduction in swelling, edema and pain. In 60 days no signs of lameness was present and in 4 months training was started. *(continued)*

75

*   <u>Tendovaginitis of the Superficial Flexor Tendon midway between the Carpus and Fetlock</u>: Case of three year old quarter horse. The magnetic foil remained on the site for 30 days at which time swelling and pain had disappeared and lameness was gone. Training commenced in 90 days.

      In most cases of severe bowed tendon, horses are not returnable to the racetrack or it takes about a year to return following surgical correction. In 24 acute cases studied here, success was replicated upon applying magnetic foil, health more quickly restorative and impressive on return to normality.

*   <u>Fetlock Area</u> (from a wind puff to sesamoiditis, tendonitis, scar tissue, sprains, strains, fractures, etc.):Case of four year old thorough-bred with subacute lameness in the right carpus showing a distention of the joint capsule in both the upper and lower joint. Radiographs revealed a low grade osteochondritis of the joint. Numerous types of therapy had been applied over to two years, including injections of steroids and hellion. Within thirty days after applying magnetic foil, the distended joint capsule disappeared both upper and lower, lameness was not apparent and the horse was totally sound at the gallop. He won his next race after this therapy, but after 48 hours noticeable distention of the joint capsule was evident so the foil therapy was continued with success.

*   <u>Subchondral Chip Fracture Third Carpal Bone</u>: Case of two year old quarter horse stallion. Radiographs revealed a small fracture that did not warrant surgery. With magnetic foil applied for 21 days, excessive joint fluid was absorbed and the knee appeared normal and not painful to the flexion of the knee upon palpation. The horse entered its assigned race and performed remarkably well.

Cases with other horses found excellent results in alleviating the following:
1. Edema and/or extra cellular fluid
2. Hematomas due to bruising
3. Interarticular pressure
4. Chondritis
5. Osteochondritis
6. Old scar tissue
7. Shin buck
8. Bone spavin
9. Ring bone
10. Post surgical healing
11. Myositis of the back
12. Sinusitis of the frontal sinus (foil placed on temporal bone between eyes over frontal bones)
13. Elbow or "shoe boil"
14. Hock

Source: Blach, Leonard P., **Magnetic Foil Trials with Energy - Pak Veterinary, Foils** (200 x 120 mm), Roswell, New Mexico; author.

Other chiropractors, such as Dr. Domenci "Nick" Capone, say they experience pain relief and healing in as much as 85 percent of their patients with magnetotherapy and do not even test for pH. Magnetic fields drive the pH towards proper balance, while good nutrition and supplements help to keep it there and get it there more quickly. Barefoot has tested subjects with pH of 6 in the evening before sleeping on a magnetic pad and by morning their pH is up to 7 or better. A regular magnetotherapy maintenance program will keep it up as will a proper intake of supplements. Remember that it may take a number of days or even weeks to drive out all the toxins, so initially a couple of hours on the magnetic pad may be right at first to hold down the stressful effects of withdrawal symptoms. If sleeping time on a magnetic pad is gradually increased, symptoms from toxin release will be less bothersome.

The new chiropractors and alternative thinkers are taking the lead in preventive medicine which includes proper nutrition, exercise, supplements, and alternatives such as magnetotherapy. More physicians are including this in their armamentarium as well. It only makes good sense.

Laying-on-of-Hands

Although the term chiropractic means "to do by hand," there are other therapists who specialize in the use of hands. Laying-on-of-hands is associated with faith or spiritual healing and the ability to heal frequently thought of as an act of God. Therapeutic touch, on the other hand, is administered in a medical or nursing context and has no correlation with spiritual healing and can be taught, learned, actualized and made to happen, says Dr. John Zimmerman, founder of the Bio-Electro-Magnetics Institute, Reno, Nevada. It also is not usually associated with chiropractors but rather with nurses who find it extremely useful. In therapeutic touch, one manipulates the bioenergy field of the body, passing excess body energies from the healer to the person being treated. It does not necessarily imply physical contact. Bioenergy field contact is enough, extending some distance away. Some laying-on-of-hands techniques are known as Johrei, Reiki, and aura balancing. Most of Western medicine has not acknowledged this treatment as valid.

Traveling around the world, Dr. Bob Beck found that all healers emitted exactly the same brain wave pattern (7.8 - 8.0 Hz) during the few moments they were in an "altered state," regardless of the society or customs or healing methods. Zimmerman emphasizes that healers engage in "centering," which is nothing more than relaxation, concentration, and quieting one's mind to the point of becoming aware of the underlying, tiny perturbations of the Earth's electric and/or magnetic fields which have been detected at the 7 to 8 Hz Schumann frequency. Physicist Dr. W. G. Schumann, in the early 1950's, mathematically predicted that oscillations occur at the Earth—ionosphere cavity, superimposed on the steady state electrical field of 100 - 150 volts per meter and on the magnetic field of about 50 micro telsa. These extremely low frequencies (ELF) were first detected ten years later by the National Bureau of Standards.

Hands seem to have a special sensitivity. If sensors are used, sensitive to either infrared or microwave radiation to examine the outstretched hand, very low frequency microwaves can be detected. The image of the hand becomes a defused blur, finally appearing like a glowing hot spot of microwave radiation near the center of the palm of the hand (BEMI Journal, 1991). The Chinese call this energy Qi that flows freely through the meridians of the body in healthy people, emitting electromagnetic radiation from the palm of the hand. Researchers insist this biomagnetic field energy does not necessarily imply physical contact but can be accomplished by the field itself, which may explain some of the strange occurrences around the world where certain pictures or statues appear to cry in the presence of a priest or certain other highly energized people. These are very possibly individuals with a high magnetic energy level and the ability to pass on magnetized fields to humans or inanimate objects to create a change in cell structure.

Nurses are particularly sensitive to laying-on-of-hands and describe the technique in their professional journals. Doctors could use more of it to demonstrate sensitivity and care for the patient which may be as important as other medication. John J. Ring, a past president of AMA, talks of the need for greater ethical concern in the medical profession and more caring for the patient. He recently cited a piece from Dr. Lewis Thomas's "The Youngest Profession," a powerful but chilling note on a changed profession that pontificates, "Medicine is no longer the laying-on-of-hands. It is more like the reading of signals from machines." Perhaps we all ought to open up a little bit, drop unsubstantiated criticism of

Information Brief

Chiropractic vs. Physical Therapy

With major structural scoliosis (curvature of the spine) of 30 degrees or more, a chiropractor is not going to help, says Thomas J. Errico, professor of Orthopedics and Neurosurgery at New York University; but, in postural scoliosis secondary to muscle spasm, he can offer great relief, he says. On the other hand, says Willibald Nagler, Chairman of Rehabilitative Medicine at New York Hospital, Cornell Medical Center, physicians who take the time can treat musculoskeletal complaints for almost any problem. Chiropractors view of health, he says, is that everything in the body is supposed to be symmetrical (line everything up); yet this theory has never been proved and overlooks normal body imperfection. Most people do not have their bodies in symmetry yet live normal, pain-free lives, he says. He cites a study of 500 men with no reported back pain, where only 28 had the symmetrical body chiropractors call normal. Significantly, the idea of subluxation, or the manipulation of spinal misalignment, is not likely the priority consideration of chiropractic any longer.

The correct combination of chiropractic and physical therapy can benefit millions of Americans who suffer from such ailments as osteoarthritis, back pain, and a variety of muscle and joint pains. Pain is a primary complaint of the elderly with osteoarthritis of the knee and affects about 10 percent of this population, says Glen E. Gresham, Chair of the Rehabilitation Medicine Department, State University of New York, at Buffalo. In a study of 80 patients, 72 experienced less pain, improved muscle strength and increased capacity in a three month program using a specially developed exercise bench which also postponed the need for artificial knee surgery. This alternative therapy, previous to this study, was not considered a viable option because of lack of evidence. Now the Arthritis Center, at Piedmont Hospital in Atlanta, says that this therapy has shown to improve the quality of life where people can go back to walking and moderate exercise that helps mobility and decreases pain.

When drugs won't do it, physicians have little choice but to refer patients to alternatives or else the patient finally troops there himself. Exercise, yoga, reflexology, chiropractic etc., all can draw magnetic fields to the site. Magnetotherapy, used by many physicians and chiropractors, has proven to draw significant amounts of negative magnetic energy to the injury for sustained healing.

Source: *Health Journal, Washington Post*, 1991; author.

methods we know little about, and, at least, be fair in our analysis regardless of what we have been previously taught.

Light Exposure and Healing

Another source of healing is light. Exposure to bright, full spectrum lighting for at least an hour upon awakening will activate the pineal gland. Activation of the pineal gland from light entering the eyes, says specialist Norman Mikesell, induces a parasympathetic healing state. Serotonin hormones increase in the brain, which in turn increase thyroid, calcitonin and growth hormone levels in the blood. The meditative healing state is reinforced and oxygen intake increases.

A number of companies sell full spectrum lighting to wake us up in the morning and to provide energy during the day by gazing into the fixture. This lighting also relieves well known depressions that some people experience during long-winter months. In this respect, we need to be cautious about tinted glasses that can eliminate a large percentage of the sun's spectrum, says Robert Barefoot, and, consequently, adversely affect us both physically and psychologically.

Information Brief

The Need for Light

Sunlight is food. Light entering the eyes influences the master glands and the pituitary and pineal glands which control the entire endocrine system, including calcium regulating parathyroid glands. Unfortunately, we spend half our lives under artificial lighting, quite different from the sun's full spectrum lighting. Artificial full spectrum lighting increases calcium absorption, plants flourish, and cows produce 15 percent more milk. Full spectrum lighting is used to treat psoriasis, neonatal jaundice and herpes simplex infection. It plays a vital role in the maintenance of a balanced hormonal system and serum calcium.

The advantages of full spectrum light and regular sunlight is that they can relieve hypertension, depression, insomnia, migraines, PMS, and carbohydrate—craving associated with metabolic imbalances. But one must take into account that too much of the wrong frequencies can create stress in adults and hyperactivity in children, especially noted under fluorescent lights in all day school settings. Halogen lights have been tested as dangerous to both humans and animals.

We need adequate exposure (neither excess nor a deficiency) of correct full spectrum lighting; otherwise, we can end up with the equivalent of malnutrition or, more appropriately, malillumination. Full spectrum lighting is only a limited part of the total and natural electromagnetic spectrum that includes all of the frequency energies.

Energy Centers are Key

Magnetotherapy can be applied to the entire body or to specific locations. The use of energy centers can make magnetotherapy even more effective. Magnets are often applied to palms and soles where a network of nerves are centered that spread over the entire body, operating at great

81

speed and activating many other centers. Magnetotherapists should become familiar with the major energy centers. Dr. Philpott is one who believes that the most important area for negative magnetic application is at the crown of the head and has designed a head board for this purpose.

Many people use a treatment technique called "zone therapy" that involves pressure massaging of various body points in order to stimulate electromagnetic fields around nerve endings to drive out toxic substances that we eat and breathe, allowing magnetic currents to flow fully again. Joseph Carvo, (U.K.) Princess Diana's massage therapist says he has been using this method successfully for years to fight off wrinkles and aging. Ameriflex, Avon, Connecticut, has a magnetic face mask (Bioflex) that they say does the same thing in effect and is used as a self-help device to reduce wrinkles, dark circles and puffy eyes without need of a therapist. It is made of hypoallergenic vinyl and non-toxic gel that molds to the curves of the face.

Reflexology and acupuncture demonstrate a high degree of effectiveness when manipulation is performed at the arch of the foot. This is where a multitude of acupuncture points are concentrated and which affect many parts of the body and body organs. In Eastern medicine, the arch is called the second heart, while the time-honored oriental practice of applying treatments on green bamboo sections, performs similarly to reflexology and acupressure. Significantly, magnetic insoles function likewise, soothing and energizing the entire body while reaching all the way up to the shoulders and other remote extremities to ease stiffness and pain and other symptoms. Magnetic fields have been proven to have a similar effect as pressing fingers or needles to relieve a particular disorder.

The center points of acupressure, like reflexology, are especially sensitive to bio-electrical impulses of the body, conducting them readily. The Chinese call this Qi and the Japanese Ki. The process relieves pain and can speed healing of broken bones. Acupressure has many effective points as described in **Acupressure Potent Points**, a guide to self-care, Michael Reed Gach, 1990. For example, the shoulder's corner refers to the point location; the Three Mile Point earned its name from the extra three miles of energy given to runners and hikers.

Proper exercise can assimilate reflexology, acupressure and other techniques that stimulate center points. The Seattle Veterans Affairs Medical Center conducted a study that showed stretching exercises reduced back pain as well as or better than the electrical nerve therapy

TENS. Lewis G. Maharam, M.D., in **Maharam's Curve** (1992), shows how exercise can maintain a pleasurable high in most people and demonstrates its value on total health and enjoyment of life. Most alternatives are interrelated and also complementary to magnetotherapy.

Most of the alternative therapies involve a magnetic influence for their effect, including naturopathy and just plain old exercise. Naturopathy, for example, is as old as civilization itself, a method of healing among the rural masses and locations of the world without doctors. Water, mud, heat, sunlight, massage and diet are its main tools. Mud plasters and mud bathing essentially make use of the curative powers of the Earth's magnetism. Naturopathy is drugless, employing the direct energy of nature. Our medical schools need to relate more to these principles in their teaching as well as to energy centers and the integrated role of proper nutrition and exercise. We had better learn quickly about the proper use of magnetotherapy since millions of people around the world are using it. Rather than an alternative, many believe it ought to be a conventional treatment and definitely part of medical education. If we fail to teach the ramifications of these alternatives, we have failed a large part of our responsibilities.

But Is It All Simply Mental ?

In respect to this wide variety of treatments, the question arises as to how much is psychosomatic. We know mental attitude has a lot to do with health and healing. A number of double-blind controlled studies are available to instruct us. What one believes about a particular method of treatment—whether it be some kind of device or a drug—seems to make little difference in the percentage of people experiencing the placebo effect. It also is quite difficult to isolate particular personalities as being more susceptible to a placebo (sham or fake) treatment than other subjects.

As reported earlier, an interesting study was conducted in 1989 by the John Hopkins Pain Treatment Center and Neurometric Laboratory, Baltimore, Maryland, to test a magnetic device for which pain-relieving qualities were claimed. In this case, the placebo response to a non-operating machine showed that 13 percent of the patients experienced relief of pain and also improved range of motion and decrease in muscle spasm (see Exhibit 3 Placebo Responses to Medical Device Therapy for Pain). Importantly, the majority of patients who actually received treatment improved their condition.

A review of numerous clinical studies dealing with placebo response to drug medication for severe acute pain reveals that about 35 percent of the subjects experienced a 50 percent decrease in perceived pain intensity, and they also experienced it for a shorter duration than the response of those who actually took analgesic drugs. Most significantly, it has been demonstrated that the number of patients who repeatedly respond to placebo treatment is no greater than 11 to 15 percent for most treatments, a figure consistent with the results of the above study on magnetic devices and reinforced by recent studies of the Japanese Ministry of Health and Welfare. The FDA concurs with these findings.

It seems likely, the investigators say, that most pain therapies will experience a placebo response around this range. Beyond this percentage, it can be said that the methodology is effective for those who claim it to be. From this, one can better judge the effectiveness of magnetic devices whose success rates claim to be effective on the greater majority of people who use them. Remember that the success rate of magnetotherapy on animals is equally high and that the placebo effect rarely comes into play, although it certainly may when the master touches and talks to his pet.

Surely, the methods and most of the cases discussed in this chapter have a great deal of merit. Little question remains that considerable benefits result from these therapies and that millions of people are satisfactorily using them. It's not some silly fad that will likely fade out and go away, even though the popularity of use has experienced cycles over the centuries. It is time to look at these techniques for a broad array of ailments.

Treatments come and go. The number of users very much depends upon the publicity generated or the marketing ability of the suppliers. It seems that it is time federal and private research agencies take these treatments more seriously and fully examine them under controlled testing so that the most effective methods can be used conventionally by all physicians.

Exhibit 2   Placebo Responses to Medical Device Therapy for Pain

> Placebo response to a functionless machine was tested in 58 patients with chronic pain. Thirteen discontinued treatment before the planned trials were complete; five did so because sham therapy worsened their pain. Forty-five patients completed three trials with a magnetic device, one trial of which was a sham. Thirteen percent of patients undergoing sham therapy experienced relief of pain, improved range of motion, and decrease in muscle spasm. The majority receiving actual treatment improved their condition. Significantly, eleven percent of the sham trials resulted in significant increase in pain. The placebo/nocebo response to sham therapy with a device is similar to that previously reported for prolonged drug treatment, but is lower than the placebo rate for short-term medication trials.
>
> **Source:** Don M. Long, Sumio Uematsu, Richard B. Kouba; Department of Neurosurgery, and Neurometrics Laboratory. John Hopkins University School of Medicine, Baltimore, MD, USA, 1989.

Dr. Stephen Barrett, psychiatrist, Allentown, Pa., and board member of the National Council Against Health Fraud, states that homeopathy is pure nonsense, yet one in four doctors in France practices it and homeopathic doctors are on the staff of the Queen of England. Dr. Wayne Jonas, M.D. of the U.S.'s own Walter Reed Army Research Institute is a specialist in homeopathy. This book has presented some science as to how it might function. But Dr. Barrett says to beware of any product that claims effectiveness against a wide-range of disorders and to ignore that which claims to strengthen the immune system, and also to beware of alternatives and testimonials. Yet isn't this precisely what proper nutrition, the mind, and good exercise do   strengthen the immune system, cure many ills, and extend a healthy life? Many of the alternative medicines are in this same category. There is plenty of fraud and malpractice to be investigated. But too often we are prepared only to understand the meaning of data and results in terms of what we already believe or have been trained to believe. There appears to be little place for innovation.

Remember the old saying that history is full of people who thought they were right, absolutely right, without a shadow of a doubt. Trained physicians should realize that medicine is neither an art or a science. It is an empirical discipline of diagnostic and therapeutic skills aided by technology. The good doctor must know his or her patients well, feel their sensitivities, respect and educate the patients, and first try all safe procedures and alternatives in a protocol of long-term care and observation. Prescribing a questionable drug or any medication or procedure that has only been tested short-term is inexcusable, just to show that you have done something. Safer, natural procedures would be better. The idea that the body is a finely tuned mechanism is simply a myth. The therapist must work on the health of the patient intensely, trying whatever might work for that individual until it is found. This effort not only includes medical alternatives but also education about lifestyle.

Dr. Bernadine Healy, former director of NIH says, "An estimated 35 percent of these deaths (cancer) may be related to diet. In fact, two-thirds of all deaths—including those caused by coronary heart diseases, strokes, or artherosclerosis, diabetes, and some types of cancer—are related to lifestyle choices, including what we eat." Interestingly, Dr. Mark Jamiesa, M.D., Haggerstown, Md., will not treat anyone who smokes. He says at least 50 percent of all illness is due to lifestyle and that it's up to the individual to become accountable for his own health care.

We have simply lost sight of proper lifestyle. It is time to come back. Alternatives will help get us there but as individuals we must take greater responsibility. And as for tests, "outcome" trials of large groups of subjects over a long-term may be more efficacious than double-blind, but limited controlled tests that fail to take into account long-term results. I believe we are approaching a new era for determining what is good or bad.

Chapter 3

How Magnetic Fields Affect our Health

Understanding Biomagnetics

From the previous discussion, we can more readily understand that we are magnetic organisms, very much affected by the Earth and sun and almost everything electrical around us. Let us look at the diagnostic and treatment sides of biomagnetics and how magnetism may be used as a medicine. We also will review how various kinds of magnetic fields and electromagnetic pollutants are damaging our bodies and environment. We need to become cognizant as to how vital all this is to our health and mental well-being. If there is a system to help us, we ought to be using it.

Applications for Biomagnetics

Observe some uses of the modern discovery of magnetism as listed below:

- The magnetoencephalogram (MEG) is a recording of magnetic brain waves which is similar to the electroencephalogram (EEG);
- Nuclear magnetic resonance (NMR), or magnetic resonance imaging (MRI), is used to take detailed images of internal body parts, and for mapping the brain, and exploratory surgery, etc., and which is rapidly replacing X-rays that place us at risk to cellular damage from adverse radiation;
- The MEG is detected with a Superconducting Quantum Interference Device (SQUID) that detects minute magnetic fields in the space around the head;

- Terafield and Diapulse electromagnetic devices for relief of pain and edema, approved or registered by the FDA in 1972 and used by more than 1,000 hospitals, colleges and health care centers throughout the United States; and
- Xomed magnetic hearing aid for conduction deafness, composed of solid-state magnets; Cadwell Magneto-Electric Stimulator; and many other devices scientifically tested and approved.

Literally thousands of research papers written by scientific professionals from all fields are available on these methods. For any one interested, one of the best sources of information is the National Medical Library of the National Institutes of Health, located in Bethesda, Maryland. Not much is available on the health benefits of permanent magnets but solid-state magnets are used in hearing aids, magnetic beds and seats, dentistry, pain relief, athletic injuries and in a growing variety of instruments and applications. For therapeutic purposes, it is possible that the benefits of permanent magnets may far outweigh the more dangerous processes of X-rays and radiation or electromagnetic (high frequency) applications.

It is well known that medical diagnosis is enhanced by magnetic fields, which are able to isolate disordered body metabolism and other malfunctions never before clearly recognized. The medical profession has strongly latched on to the application of magnetism for diagnostic purposes but, so far, has pretty much shied away from use for therapeutic purposes, mostly from lack of knowledge and support from the medical associations.

Nevertheless, Magnetic Resonance Imagery has benefited the therapeutic application of permanent magnetic fields. MRI has been in the forefront of introducing magnetic resonance into conventional scientific medicine. Studies on toxicity prior to marketing MRI convinced the FDA to declare magnetics in human diagnosis and therapy as "not essentially harmful," leading to further study and trials in medical magnetics without the need of additional toxicity evaluation (**Investigational Devices Exemptions**, *H.H.S. Publication, FDA 89-415*, Rockville, Md. 20857, Aug. 1989).

To advance further the therapeutic use of permanent magnetic fields, the Bio-Electro-Magnetics Institute has set up an Institutional Review Board which qualifies for FDA approval in all states for acceptable and ethical data gathering research in preparation for definitive publications in peer review scientific literature. The goal of the Magnetic Resonance Therapeutic Research Project (MRTRP) is to firmly establish magnetic resonance therapy in professional clinical medical practice as a self-help treatment for preventive and health maintenance.

Application to participate or commence a research project may come from physicians or other interested parties by communicating with BEMI. The physician's agreement requires a report three times annually and an agreed monitoring format and treatment follow-up. The patient's agreement does not promise symptom relief or a cure. It does require a monitoring protocol and accurate record-keeping.

Exhibit 3   Magnetic Resonance Imaging for Breast Cancer

> Magnetic fields for diagnostic purposes have become very important. The much more sensitive three-dimensional pictures produced from magnetic resonance imaging can find almost 100 percent of breast tumors compared to about 64 percent from mammography's two-dimensional image. Mammography misses from 5 to 60 percent of additional tumors; but its per test price is $55 compared to nearly $1,000 for MRI. Costs could be cut substantially through the use of cooperative, regional non-profit testing centers, if the nation is truly interested in saving women's lives.
>
> **Source:**   *Washington Post, Health Journal,* Dec. 17, 1991; and author.

Freedom of Choice

It is interesting to note that major changes were called for in our national health care insurance system by Dr. Alan R. Nelson, past president of the American Medical Association, in March of 1990, to insure patient freedom to choose providers. Dr. Nelson stated that "the individual's freedom of choice remains a cornerstone of the American system." Yet he failed to say that the system pressures to allow the patient the choice of doctors but not the doctor and his patient the choice of treatments, even when that treatment is safe and reliable. Too many physicians neglect even to discuss the choices of treatment, leaving patients in the dark. And insurance providers play along with this game even as they call for less expensive methods and better care, protecting conventional choices at the expense of innovation. Tens of billions of dollars are at stake in a system not so free. As the structure leans towards bankruptcy, less and less choice is evident. The paper work is outrageous and some of the best medicine is ignored. Private administrative costs hover at 20 percent of the medical bills compared to three percent for the single payer Medicare and Medicaid system. The vast majority of excellent doctors need to stand up courageously to the system regardless of stated policy, and demand that the best treatment possible be made available to the public in the most cost effective way. The system doesn't need competition in insurance sales but rather in doctoring, which will maintain the strength of free enterprise.

Alternative treatments are on the increase, magnetotherapy being one of them. Countless references exist for uses of magnetic medicine. A review in just one field, **Magnetism: A New Method for Stimulation of Nerve and Brain**, the *Journal of the American Medical Association*, July 1989, listed over 30 articles from various medical journals on magnetic energy involving nerve testing. Over 1,000 scientific articles have been written on the subjects of bone fusion, edema, muscular stimulation, pain relief and other types of ailments treated by magnetic energy. Numerous articles exist on the treatment of the total human biological system, including strengthening the immune system by magnetotherapy.

Nevertheless, much more needs to be done in research, controlled studies, and clinical observation of the benefits and risks of magnetic fields. If it is not approached sensibly with proper testing and validation, this extraordinary method of healing may be relegated once again to the grave yard of history. We must reach the stage where magnetotherapy is not considered an alternative but a most fundamental, conventional treatment. It has a poor historical connotation that the wisest of the profession must overcome.

Although the medical profession feels more comfortable with double-blind, controlled studies to prove efficacy, the vast majority of drugs, for example, have not been fully tested or have shown little treatment value. Although some drugs have proved highly effective, many are highly toxic. In the treatment of cancer, to take just one drug, Fluorouracil prescribed against colon cancer continues to be used in the United States despite a failure to demonstrate efficacy in placebo-controlled trials, as reported by Harrison Salisbury, **The Uncertainty of Medicine**.

"Doctors still don't know what works." This statement was made by Dr. Robert M. Centor, before a congressional committee, June 1989, on behalf of the 65,000 members of the American College of Physicians. Dr. Dennis O'Leary, president of the Joint Committee on Accreditation of Health Care Organizations points out that, "uncertainty of the most effective diagnostic and therapeutic approaches is pervasive." The Institute of Medicine reports that as much as one-fourth to one-third of medical services may be of little or no benefit to patients. For over one-third of Americans, it makes little or no difference whether they get any medical care or not. With conventional care, nothing really can be done for many symptoms. Prescribed drugs or chemicals are essentially a waste of resources in many cases, yet the doctor feels that he's got to do something. If he understood alternatives, he might very well be able to offer something worthwhile.

How many of us would consider undertaking serious chemotherapy treatment knowing that our good cells are very likely to be killed off while we suffer extensively for perhaps the last days of our lives? Of course, many lives have been extended, but almost all of us can recite examples where lives have been ruined. Chemotherapy and drugs have their place, but so do less invasive and less dangerous alternatives.

Support for Alternatives

Movement is afoot more strongly than ever in the direction of alternatives. Now a half dozen or more bioelectromagnetic organizations are in existence. Some have close to 1,000 members composed of professionals, doctors, physicists, scientists, therapists, etc. They hold annual conferences with thousands more in attendance and hundreds of papers presented. Also acupuncturists, homeopathics, naturalists, diverse medical practitioners and a variety of others number in the tens of thousands and have extensive association memberships. The American Holistic Medical Association climbed in membership from 220 members to 2,000 from 1978 to 1980 and has expanded greatly since. Over 20,000 physicians are closet progressives who recognize the system as faulty but who aren't up to challenging the establishment, even though they admit that medicine is having only a minimal effect on health and longevity.

No system has a monopoly on cures or failures, says Andrew Weil, M.D. Every treatment he has examined has failed to work sometime. The true art of medicine is the ability to prevent, select and find the best cure. Medicine, Dr. Weil says, can never be a science like physics or chemistry because it is so close to the basic mysteries of our existence. Perhaps a greater understanding of the DNA will help in this respect. Healing, Weil believes, involves the innate capacity of the body to find solutions as compared to something outside the body.

Too much bad research and too few good articles in the medical journals contribute to the cause of thoughtful prevention or treatment. Papers appear scientific in their use of technical jargon, graphs and titles, but that is where it usually ends. The lay person ought to insist that any paper using outrageous, unnecessarily complex language that intelligent people can't understand, ought to be discarded. We are tired of being fooled and professionals are tired of being used in order to maintain status among their peers by pouring out papers every year of questionable value.

Magnetism and the Functions of our Bodily Systems

Look briefly at how biomagnetism works. It functions in marvelous ways. Medical texts tell us that if blood circulation is interrupted or impaired, required nutrients and oxygen will not be supplied to our tissues. Waste products and carbon dioxide will remain and accumulate to foul up the system. Proper contraction and expansion of blood vessels helps the blood flow smoothly. If the autonomic nervous system is impaired, the blood vessels will soon fail in sporadic contraction.

Studies conducted in several countries show that magnetic contact with the human blood supply activates the iron content and creates a weak current. An increase in the number of centers of crystallization occurs, directly proportionate to the strength of the field, reports Dr. Bansal. He believes also that the process of ionization is hastened which alleviates the danger of blood clotting and stimulates the flow of blood to the arteries and veins. Magnetic flux in the blood increases the number of red corpuscles and strengthens inactive and decayed arteries; the movement of hemoglobin is accelerated and calcium and cholesterol deposits are held to a minimum, all of these clinically observed by Dr. Bansal and associates. Magnetism has been demonstrated to stimulate other fluids in the body as well (Bansal, 1983, 1990).

Dr. Bansal enumerates effects of magnetic fields on the biological system:

1. Secretion of hormones and other fluids is promoted and a positive effect is exercised on the working of the glands in the entire secretory apparatus;
2. Function of the autonomic nerves are normalized and strengthened, improving the functioning of all internal organs;
3. Build up of new cells and rejuvenation of tissues; and
4. A stabilizing of the genetic code.

Figure 2   Blood cell going through a capillary

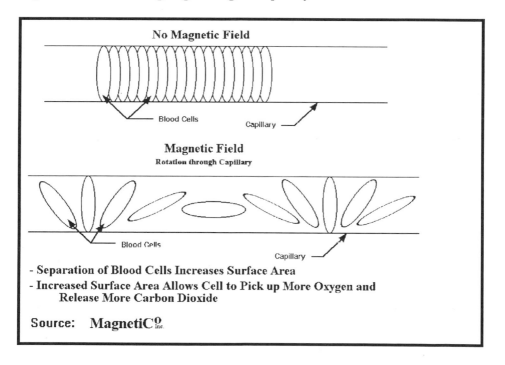

No Magnetic Field

Blood Cells

Capillary

Magnetic Field
Rotation through Capillary

Blood Cells

Capillary

- **Separation of Blood Cells Increases Surface Area**
- **Increased Surface Area Allows Cell to Pick up More Oxygen and Release More Carbon Dioxide**

Source: MagnetiCo.

Magnetic Fields and Living Organisms

Physicist and psychologist, Dr. Buryl Payne, formerly a Professor at Boston University and Goddard College, reports in **The Body Magnetic** and **Getting Started in Magnetic Healing**, various ways magnetic fields affect living organisms:

1. Increases blood flow with resultant increased oxygen-carrying capacity, both of which are basic to helping the body heal itself.

2. Changes in migration of calcium ions which can either bring calcium ions to heal a broken bone in half the usual time or can help move calcium away from painful arthritic joints.

3. The pH balance (acid-alkaline) of various body fluids (often out of balance in conjunction with illness or abnormal condition) can be altered by magnetic fields.

4. Hormone production from the endocrine glands can be either increased or decreased by magnetic stimulation. He cites documented changes to the body that includes electricity generated in the blood vessels, ionized particles increased in the blood, autonomic nerves excited, and improved circulation.

Barnothy in **Biological Effects of Magnetic Fields** (New York 1964) explains a thermomagnetic effect and an electromotive force created by electromagnetic induction in a liquid, probably exerting its strongest action on the blood. Also, researchers P. Fabre and A. Collin (cited in Nakagawa's study) discuss a similar force involving a magnetic-hydrodynamic effect on circulation.

Other effects take place as well. Dr. Robert O. Becker, for instance, believes that the negative polarity is that which heals and arrests infectious cell growth, and that it only takes microamperes of electric current to affect the body system dramatically. Melatonin secretion can be changed at will by exposure to steady magnetic fields of the same strength as the rather low geomagnetic field. Any deficiency or disorganization of energy results in disease. All organs and systems of the body depend on magnetic energy and also on magnetic frequencies that can be increased with the positive field and decreased with the negative polarity. The pineal gland, in the center of the head, is a magnetic organ containing magnetite crystals and is responsible for the production of melatonin, the master controller of our hormones, enzymes, immune system, metabolism and cyclic patterns. Magnetic energy can be directed into the crown of the head in order to stimulate the pineal gland.

The principle behind diathermy, Dr. Bansal informs us, is the same as magnetotherapy. Both affect the electrons and the nuclei of the atom. The major difference and advantage for magnetotherapy, Bansal believes, is that magnetism is far milder than the lowest electric current used in diathermy (which is also short-lived). Magnetism by virtue of its low density causes no trauma and provides a sustained and stable effect. Magnets of the proper strength, applied for the correct duration can be given with no danger to cells, tissues, or nerves and without fear of aggravation, Dr. Bansal believes. He supports the application of either polarity or both polarities together, but acknowledges that the polarities function differently, without the mention of the possible adverse effects from extended use of the positive pole. He does not discuss the counter-irritant effect of the positive polarity or of dual polarities that makes this methodology respond more like diathermy, drawing negative energy to the locale in order to counteract the positive field. Experiments of Dr. Becker show that the electrically negative polarity responds quite differently, as it places the healing negative energy directly at the source.

Scientific research reveals that our biological energies come from a variety of sources including (Becker; Philpott; Semm):

- Food and water through the digestive system
- Sleep that recharges our negative ions
- Absorption of the Earth's magnetism
- Piezoelectric energy from bone stress and exercise

Many practitioners believe that both magnetic polarities are healing and that if a stressful point is reached in therapy, simply stop using these medical tools until the body has had a chance to rest or recuperate and rebalance itself. Dr. Kyoeche Nakayawa, M.D., Director of Isuzu Hospital, Tokyo, Japan, has identified a magnetic field deficiency syndrome that results in stiffness to the shoulders, back and neck, and causes chest pain, habitual constipation, and general lassitude. He prescribes the dual magnetotherapy approach for these and a great variety of illnesses. He does not discuss the long-range consequences of the positive polarity.

Channel Openings

The opening and closing of ion channels stimulates bioelectrical fields that send electric signals to the muscles which, in turn, generate cell secretion and motion. Magnets act as regulators by changing the intensity of the electrical fields and corresponding magnetic fields. Barefoot, Reich, and Richard Broeringmeyer state that magnetic fields cause bicarbonate bonding to bend and break, producing hydroxides that create a negative (or alkaline) pH and extra cellular fluid capable of absorbing far more oxygen than a (low pH) positive fluid. The magnetic fields also raise the potential difference between the external and internal fluids, allowing the nutrient channel to open more readily. They find that this is a temporary but healthy purging of the body. On the other equation, they caution against the adverse effects of abnormal frequencies from electromagnetic pollution that hit us from such things as high power lines and a multiple of electrical gadgets.

A wide range of frequencies and currents affects the human body. Healing of wounds has been observed at electrical potential differences as little as 0.00006 volts, according to Barefoot, and exposure to radio waves with amplitude modulated at 16 hertz dramatically increases the flow of calcium from brain cells, interfering with impulse transmission and brain function. ELF fields have been shown to change brain stem levels of the neurotransmitter, known as acetylcholine. Barefoot observes that human cancer cells exposed to 60 hertz electromagnetic fields for 24 hours experience a six-fold increase in growth rate in one week. Also, decreases in red blood cell counts and changes in the number and types of white blood cells under ELF fields have been observed. Ionic calcium is also seriously affected.

The Earth's magnetic field causes the pH of extra cellular fluids to "gently rise" as bicarbonates and carbonates are converted to hydroxides and soluble carbon dioxide, as described by Barefoot and Reich. Magnetic beds create the same effect. Water at pH 7.5 when passed through a 7,000 gauss magnetic field rises to 9.2 pH. William Reed, Colorado, researcher and engineer, has used soft iron magnetic balls of 20,000 gauss to raise water pH from 7.5 to approximately 8.4 by simply passing water over the bipolar magnetic pieces. The moon's micropulsations—from 0.1 to 35 hertz—are in perfect harmony with the electrobiochemical impulses of man that they helped to develop during evolution. And the sun provides the necessary radiant stimulus through the pituitary gland that controls the production of calcium and vitamin D.

Exhibit 4   Opening Cell Channels

> Two German physiologists, Ervin Neher and Bert Sakmann, of the Max Planck Institute for Bio-Physical Chemistry in Gottingen, Germany, won the 1991 Nobel Prize for Medicine for perfecting the study of chemical traffic that takes place through pores on the surfaces of living cells. It has long been known that muscle cells, like nerve cells, carry electric charges, and that sudden changes in their charge is the way these cells "fire." Electric current comes from the rapid movement of charged atoms, such as sodium, potassium and chlorine, through "ion channels" of the cell membrane.
>
> With an advanced technique of using a hollow glass tube, 1/25,000th of an inch wide against the cell membrane, a few channels can be trapped without disrupting the cell. Neher and Sakmann detected channels that do a variety of things:
>
> 1. Show voltage changes in different environments
> 2. Are stimulated by neurotransmitters
> 3. Appear to be plugged and unplugged by other molecules
>
> They believe this shows that cells in the pancreas, kidney, blood and other tissues use ion channels to communicate. Some of the diseases that involve these ion channels are diabetes, cystic fibrosis and a number of other muscular disorders. Hypothetically, magnetic fields can open up these ion channels to allow nutrients stacked on the cell wall to enter.
> **Source:** *Washington Post*, Oct. 8, 1991, First Section, David Brown and Marc Fisher; author.

The loss of energy from natural magnetic fields means that cellular calcium is not maintained in an active ionized state and so reverts to its inert molecular state and is deposited as a solid substance on cells. The benefit of magnetotherapy is the ability of its magnetic fields to raise pH and thereby ionize the calcium, converting it into biologically active calcium ions, Barefoot reports.

Figure 3   Magnetically Induced Chemical Reaction in Fluid

$Ca(HCO_3)_2$ Calcium bicarbonate	Magnetic $\longrightarrow$ Field	$Ca(OH)_2$ Calcium Hydroxide	$2CO_2$ Carbon dioxide
pH7.5	Magnetic $\longrightarrow$ Field	pH9.2	Water
pH 7.2	Magnetic $\longrightarrow$ Field	pH 7.5	Blood
pH 6.2	Magnetic $\longrightarrow$ Field	pH 7.4	Cellular Fluid

Structural Charge Oriented Representation

Molecular orientation without magnetic field	Molecular orientation with magnetic field	Reorganization of molecular bonding

Calcium bicarbonate normal straight chain form	Negative magnetic field reorganizes structure of calcium bicarbonate	Calcium bicarbonate breaks into calcium hydroxide and carbon dioxide

With the loss of magnetic energy, the following sequence of events occurs in the cell, according to Dr. Reich's findings:

1. Deposition of solid molecular calcium in various sites of body cells, creating ionic calcium deficiency

2. Cellular energy starvation

3. Declining cellular, organ, and total body function

4. Occurrence of symptoms

5. Organ adaptation to this deficiency which may result in exhaustion and deterioration of the function

6. Occurrence of adaptive disease

7. Increased acidity of the cell and body fluid.

Energy starvation can result in ailments to ligaments, bones, muscles, intestines, lungs and nerve tissues, as well as produce a general decline in body function expressed as chronic fatigue, irritability and depression.

Barefoot and Reich explain that the difference in voltage between the outer (negative) and inner (positive) sides of the cell membrane is about 70 millivolts. This is enough to exert a pull at each end of the charged proteins (blocking the channel) to cause them to stretch and open repeatedly like breathing. The upper (negative) polar nutrients are attracted to the positive charges within the cell, causing the stacked nutrients to break and rush through the channels into the cells. This electrical energy activates all biological processes responsible for cell nerve stimulus. In this respect, the potential difference of 70 millivolts can be created whenever internal ionization is greater than the external, regardless of pH. This means that an unhealthy cell with a positive external pH of 6.5 can create 70 millivolts from internal positive cell ionization, making the internal pH even more positive and disease oriented. And natures second buffer mechanism that involves getting the large potassium ion to leave the cell performs only modestly. Remember *that low pH produces toxic enzyme cell breakdown, reflected in diseases, the aging process and mutation.   As stated previously, cell potential difference is important but only a small part of the process.**

Natural Flow of Electrons

Much of the medical establishment has yet to accept that magnetotherapy heals disease.   Consider that Robert O. Becker has measured the natural flow of electrons from new wounds in what he calls "a current of injury proportional to comparative growth," allowing wounds to heal from this natural energy.   Clear evidence shows that electrical and magnetic stimulation encourage more rapid regrowth.   In the early 1970's, surgeon Cynthia Illingworth, of the Sheffield Children's Hospital in England, found that when a young child's finger is sheared off beyond the outermost crease (last joint) and the wound is dressed but not closed (allowing it to remain electrically negative), the finger will grow back perfectly within three months.   Hundreds of such cases have been documented.   Pediatric surgeons, like Dr. Michael Bleither of New York's Mount Sinai Hospital, have become confident of the infallibility of the process.   Yet few hospitals or doctors accept this natural replacement flow of electrons because it is not endorsed by the establishment and not understood, Barefoot laments.

Similar magnetic field effects have been experienced by astronauts. Barefoot informs us that decalcification of up to eight percent of the body's bone mass (osteoporosis) has occurred after only a few weeks in orbit, caused by magnetic deficiency and possibly the effects of gravity from being outside the Earth's field. Calcium is dissolved from the bone and transferred into the muscle cells to maintain the 60 millivolts intercellular potential needed to maintain life. Tissue repair—that depends on regulated cell division—is synchronized with the Earth's magnetic field.   In the 1960s, scientists overcame space osteoporosis by strapping on electromagnetic coils that approximated normal magnetic field signals.

---

* The italicized text refers to more complex information.

Figure 4   Cell

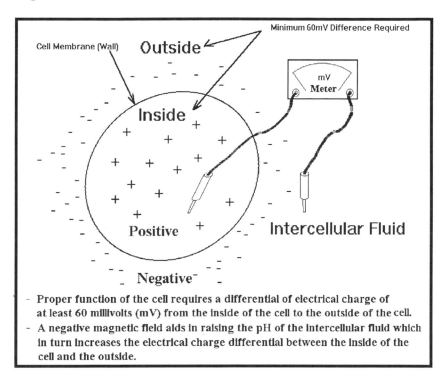

Minimum 60mV Difference Required

Cell Membrane (Wall)   Outside

mV Meter

Inside

Positive

Intercellular Fluid

Negative

- Proper function of the cell requires a differential of electrical charge of at least 60 millivolts (mV) from the inside of the cell to the outside of the cell.
- A negative magnetic field aids in raising the pH of the intercellular fluid which in turn increases the electrical charge differential between the inside of the cell and the outside.

Later in this chapter, the adverse effects of radiation are discussed. Here it is enough to say that flying can be hazardous to your health. **It has been estimated that flying at 40,000 feet exposes the body to 200 times more cosmic radiation than at ground level—or the equivalent of one chest X-ray after flying five hours. The airline industry and pilot associations need to evaluate this more closely. The industry would more likely want to keep it a secret, whereas various steps in construction of airplanes could very well correct much of the problem.** It is time we took seriously the consequences of man-made interference and lack of knowledge about the natural flow of electrons.

Alkaline versus Acidic Cells

The pH test serves as a very valuable visual incentive to improve health and prevent various diseases for many people. The FDA could provide instruction pamphlets on the use of litmus paper and proper diet

SCIENTIFIC DIGEST

The Value of Testing for pH

Researchers Barefoot and Reich discovered in the early 1970s that the acidic state of saliva was an outstanding manifestation of calcium ion deficiency and magnetic imbalance. A simple, 10 cent, three second test from litmus paper placed on the tongue, can determine calcium deficiency by measuring the pH level of an individual. When the pH of saliva is slightly alkaline at 7.5 to neutral at 7.0, body excretion tends to be acidic, throwing off toxins. When a patient is ionic calcium deficient, pH is acidic at 6.4 to 4.6, and body excretions tend to be alkaline. People with ailments fall into the lower range. But after only a few weeks or months of dietary changes—along with vitamin and mineral supplements—the saliva pH slowly rises to 7.0 and impairments are dramatically improved or eliminated.

A change of just one pH unit reflects a 10 fold shift in the hydrogen ion or the hydroxyl ion concentration. A drop of 7.0 to 4.0 pH, for example, is a 1,000 fold difference. From this we can begin to recognize the significance of the acidic state that causes the body to self-digest. Most children show dark blue (7.5 pH) on the litmus paper, over half of adults show blue green (6.5 pH or lower), while cancer patients usually show yellow (4.5 pH). Acidic pH is usually exhibited by anxious or depressed adults, hyperactive children, and rebellious or delinquent adolescents. Psychologically, Barefoot says, individuals will do almost anything "to get blue" (or healthy). Skin cancer from the sun or cancer from smoking can be reduced sharply by keeping pH in proper balance, which has the effect of starving the carcinogens of the electrons they so vitally need.

Source: The Calcium Factor: The Scientific Secret of Health and Youth, Robert R. Barefoot and Carl J. Reich, M.D., Boker Consultants Inc., Publishers, P.O. Box 21270, Wickerburg, Az., 1992.

and nutrition to effect the proper pH balance. In sampling saliva, results can be influenced by recently consumed food, giving a false positive test, therefore waiting two hours after putting the litmus paper in the mouth, is recommended. The patient should also draw fresh saliva into his mouth and swallow it several times before taking the test. Several tests to ensure quality over a period of hours or days should confirm the accurate pH. Taking the test when one arises in the morning is probably the best time to get the most accurate reading. A proper, non-acidic diet with needed supplements, plus exercise and magnetotherapy are recommended among other measures to correct low pH.

Both Barefoot and Reich say that negative magnetic field treatment will speed up the above pH process but will be better maintained with the appropriate intake of calcium as well as other deficient minerals. In some cases, magnetotherapy can improve symptoms in minutes without changes in diet or lifestyle, since the negative magnetic fields release the nutrients already stacked on the cell walls and, as already pointed out, add negative energy to the site almost instantly.

Dr. Kenneth Bernd, mentioned earlier, says that he had found better results in patients whose pH levels were already in the healthy range of 7.0 or above. When pH is too low, its like "beating a dead horse," he believes. This may be true if one is substantially depleted of ionic calcium and other minerals with little left to allow the magnetic fields to stimulate cell walls. It may be one reason why some people do not react to magnetotherapy, at least initially.

Barefoot has tested the pH of subjects before sleeping on a negative, magnetic pad and after arising in the morning. In cases where the pH tested was low (6.0 pH) in the evening—after a night on the magnetic pad—the pH had climbed to 7.3 or greater, which had not occurred without the pad. The pH might drop again during the day. With continual magnetic use and proper nutrition pH should stay up as toxins are sucked out over a period of time.

It appears that these treatments work best side-by-side, with the practitioner determining the best art for the human condition at hand. A therapist might apply magnetic treatment as a priority option to get immediate results for most patients or after waiting a period of time for one's nutritional level to improve in order to gain a higher peretage of success, knowing that a full 30 perent of the body's energy comes from non-nutritional sources.

Case histories show that over 70 percent of magnetotherapy users realize effect in short order, which may indicate that this group is in a state whereby health can be regenerated readily from existing body nutrients. Few will disagree that proper nutrition benefits the process. Dr. Bernd encourages providers of magnetotherapy and chiropractors and other users to supplement their treatment with sound nutrition. Conversely, suppliers of nutritional products are encouraged to combine their supplements with magnetotherapy. The effective integration of appropriate, non-invasive, alternative therapies is the best course of action for the patient.

Adverse Effects of Electromagnetism

Different electric and magnetic fields will have varying effects on our health. If used properly, they can improve health, possibly extend life span and heal many diseases. Improper use can damage cells, inflict pain on our bodies, produce headaches and dizziness, or create insomnia and a whole host of ill effects. Used properly, magnetic fields can be one of the safest therapies essentially without side effects.

Now that we realize a little more how magnetism can assist our bodily systems, we must become more cognizant as to how it might adversely affect us. If we get too little magnetic force, too much or the wrong polarities, we may suffer. Remember that the Earth's geomagnetic energy can be severely cut back or even blocked by elements in our environment, causing a variety of problems from headaches and fatigue to tumor and circulatory disorders. Society's escalating alternating current (A.C.) and electronic technology are creating interference with the Earth's natural magnetic fields. In the average home and workplace, A.C. magnetic fields can be strong enough to redirect the natural magnetic field or influence cell function. In buildings with reinforced concrete and steel rods, and homes with cinder block construction, the Earth's natural magnetic field can be cut by more than half. This is true of the automobile as well with which we have a love affair. An elevator can almost completely block out the field. Harmful effects that dampen out the desirable magnetic fields also come from the "electronic smog" of television and radio waves, radar, electric blankets and shavers, water bed heaters, household appliances, power lines and a variety of other sources.

Our world has changed radically and we are warned by consumer groups, researchers, and the United States Surgeon General of these adverse conditions. But until our loved ones get sick, we seem to take little action. Ominous conditions are occurring at the same time that the Earth's magnetic field continues to lessen year by year, preventing us from getting the normal level of magnetic energy.

Consider the effects of radio and television waves. The density of radio waves around us is now 100 to 200 million times the natural level of similar frequencies reaching us from the sun. There are 35 million CB radios, plus short wave ham operators, air and sea navigation systems, high power global communication military and spy satellites, police and taxi auto radios, UHF and cellular telephone and FM receivers, 10,000 commercial radio and TV stations, seven million radio transmitters, walkie talkies, 250,000 microwave phone and TV relay towers, 10 million microwave ovens, and more. New superconducting power lines will increase intensity 10 or 20 times. Certainly we ought to study these effects further.

Radar Guns, Video Display Terminals, Other Agents

Most recently a number of police departments around the country decided to limit the use of radar guns that emit magnetic radiation. In the case of St. Petersburg, Florida, the chief of police ordered the discontinuance of all radar guns because of their potential hazards. Police officers of Pataluma, California, have documented a considerably higher rate of cancer in their officers, as they approach middle age, due to holding a radar gun on their laps for eight hours a day. Officers in the State of Connecticut have sued their department for the same reason, and similar cases have arisen all over the nation. The National Standards Association, who represent the manufacturers of these devices, say that these instruments are safe and that it is all simply a phobia in the minds of these officers, who incidentally hail from many different parts of the nation. They say they would be willing to have their families or friends sit in a radar car all day with these units on their laps. But when angry police associations take up this issue, a new way to track speeders may have to be found. Hand held speed detectors using laser technology and optics instead of radio waves have been developed and are in use in some areas. Since it is not very expensive to pull radar guns from use, the nation may be able to solve this particular problem. But what about transmission lines that cost billions of dollars to replace as just one expensive example? The question is do we have the will to change or will we let our children suffer slowly!

Another serious problem is computer terminals. International Business Machines (IBM) recently announced a program to reduce the electromagnetic fields generated by its video display terminals (VDTs), although they will not admit that they are unsafe. Other manufacturers are taking similar steps. Sigma Systems and Tandberg Data also stated they will soon sell monitors with reduced ELF emissions. Over 40 million VDTs are used in the U.S. Clusters of miscarriages and other problems have been reported for years among users. It appears that the very long wave lengths which VDTs emit are worth worrying about.

On the corrective side, a new company in Needham Massachusetts, Safe Computing Company, has developed a computer terminal that they say emits virtually no radiation or electromagnetic fields. A common misconception is that electromagnetic energy is given off only by the screen; however, magnetic fields are generated within the circuitry of the entire set and the cabinet is transparent to this condition. If placed against the wall, the pollution will penetrate into the next room. And at this stage, we have no rules or recommendations for official recognition for computer use in schools, for example, even when our children are at risk.

Concerning ELF fields, Dr. David Carpenter, dean of the School of Public Health at State University of New York, Albany, once a skeptic now says, "this is really harming people. In my judgment the present state of affairs is like the correlation between smoking and lung cancer was clearly demonstrated only with extensive cellular and animal studies not yet done with ELF fields." (Fortune, Dec. 31) Carpenter says that based on the Savitz studies, up to 30 percent of all childhood cancer may be attributable to ELF fields, and "that's conservative."

Children are suffering from a host of pollution problems, including electromagnetic fields, chemicals and asbestos. Fluorescent lights, for instance, are in the very small range of the visible light spectrum that function not by filament but rather by a coating of chemicals on the interior of the tube that are excited by high voltage discharge. This causes the lights to flicker on and off faster than we can perceive but at a rate detectable by brain and visual system. The harmful effects from fluorescent is 20 times greater than from incandescent lights but fluorescent lights save more energy. Dr. John Ott is convinced that behavior disturbances that run in the classroom are very much affected by improper lighting. Children are constantly under exposure from adverse electromagnetic fields from the ballast transformers in the fluorescent lighting units.

Research indicates that ordinary 60-cycle household A.C. electricity, and also higher frequencies from such things as radio and radar waves, can cause memory loss, headaches, changes in heart rate and blood chemistry and general malaise. Furthermore, exposure is cumulative, further contributing to sluggishness, digestive and other problems.

We know about the possible dangers of electric blankets. The FDA has conducted major reviews of these devices. They say that it is better to heat blankets first, unplug the blankets, then use them rather than lie there all night in the emanation of their fields. But the plug must be taken out of the socket, otherwise some blankets still produce an electric field. Dr. Nancy Werthemer of the University of Colorado in Boulder, found the incidence of miscarriages much higher among pregnant women who use electric blankets than those who do not. Dr. David Savitz and colleagues, University of North Carolina, in the *American Journal of Epidemiology (Vol 131: pp763-77, May, 1990)*, provided further evidence and reason to avoid electric blankets and pads. Mothers who used electric blankets during pregnancy increased the risk to their offspring of brain tumors and leukemia, according to Savitz. FDA's Center for Devices and Radiological Health (CDRH) has concluded that evidence from various sources so far does not warrant regulatory action, although the design of electric blankets has changed and techniques are being developed to reduce magnetic fields by 95 percent.

In 1991, Congress passed the National Electromagnetic Fields Research and Public Information Dissemination Act which is incorporated into the nation's energy policy to coordinate ELF research and public information. Eventually we may learn considerably more, meanwhile we can only work with the data available.

Comparative data show that electric heaters in our homes and offices may be a menace. A four foot-long baseboard electric heater produces 23 milligauss of varying magnetic fields at a distance of six inches. Heat cables in the ceiling can produce this level of power over the entire room. Significant magnetic field levels can be produced by ground currents from the plumbing system, wiring irregularities, or the type of electrical distribution system employed in the community. Sometimes underground distribution lines run very close to homes, and since the Earth provides no shielding from fields, high levels of magnetic fields enter the house—a special problem in townhouse developments. Dr. Wertheimer indicates that the miscarriage rate among pregnant women in homes under these conditions is higher. Certain research shows it is not the strength of the magnetic fields that causes the damage but rather the bipolar frequencies. Some believe the polarity is irrelevant since in a 60 Hz frequency the field changes 60 times per second. Importantly, this frequency injects itself into the body in adverse manners.

Are we able to avoid dangerous frequencies? In respect to aluminum siding protecting our homes, for example, it won't shield your house from internal or external pollution. It is a practical impossibility, Dr. Becker wants us to know. Every piece of siding needs to be carefully bonded together and well grounded; otherwise, it is useless for protective purposes and would provide minimal shielding at the magnetic field component. Becker has documented evidence of electromagnetic pollution that causes some cancer and possibly contributes to such maladies as Reye's Syndrome, Lyme disease, Legionnaire's disease, and AIDS. Electromagnetic pollution can weaken our immune system and make us vulnerable to many diseases.

An interesting finding was discovered by Dr. Philpott. He tested the ear piece in the phones that we all use and determined that they are putting out 800 gauss of magnetic energy into our heads. And rather fascinating, the AT&T phones tested were emitting positive magnetic energy, while the Bell Company phones were giving off negative fields. He cites an interesting case where an individual continually experiences a paralytic flare-up every time he uses the phone.

The only way we communicate involves electromagnetic fields, which are not the same frequency as our brains. We find them in cordless phones, cellular phones, security systems, radios, controlled electric toys and a whole host of electronic devices. The incidence of leukemia has been found to be significantly higher among amateur radio operators. It would appear tests are in order to determine whether our phone systems ought to be emitting the more benign negative rather than positive magnetic fields. A vast disagreement exists among the experts on this, therefore we need some immediate answers. Walkmans and phones may be driving us "batty." What better way to spend our research monies than to determine what polarity and frequency is best for us? Some in science have already said that these differences have little effect.

It is also fascinating that laboratory experiments by Kenneth Ring, Ph.D., described in his book, **The Omega Project**, demonstrate a common neurological mechanism at work involving electrical current induction and increased magnetic field response to the body's temporal region for such largely unexplained activities as out-of-body experiences, feeling as though the body is floating or being pulled towards a powerful light, hearing strange music, visits or sightings of people from unidentified flying objects, near death experiences and other unusual phenomena.

A 1982 Gallup Poll showed that one in seven Americans had a near death experience (NDE). People who experience NDEs or UFOs and similar encounters, Ring states, are as much as four times likelier than the general population to:

- Be usually sensitive to electrical fields, light, sound and other environmental influences;
- Have unusual sleep patterns;
- Undergo powerful mood swings and depression;
- Have other paranormal abilities, such as telepathy.

Ring says that there is little doubt that the above experiences can be correlated to temporal-lobe activity. Also he finds moderate intercorrelation between temporal-lobe epilepsy, multiple personality, and early child abuse, specifying that certain types of people are more prone to electrical microseizures. Dr. David Fish, National Society of Epilepsy, states he believes that computer games carry unusual electromagnetic fields that can adversely effect epileptics as well as other persons.

The concept of the computerized Virtual Reality that brings people into an entirely new world of realistic experience also plays on the brain's electromagnetic fields. We can program and stimulate the brain to imagine almost any experience we desire from floating in space or a drug high to having an unbelievable sexual encounter. If you don't believe it, simply place one of these $50,000 units on your head. As the price drops, they may be in every home and the question arises—will this be good or bad for our mental health and more electrical pollution?

Homes, Offices and Schools

We are affected from so many sources, it is hard to keep track of them. Dental amalgam fillings, for example, set up a measurable direct flow of current between the fillings. The D.C. positive force encourages microorganism replication, and for some people a ringing has been observed in their heads. But most studies show that there is little danger from dissipation of amalgam into the body, perhaps because of the amount used.

Chemicals in a typical mall are big culprits—fabric dyes, synthetic carpet materials, insecticides, plastics, building materials, paint, detergents, cleaning supplies, and cigarette smoke. National TV networks have shown us examples of people—total numbers believed to be in the hundreds of thousands who suffer from chemical reactions and cannot go near any chemical, plastic, gas or oil products. Many people must wear face masks wherever they go and some cannot ever leave their residences for fear of an attack. Healthy individuals who have been exposed to chemical spills have been so affected that the symptoms last for years from just one incident. The body becomes chemically or electrically unbalanced and a variety of treatments may become necessary, including stimulating the immune system with appropriate magnetic fields.

Military Defense

Another fascinating verification of pollution's effects and the consequences that the nation and the world face is the new military defense "killing fields" of electromagnetic weapons (EMP) which reportedly can be as dangerous and damaging as nuclear explosions.

If EMP is produced and released 100 miles above an urban area, it would shut off all electric power systems, destroy all computers and magnetic disks and blank out the guidance systems of missiles and communication apparatus of aircraft and other radio systems across the entire nation.

The GWEN communication system, with towers planned across the country, would be stymied as well. The GWEN system, designed to function even after a major attack at the low frequency (LF) range (150 - 175 kHz) hugs the ground rather than radiating through the higher atmosphere. Many scientists believe that it will be very dangerous to our health and behavior patterns and probably would be blasted away in any case after an EMP explosion. Over 300 towers—up to 500 feet high—were initially planned to be completed sometime in the 1990's, even though the military threat from a major foreign power has virtually waned. The full system now would be about 98 ground stations operating in the 150-175 kHz and 225-440 MHz range. The latest study mandated by Congress in 1990 and completed in May, 1993 by the National Academy of Sciences, **Assessment of the Possible Health Effects of Ground Wave Emergency Network**, National Academy Press, states that GWEN fields should have only a minimal, and probably undetectable, impact on public health. Because there is little information about the effects of low frequency signals, the review committee used information from AM broadcasting to establish an upper-bound estimate of cancer risk which they found to be less than one additional death over a 70-year period for persons living within 10 km of the entire system of sites. However, other effects associated with depression, hyperactivity, chronic fatigue syndrome and a host of related problems were hardly addressed. Cancer seems to be the prevalent issue when there are so many other pressing problems that adults and particularly children must live with everyday of their lives. If one additional person dies of cancer or his life is shortened by several years, this is almost insignificant to living with chronic fatigue for a lifetime. Perhaps a new study will be conducted. After all, this analysis simply reviewed existing literature which may have been flawed. No additional insight was brought to the question.

Also under study are HPMs (high power pulse micro waves) that produce intense, extremely short pulses of microwaves from 1,200 MHz to 35 GHz and up to 1,000 megawatts. The Microwave Research Department, Walter Read Army Institute of Research, states that a microwave of one to five GHz penetrates the entire bodily system and can kill, control behavior or simply interfere with one's work. This we are still planning to do to some enemy in some future war. But the enemy appears to be the human race. These plans are generally kept secret from the American public, otherwise there would be an uproar. And believe it or not, even with the massive federal deficit, the Center for Defense Information reports that the Department of Defense will spend $150 billion over the next decade on atomic weapons even without a superpower enemy. The public can get a little discouraged with this when our health needs are not being adequately addressed.

Recent Evaluations of Electromagnetic Pollution

Environmental Protection Agency Reports

A number of reports have come out of the Department of Energy (DOE) and the Office of Technology Assessment (OTA) concerning electromagnetic pollution. A 1989 study by Carnegie Mellon University, Pittsburg, with a grant from OTA, Biological Effects of Power Frequency Electric and Magnetic Fields, which stated that "... There are no significant transfers of energy from magnetic fields to biological systems, unlike X-rays and microwaves, and secondly, that natural occurring fields are at least 100 times more intense on cell membranes than those induced from commercial power frequencies." Nevertheless, they reported that "it has been demonstrated unequivocally that cell membranes are sensitive to weak fields and can cause modulation of ion flows; can cause interference with DNA synthesis and RNA transportation, interact with hormone and neurotransmission; and can cause interaction with the biochemical kinetics of cancer cells." Evidence indicates that even a minute 0.00005 milligauss of magnetic energy can effect the human system. They did conclude that "we can no longer categorically assert that there are no risks."

Later in 1991, OTA stated that "there is now a very large volume of scientific findings based on experiments at the cellular level and from studies with animals and people which clearly establish that low frequency magnetic fields can interact with, and produce changes in, biological systems." This new report states that developing nervous systems may be particularly susceptible and effects may be latent, manifested only in specific situations or later in time. OTA reports that ELF fields, more than any other agents known, except perhaps some psychotropic drugs, are specific to the response of brain tissue effected and point of influence in the circadian rhythm. They concluded that they are not likely initiators of cancer but can affect the cell membrane and increase cancer promoting ornithine decarboxylase (ODC) activity.

OTA also acknowledges that ELF fields may have an effect on tumor growth to the extent of altering protein synthesis, immunological and hormone status, and metabolic competence via circadian shifts. These fields also depress pineal melatonin associated with cancer growth, and show a weak association to nervous system cancer and leukemia. In fiscal 1988, the DOE awarded over two million dollars for the study of ELF fields on such things as pineal gland melatonin, circadian rhythms, human response to 60 hertz fields, cellular mechanisms, cyclotron resonance, and leukemia cell reaction. They conclude that more study is needed on psychological effects, such as chronic depression. But some progress is being made. DOE has been funded for $65 million over a five year period. Also the private Electric Power Research Institute is spending $15 million annually to study many of these problems.

Information Brief

Suppressing the Bad News of Radiation

Review of 124 studies, representing most of which is publicly known about the health of some 600,000 Americans who have worked in bomb factories over the last half century, shows flawed data, inconsistent measuring techniques, and suppression of unwanted findings, according to H. Jack Geiger, Epidemiologist, City University of New York, and David Rush, Tufts University. As a result, independent scientists lack the information they need in order to assess health risks of exposure to low levels of radiation to be able to set appropriate exposure limits. For 40 years the energy department and its predecessors restricted access to health data on national security grounds. This analysis, sponsored by Physicians for Social Responsibility (25,000 medical professionals), concludes that the studies were found to be "lousy research done in private...DOE shows a lack of curiosity. Clues weren't followed. Scientists seen as troublesome disappeared from the folds of DOE research." The authors state that this inevitably led DOE to minimize or suppress indication that radiation was producing elevated rates of cancer and leukemia among workers. Furthermore, the politics of suppression has permeated many of our most trusted federal agencies in respect to the hazards of radiation and electromagnetic pollution.

Source: Physicians for Social Responsibility; *Washington Post*, May 8, 1992, Thomas W. Lippman; author.

Certain state governments are not waiting for DOE or congressional action. At least seven states have passed laws to limit the intensity of electric and magnetic fields on transmission rights-of-way. In order to prevent new line construction from exceeding existing field levels so that at least the utility industry can proceed with construction. However, their limits have no realistic association with safety standards. A brief summary is shown in Exhibit 5.

When Rolf Lindgren, EMF manager for the state power company, Vattenfall, Sweden, was asked whether Sweden would adopt a 2 mG occupational standard, he replied that such a limit "would bring an end to industrial society in Sweden." A 2 - 4 mG standard would be about 100 times more stringent than standards adopted by New York State and Florida. Yet many believe that this is the RoW standard necessary to protect society.

Exhibit 5   State Regulations Limiting Field Strength on Transmission Rights-of Way (RoW)

State Field Limit

State	Field Limit
Montana.............	1 kV/m at edge of RoW in residential areas
Minnesota............	8 kV/m maximum in RoW
New Jersey..........	3 kV/m at edge of RoW
New York.............	1.6 kV/m at edge of RoW
North Dakota........	9 kV/m maximum in RoW
Oregon...............	9 kV/m maximum in RoW
Florida..............	10 kV/m maximum for 500 kV lines in RoW

2 kV/m maximum for 500 kV line at RoW
8 kV/m maximum for 230 kV smaller lines in RoW
2 kV/m maximum for 230 kV and smaller lines at edge of RoW
200 mG for 500 kV lines at edge of RoW
250 mG for double circuit 500 kV lines at edge of RoW
150 mG for 230 kV and smaller lines at edge of RoW

Source: **Regulatory Activity and Exposure Standards**, 1989, Department of Energy.

In March, 1990, the Environmental Protection Agency released a controversial draft of a report (EPA#600/6-90/00513) on the possible hazards of electromagnetic fields (EMF). Because of the usual unwillingness to release adverse information, as well as some problems of report quality, according to William Farland, Director of the Office of Health and Environmental Assessment in EPA's Office of Research and Development, EPA is delaying the report's release for another year. He stated that, in any case, "it will probably not move us substantially towards a definitive answer" to possible human dangers. It very likely will link EMF and health effects but, as most of these reports have done, will simply recommend more research while our population is at risk.

The draft report, **Evaluation of the Potential Carcinogenicity of Electromagnetic Fields**, concluded that several studies show "a consistent pattern of response, which suggests a casual link" between certain kinds of EMF to various types of "leukemia, lymphoma, and cancer of the nervous system." The Bush White House Science Advisor called for a separate review by the Federal Coordinating Committee on Interagency Radiation Research and Policy Coordination.

EPA states that biological effects do occur but that more information is needed to differentiate the effects of low frequency household EMF from those of high frequency, such as radio waves. Also EPA says it has not properly evaluated the findings on biological effects and field-tissue interaction mechanisms, as well as the values of magnetic field strength that may be hazardous to human health. Meanwhile, utilities are left without federal guidelines for construction and safe maintenance of their facilities.

The *Microwave News*, respected newsletter on bioelectromagnetism, revealed, in the May 1990 issue, that the Office of Technology Assessment forced a change in the wording of a key paragraph in the EPA report. The following paragraph was omitted:

> **"Concerning exposure to fields associated with 60 Hz electrical power distribution, the conclusion reached by EPA staff members in this document is that such exposure is a probable carcinogen risk factor corresponding to a B-1, degree of evidence that it is a risk factor. This conclusion is based on limited evidence of carcinogenicity in humans which is supported by laboratory research indicating that the carcinogenic response observed in humans has a biological basis, although the precise mechanisms are only vaguely understood."**

Some highly ranking persons were at the meeting, including William Farland and William Reilly, former administrator of the EPA. At least two of the organizations in attendance, says Paul Brodeur of the *New Yorker*, have been involved in attempts to deny that ELFs pose a biological hazard. Dr. James Wyngarden was also present who, in 1989 as director of the National Institutes of Health, was persuaded by adverse publicity to initiate a review of why three NIH scientists had testified in a court trial on behalf of the New York Power Authority that there was no scientific basis for concluding that ELFs from power lines could cause cancer. Brodeur stated that these scientists received payments from the power authority that far exceeded NIH regulations. In addition, several top level scientists at the

116

National Cancer Institute, over the past several years, have testified in legal proceedings that power frequency electromagnetic fields have no biological effects and that exposure to them is absolutely harmless.

Also, in this regard, Centers for Disease Control epidemiologists dismiss the possibility that there is any connection between miscarriages and birth defects by women exposed to low frequency ELFs given off by video display terminals. Dr. Zimmerman, Dr. Becker, and Laurence F. Herbert (and others) believe that the establishment is unwilling or fearful to speak out. They say evidence exists of a conspiracy or cover-up by at least part of the scientific community who are awarded the lucrative contracts to provide counsel to the manufacturers who produce these harmful products. The experts sit on the boards while those who raise their voices in disagreement are discredited. Pressure is at hand to withhold vital information or, at a minimum, a conspiracy of ignorance exists, they believe. Yet the public has no place to hide, while acting as guinea pigs.

Colorado Public Utilities Commission Hearing

Lawrence F. Herbert, in the winter 1990-91 BEMI journal, recounts testimony before the Colorado Public Utilities Commission concerning magnetic fields and human health. Expert witnesses verified the close relationship of electric and magnetic field frequencies to man-made, human body frequencies:

> *It is general knowledge that most of our normal brain wave frequencies are in the electromagnetic spectrum of ultra low frequencies of 1 Hz and up to 30 Hz. Brain wave frequencies are as low as 0.5 Hz and as high 100 Hz, with most between 1 and 20 Hz. Low brain wave frequencies (0.5 - 7 Hz) are associated with sleep and drowsiness; high frequencies (8 - 20 Hz) with wakefulness and alertness.*

> *Our muscle actions generate alternating current at frequencies between 10 Hz and 10,000 Hz, yet the peak power of muscle activity is the same frequency as the power frequency of 60 Hz. Amplitude ranges from less than one microvolt to hundreds of microvolts. The nervous system*

response to sub-threshold electric fields is too small to cause nerve firing but the fields cause changes in the cells electropotential, called Transmembrane Potential Difference. An increase in this potential is called hyper-polarization while a decrease is called depolarization. The 60 Hz electrical activity, with less than one millionth of a volt, is associated with physiological effects in the human body. Calcium, for example, regulates the contraction and relaxation of muscle fibers, assists nerve conduction and the beating of the heart, and importantly is in a cyclotron residence frequency of approximately 60 Hz, the same as our power frequencies.*

These harmonious frequencies of body and power lines, as verified by utilities commission experts, result in a stress response to which the body adapts after a short period. But after continuous exposure, the immune system begins to weaken, leading to exhaustion and eventual depletion. Studies also show calcium afflux from cells exposed to extremely low frequency fields, discussed in the OTA report. Finding a balancing magnetic force that could counteract adverse forces would be highly significant.

Serotonin or melatonin metabolism is not compatible with 60 Hz electromagnetic fields. The pineal gland is located in the center of the brain, once called the "seat of the soul," where Dr. Philpott concentrates negative energy applications to counter adverse effects from various sources of pollution. Serotonin is metabolized into melatonin, which, in excessive amounts, causes depression and sexual dysfunction. Melatonin is synthesized from many parts of the body and especially secreted by the pineal gland, an important regulatory organ for our biological rhythms. The pineal gland is also a feedback modulator of the circadian rhythms of our 24 hour body clock of sleep and wakefulness. It also controls dozens of other bodily rhythms, involving blood pressure, heart and respiratory rates, and urine secretion. At the other extreme, low levels of melatonin have been associated with cancer in some people. The evidence shows that the 60 Hz field affects melatonin production in our pineal glands, an

---

* The italicized text refers to more complex information.

imbalance of which can make us feel like we are in jet lag or can influence
our pain thresholds and attention span. *

Solutions

What can we do about these problems ? Not all is lost. The nation's pollution could at least be reduced if local governments and power companies would take certain steps for energy efficiency or utilize more solar systems, for example. Burial of lines appears too expensive in most cases. However, it is estimated that proper preparation of the lines can cut emissions as much or more than if they were placed underground. Herbert says that one way to reduce magnetic fields 50 percent is to balance the loads on each line more accurately to effect a natural self-cancellation of magnetic fields of nearby lines. Companies can also change the phasing of lines. Three current-carrying lines wrapped in a metal conduit twisted around each other can reduce the field 70 to 90 percent. Another method for a 50 percent reduction is to double the voltage in distribution lines which reduces the required current in the line and, in turn, its magnetic fields, while still maintaining the same power. On-site generation of power is another alternative. So there are solutions, some of which are financially feasible and beneficial energy-wise. All is not hopeless even in such a complex and costly field. We simply need the will to act.

Biological Effects of
Electromagnetic Pollution

Effects of Different Levels of Frequencies

Electromagnetic field frequency rates and shapes of wave form have important implications on our body's reception of magnetic radiation. Yet our bodies are so adept that they can accept almost any level or type of

---

* The italicized text refers to more complex information.

electric or magnetic fields; therefore, we must learn how to offset any adverse impact.

Dr. P. Z. Sanker Narayan (Bioelectromagnetics Journal of the Madras Institute of Magnetobiology, India, December 1988), believes that the most important elements of the body's ability to accept magnetic fields are the actual waveform shape and its time-varying rate. A square wave (similar effect also for a saw tooth wave) with a pulse repetition rate as low as one Hz can have a rise time or fall time as small as one millionth of a second or smaller, meaning a very high time-rate of change of magnetic field. A sine wave will have a rise or fall time a few hundred times longer, so would induce a smaller voltage in biological tissue and have a much smaller effect.

Fields with frequencies up to 100 Hz and strengths up to a few milli-Teslas can induce ionic current densities of about one $MA/meter^2$ in the tissue. Many believe that the shape of waves has a great deal to do with the effect on the human system. In the case of permanent magnets, frequency or waveform is non-existent but we still get a whole range of effects based on polarity and strength.

The above levels, says Dr. Narayan, do not have any direct effect on the brain's electric patterns as revealed by the ordinary EEG, but this is based on the entire cranial volume involvement and not just parts of it, which may have different electroconductivity. So particular parts of the body, perhaps more sensitive than others, can be more profoundly affected than other sites. Therefore, the measuring of effect on the entire body may not be as important as testing specific parts of the brain or nervous system. Changes in EEG activity in response to ELF magnetic field exposure has been demonstrated by researchers at Louisiana State University Medical Center. Yet there appears to be an interaction between the brain and extremely weak magnetic fields that could influence our neural activity and thinking processes. Resonance is defined as a process involving the frequency of an applied force achieving the natural frequency of a vibrating body organ. Understanding how resonance works is fascinating and very revealing. By resonance our bodies are able to modulate or accept certain electromagnetic frequencies. If the pulse repetition rate of an external magnetic field is tuned to match exactly the beat frequency of the heart, it is possible, says Narayan, that the cardiac rhythm could go into sympathetic resonance with the pulsations of the external magnetic fields. The amplitude of the biological rhythm can be expected to increase and out-of-step beats or systoles can occur. These changes can cause stroke or other cardiac disturbances, as we especially note during solar storms, as just one example.

Microwaves oscillate at hundreds of millions of times per second and even higher, while normal power frequencies oscillate at less than 100 times per second, yet, says Dr. Becker, the biological effects are virtually identical. The body can demodulate signals from a modulated radio frequency, as an example. An AM radio is amplitude modulated. The biological effects produced by ELF frequencies can cause the body to turn these man-made signals into natural frequencies between 0 and 30 Hz. [*]

Information Brief

Resonance Theory

The resonance theory is based on frequency, not power. Cyclotron resonance, as one case, has the ability to transfer the energy of ions and to cause them to move rapidly, changing the function of living cells and enabling the ions to pass through cell membranes more effectively and in greater numbers. As the strength of steady-state magnetic fields decreases, the frequency of the oscillating electric or magnetic fields needed to produce resonance also decreases.

Years ago, virtually all of our electro-magnetic radiation came from the sun. This is broad-band, incoherent radiation. Now we have man-made, coherent radiation, both spatially and temporally repetitive. Coherent radiation is exemplified by Radio Frequency Interference (RFI) which can cause a variety of symptoms, reports William Van Bise, chief research scientist of the Pacific Northwest Center for the Study of Non-Ionizing Radiation. To reinforce this effect, the former Soviet and East European nations have cited non-thermal microwave induced disturbances as detrimental to the nervous system, referred to as "neuroasthentic syndrome." Apparently, they have been studying this problem a lot longer than the U.S. and taking it more seriously.

Radio frequency power of about 100,000 microwatts per square centimeter can produce thermal effects. U.S. standards were set only 10

---

[*] The italicized text refers to more complex information.

times less than this intensity but are 100 times greater than safe levels established by Eastern Europe, as though they know something the U.S. doesn't. Van Bise reports that the effects of radio frequency radiation through heating tissue is in direct proportion to the power density. Thermal effects include such things as cataracts; change in EEG brain waves and electrocardiogram and blood flow; and disturbances of the endocrine glands and alimentary tract. The organs most susceptible to electromagnetic induced heat—which tend to retain heat—are the lungs, eyes, testes, gall bladder and the lumen of the intestinal tract. The combination of ionizing radiation (X-ray or gamma rays) and non-ionizing radiation (radio waves) is even more devastating.

Cancer Incidence

Another study, conducted over four years, that lends credibility to the adverse effects of power lines is reported by Dr. Genevieve Matanoski involving 50,000 New York State telephone linemen who work very near high power cables. Before the study, Matanoski thought the theory of any connection between cancer and power lines was wrong. Since then, the results she obtained in the study have changed her initial doubts. She found the incidence of all types of cancer higher to exposed linemen compared to a controlled, non-exposed group of telephone workers.

A second critical association was found among male technicians, who work telephone switching equipment that produces low level, non-ionizing, pulsed electromagnetic radiation. Normally, the incidence of breast cancer in males is about one in one million. In this case, reports Dr. Matanoski, of 9,500 central office technicians, the breast cancer rate was an astonishing 1 out of 4,250.

Informative reports have been prepared by the Congressional Office of Technology Assessment such as **Biological Effects of Power Frequency Electric and Magnetic Fields**, and the House of Representatives Subcommittee on Water and Power Resources report, **Health Effects of Transmission Lines**. These studies show definite health relationships. Also, the State of Hawaii's department of Health, in a 1986 report, entitled **Cancer Incidence in Census Tracts With Broadcasting Towers in Honolulu**, found that in the tracts were broadcasting towers are located, cancer of all types was significantly higher than in adjacent areas were towers were not located. However, the state took no action.

In a related test, Dr. Daniel B. Lyle of the Jerry L. Pettis Memorial Veterans Hospital in Loma Linda, California, reported that when exposed to 60 Hz magnetic fields for 48 hours, T-cell lymphocyte cytotoxic function is depressed significantly in its fighting ability against foreign cells. Biological effects are present in all man-made electromagnetic fields, regardless of frequency, reports Dr. Robert O. Becker. If electromagnetic fields are applied properly for therapeutic purposes, using correct frequencies and duration of use, they can be beneficial. On the other hand, adverse electromagnetic fields can be cancer promoting but not necessarily cancer causing, Becker states as he describes the effects:

1. Increase in the rate of cell division
2. Increases in the incidence of certain cancers
3. Developmental abnormalities in embryos
4. Alteration in neurochemicals, resulting in behavioral abnormalities, such as suicide
5. Alteration in biological cycles
6. Stress responses in exposed animals that if prolonged, lead to a decline in the immune system efficiency
7. Changes in learning ability

Why are most cancers increasing rather than decreasing? The National Cancer Institute's Division of Surveillance Epidemiology reveals an 80 percent increase in the incidence of melanoma in the U.S. between 1973 and 1980. Dr. Thomas B. Fitzpatrick of Harvard Medical School says, "it's epidemic," not only the fastest growing of all cancers but also affecting more of the younger age groups. Dr. Mark H. Green of the NCI states that the "incidence of cutaneous, malignant melanoma is rising rapidly throughout the world." Significantly, any link of melanoma to a decline in the atmospheric ozone level is unlikely because the increased cancer rate came well before the reported decline in ozone, which was limited to the "ozone holes" found over the Arctic regions, but now seems to be spreading globally.

Exhibit 6 Incidence of Leukemia and Brain Tumors in Finnish Workers Exposed to ELF Magnetic Fields

Several epidemiological studies have suggested that employment in various electrical occupations is associated with an increased risk of leukemia and brain tumors.

A Finnish study researched the relative incidence of leukemia, acute myeloid leukemia (AML) and central nervous system (CNS) tumors among workers, presumably exposed to extremely low frequency (ELF) magnetic fields (MFs). The study population consisted of all male industrial workers in Finland aged 25 to 64 years during 1971 - 1980 according to the Population Census in 1970. The occupations were grouped into three exposure categories according to the probability of exposure. The category of "probable" exposure included electrical occupations while the category of "possible" exposure included occupations where electric motors or welding are common. All other occupations were included in the category of "no exposure." Cancer incidence rates in different occupational groups, during 1971 - 1980, were obtained after linking the census records with the national death certificates and the files of the Finnish Cancer Registry. The adjusted relative risks had a 95 percent confidence limit. Findings showed a small but significant increase in the incidence of leukemia and less certainty concerning brain tumors.

Two other Scandinavian epidemiological studies point to an EMF cancer risk. Dr. Tore Tynes, Aage Andersen and Froydis Langmark of the Cancer Registry of Norway in Oslo reported in an investigation of 38,000 employees that male electrical workers with a "long duration of employment" had a statistically significant 40 percent increase in acute and chronic leukemia. The highest risks were among radio and TV repairmen, radio and telegraph operator, and power line workers.

Also, Dr. Jorgen Olsen of the Danish Cancer Registry in Copenhagen stated that children living near high voltage power lines with magnetic field exposures of 1mG or more had a five-fold elevated risk of lymphoma, compared to controls.

Sources: Jukka Juutilainen, Esa Laara, and Eero Pukkala Department of Environmental Sciences, University of Kuopio, P.O. Box 6, SF-70211 Kuopio, Finland. Department of Applied Mathematics and Statistics, University of Oslo, SF-90570 Oslo, Finland. Finnish Cancer Registry, Liisankatu 21 B, SF-00170 Helsinki, Finland; Sheikh 1986; Savitz and Calle 1987; Thomas et al. 1987; Coleman and Beral 1988; Speers et al. 1989; *American Journal of Epidemiology* (136, p.88, 1992); *Micro Wave News*, Vol. XII No.5, No.6, Sept./Oct./Nov./Dec. 1992.

Information Brief

Male Sperm and Children

We must not forget that exposure of a male to certain adverse elements may eventually influence the health of children he is yet to conceive. The health of the unborn may be affected by various exposures of the father from such things as alcohol, drugs, workplace chemicals and electromagnetic fields. Birth defects occur in 250,000 of the three million babies born in the U.S. every year. Pregnant women are urged to take great cautions, yet men are virtually ignored. Various exposures may cause damage to the male's sperm count, sperm shape and mobility, or genetic makeup. Andrew Wyrobek, molecular biologist at California's Lawrence Livermore Laboratory, estimates that 25 percent of Down Syndrome cases are caused by chromosome defects in the father's sperm.

Men are more likely than women to be exposed to toxins in the workplace that raise the chance of children being stillborn, premature or underweight. Men exposed to electromagnetic fields, such as electricians, power company line repairers and utility employees and welders, may be twice as likely to father babies who develop a nervous system tumor called neuroblastoma.

Also, ionizing radiation in nuclear power plants and regular exposure to chemical solvents have been shown to increase risk to the offspring as much as six times for leukemia, cancer and brain tumors. Men who smoke before children are born are 40 to 60 percent more likely to have children who get leukemia or cancer. Fathers who have two or more drinks of alcohol daily in the month before they conceive children are more likely to experience underweight children.

Recent reports of the adverse effects of second hand smoke, (causing some 3,000 deaths annually) have been devastating to the tobacco industry. Reports that men—not only women carrying a fetus—who smoke are more likely to have diseased children may be even more revealing of the many things that affect our children and the nation's health. Greater attention to the male is certainly in order.

Source: Andrew Wyrobek, Lawrence Livermore Laboratory, California; *Washington Post Health Journal*, Aug. 20, 1991; author.

Evidence is absolutely conclusive says Dr. Wendel Winter, University of Texas, and Dr. Jerry Phillips of the Cancer Research and Treatment Center, San Antonio, Texas, that 60 Hz magnetic fields cause human cancer cells to permanently increase their rate of growth as much as 1600 percent, developing more malignant characteristics. Another researcher, M. Speers, University of Texas Medical Branch, Galveston,

Department of Preventive Medicine, reported a 13 fold increase in brain tumors among electric utility workers.

All of the above cancers are in tissues with continuous rates of cell division, emphasizes Dr. Becker. He believes that the pollution around us has much to do with this disaster. Dr. Sam Koslar, Director of Applied Physics Laboratory at John Hopkins University, states that microwave exposure has a definite link to Alzheimer's disease of which millions of Americans are inflicted. Dr. Darrel Regier tells us 20 percent of U.S. mental disorders are severe enough to require psychiatric treatment and that for persons under the age of 45 the rate is twice as high as those over the age of 45. There is anecdotal evidence that cancer of the female breast is more common among beauticians than the general population because of the extensive use of hair dryers and chemicals.

Two new Swedish studies, released September, 1992, have caused Sweden's National Board for Industrial and Technical Development to state that henceforth it would "act on the assumption that there is a connection between exposure to power frequency magnetic fields and cancer, in particular childhood cancer." These studies cost a little more than two million dollars over five years. Compare that to the $100 million plus the U.S. and state governments are spending on these same questions. Hopefully, results will be even more efficacious.

One of the studies looked at all of the 500,000 children and adults in Sweden who were exposed to magnetic fields in their homes because they lived near high-voltage power transmission lines. Researchers found that children who lived near fields greater than 3 milligauss (mG) were four times as likely to develop leukemia (twice the risk other studies found) and that there appears to be a dose response relationship between exposure and leukemia in children. Risks to adults were smaller (about 1.7). The corridor of study was wide enough to include both exposed and unexposed homes.

The other study looked at 1,662 people, including 250 with leukemia and 261 with brain tumors, who were exposed to magnetic fields on their jobs. Men were three times as likely to develop leukemia if the average magnetic field on the job was 2.9 mG or more. Results were mixed for brain tumors. It is unlikely that results were influenced by confounding (mixed consequences) from benzene, ionizing radiation, pesticides, solvents or smoking.

Importantly, any wires that carry electricity, such as transmission lines, household wiring, wiring in electric blankets, etc. produce a magnetic field. Louis Slesin of Microwave News says the case is convincing enough that it's time to start protecting people by minimizing exposure.

These studies are significant because they counter criticisms or flaws in some of the past studies. Dr. David Savitz, epidemiologist at the University of North Carolina, Chapel Hill, stated. "The results are very suggestive of a real association with childhood leukemia." And Dr. Richard Stevens of the Battelle Pacific Northwest Laboratory in Richland, Washington, said, "It is hard to imagine what obvious problem could account for these results other than magnetic fields." (High power electromagnetic fields.)

Furthermore, the Ahlbarn-Feychting Swedish study found that childhood leukemia rates rose with increasing magnetic field exposures (such as from power lines and other frequency fields), a clear dose-response relationship. Children exposed to 1 mG had twice, more than 2 mG three times, and more than 3 mG had nearly four times the incidence of leukemia as those exposed to less than 1 mG. The researchers found similar results when exposure was defined by proximity to power lines. They also noted that controlling "for confounding from air pollution or socioeconomic status did not change the results."

A summary follows of studies that show an increased disease rate from double to seven times:

Exposure to Power Lines and Childhood Cancers
• Wertheimer and Leeper, 1979, Denver, Co.
• A. Meyers and co-workers, Leeds, U.K.
• L. Tomenius, Sweden
• D. Savitz and co-workers, Denver, Co.
• S. London and co-workers, Leeds, U.K.
• M. Feychting and A. Ahlbarn, Sweden
• Olsen and co-workers, Denmark

Exposure to Power Frequencies and Adult Cancers
• Wertheimer and Leeper, Denver, Co.
• Coleman et al.
• McDowall and co-workers, U.K.
• Stevens and co-workers
• Steverson et al.
• Floderus and co-workers, Swedish occupational study

The Disclaimers

On the doubting side, Michael Fumento in his book **Science Under Siege** (1993) disclaims most of the findings of environmentalists, chemical and toxic waste watchers, and electromagnetic pollution believers. When studies record a higher rate of miscarriages or birth defects, he says these conditions are common and unexplained. Fumento believes that epidemiology is an inexact science and that clusters of defects in people almost always mean absolutely nothing, "simply an elevated incidence of disease or other problems in a given population." Larger study groups are needed or whole populations, not some cluster from part of a group, he says. Of course, this is precisely what the Swedish study cited here has done, having looked at all of the 500,000 children and adults in Sweden who were exposed to high-voltage magnetic fields.

It may be "electrophobia." Few studies show an effect that can be duplicated, says Fumento. When someone else tries it—it disappears. EPA states that studies have consistently found modest elevated risks (some statistically significant) of leukemia, cancer of the nervous system, and lymphomas; and the results do not seem attributable to confounding factors or biases generated by study design. It is generally accepted that the latest Swedish studies have the most reliable study design, although all studies have some flaws that might include recall bias, lack of case controls, improper electro-field measurement, and different immune system functioning. Some people may drink coffee, smoke, or be under a higher degree of stress. Large sampling helps to dissipate much of this.

In regards to the earlier studies on the effects of magnetic fields from power lines, Imre Gynk, Ph.D., program manager of DOE's Biomagnetics Research Division, Washington D.C. says, "I believe it is a potential health hazard and though statistically small, the risks warrant further investigation. And other devices in the home-appliances, wiring, fluorescent lights, etc. may pose an equal or greater hazard."

Fumento says that people like Paul Brodeur, a strong exponent of electromagnetism's adverse effects, refer to studies showing effect but not to the hundreds that show no effect. Of the opposite view is Martin Halper, EPA, director of the analysis and support division in the Office of Radiation Programs, plus many years with the Office of Toxic Substances, who says, "In all my years of looking at chemicals, I have never seen a set of epidemiological studies that remotely approached the weight of evidence that we're seeing with ELF electromagnetic fields. Clearly there is something here."

The critics find fault with the studies saying confounding factors may be at play such as traffic fumes or carcinogenic solvents. Halper says, "If people want to be nay-sayers, they'll never talk about the 60-some studies together. They'll pick out each one and fault it individually. But when you have this number of studies, it is improbable, if not impossible, that a confounding factor could have invalidated all of them."

In the frequently quoted New York State Power Lines Project, researchers reported that cancer cells reproduced faster after exposure to electromagnetic fields. Researchers believe that the fields increase the activity of ornithine decarboxylase, an enzyme involved in DNA synthesis and cell growth (*J. Electroanal Chem*, 1986, 211:447-456).

Exposure may also alter cancer cell membranes and make cells more resistant to action by the immune system. In a Texas study, adenocarcinoma cells exposed to electromagnetic fields were less vulnerable to onslaughts by natural killer cells (*Immunal Lett*, 1986, 13:295-299). The researchers hypothesize that natural killer cell cytolysis is decreased in cells with greater numbers of transferrin receptors, which are found on the cell membrane. Cells exposed to the fields were found to have large numbers of these receptors.

Dr. Ross Adey, neurologist, says. "We have found that the cell membrane is indeed a very powerful amplifier of the energy in these very weak fields. It's a physical, not chemical, process."

An additional argument that 60 Hz fields do not have an adverse effect is in assuming that their energy is too small to directly break molecular or chemical bonds or to heat tissue. But magnetic fields may induce harm in different ways by interfering with the timing of cell operations or disturbing the electron balance at the membrane of the cell. As just one consideration, the positive field may have opposite effects on cell structure as compared to the negative field.

However, intensity may be less of a factor than frequency. With solid state magnets, we can apply 1000 or 14,500 gauss negative oriented magnets directly on the body without adverse effects. Long-term application of the positive polarity of such strength could well have adverse consequences. So polarity is important with permanent magnets and may well be with frequency changing electromagnets also. The effects of frequency and intensity need to be studied more carefully.

The New York study mentioned above, reports that cancer cells reproduce faster after exposure to electromagnetic fields. Another study shows that exposure may alter cancer cell membranes and make cells more resistant to the immune system. The Lawrence Berkeley Laboratory suggests that the immune system can be influenced by ELF electromagnetic fields too weak in intensity to act through any thermal mechanism.

SCIENTIFIC DIGEST

Electromagnetic Field Effects on Cells of the Immune System: Role of Calcium Signaling

Considerable evidence exists in support of the existence of low-frequency EMF effects in cells of the immune system and mechanisms involving Ca^{2+}. These dependent signal transduction mechanisms are probably participating in the mediation of weak field effects on immune cells. The apparent existence of such cellular EMF effects represents a remarkable discovery for immunology. These in-vitro results, together with the immunological effects in organisms observed after in-vivo exposures, suggest that the immune system can be influenced by ELFs and EMFs too weak in intensity to act through any thermal mechanism. A similar responsiveness to weak EMFs has also been documented for cells and tissues of the neuroendocrine and musculoskeletal system, indicating that EMF sensitivity might be a general property of biological systems.

Source: Walleczek, Jan; Research Medicine Radiation Biophysics Division, Lawrence Berkeley Laboratory, University of California, Berkeley, California, Oct. 1992.

So what of intensity? Garbage disposals throw out fields from 1 to 5 milligauss (mG) several feet away and a maximum of 33 mG by direct contact. For an electric kitchen range it is 1 - 80 and maximum 625; electric can opener 30-225 and maximum 2,750; electric razor 50 - 300 and maximum 6,875; electric alarm clock 1 - 12 and maximum 450 and so it goes. Charles M. Keen, Magnetic Safety Consulting, Gaithersburg, Md., who measures electromagnetic fields and provides safety tips says these intensities mean little because of the short exposure time and limited body coverage. One can control these devices by keeping the body at a distance or using them only for short periods of time. Keen says it's the massive structures running through house wiring, plumbing, and outside transmission lines that are the culprits because they are constantly around the body; and the greater the intensity, the more serious the problem.

A good point is made by Fumento, quoting Dr. Raymond Neutra, epidemiologist with the California Department of Health and Services, who says that doubling the cancer rate from one child per 10,000 to two is insignificant—that cluster rates need to be 20 or higher before fear sets in. But remember, cancer and miscarriages are not the only concerns. Much of society suffers more from hyperactivity, chronic fatigue syndrome, stress, prolonged headaches, strain, vision problems, musculoskeletal defects, and a whole list of apparent new, more serious symptoms. Electromagnetic pollution may be part of the cause.

One thing that we need to look at in addition to spending billions of dollars on changing transmission lines and improving electric products is preventive health. We need to study in greater detail various safety methods and whether permanent magnetic treatments might counteract adverse magnetic influence and actually increase energy levels to improve immune system function. New answers from old practices await us. A million dollars spent on preventive health might be worth more than a billion dollars spent on putting lines underground.

The latest DOE money to investigate the effects of electromagnetic fields is to be matched equally with private funds and is monitored by one of its divisions, the National Institute of Environmental Health Services (NIEHS). In 1992, Florida State University, Tallahasse, Fl., was awarded $60 million of the funds to be used over the next five years and is matching it with expenditures from state and local funds for buildings, other capital expenditures and staff. One million dollars per year is for communications to allow any and all interested parties access to the studies and results. A new, open-door policy to conduct certain private research and to have access to all reports seems to have emerged. A final report to Congress is due September 30, 1997.

The National Institute of Environmental Health Sciences also awarded, September 1992, a 56-month $8,292,397 contract to the Chicago based IIT Research Institute for the study of the possible carcinogenic and reproductive effects of 60 Hz magnetic fields on laboratory animals. Three generations of some 2000 rats and mice will be exposed to continuous 20 mG, 2 G or 10 G magnetic fields or to intermittent 10 G magnetic fields for up to two years.

Effects of Magnetic Beds

It was stated earlier that Dr. Elizabeth Rauscher and William Van Bise feel that permanent magnets may actually be deleterious to the human body by enhancing any adverse effects from electromagnetic fields from high power lines and other sources. However, they conclude that this is a very mixed picture with many variables of strength and direction and other factors. It might seem scientifically logical that magnets in a magnetic bed, for example, could attract opposite or bipolar EMF polarities. However, attraction would depend on field strength, direction, impediments, and other factors. The direction of the Earth's field is assumed to play a role. The power from transmission lines and house currents is relatively small compared to the four or more gauss strength realized against the body in a magnetic bed.

Charles Keen, as an on-hands practitioner in the field, has taken numerous readings of electromagnetic fields under, over and around magnetic beds in different positions and locations and has found virtually no difference in readings. In some cases, a slight variation was noted but relatively insignificant. Ironically, he says, magnetic beds appear not to attract or deflect EMF energies. In his latest study, I let him use an extra-strength magnetic bed with 297 magnets of 850 gauss each, spaced one inch apart. This bed like the others had no effect on blocking or increasing the EMF field strength or direction of flux when tested under varying conditions and locations.

Some variation may be found because metal bed frames themselves can redirect EMF fields similarly to automobile frames or elevators (although autos have a very mixed effect because of their large window areas). It takes heavier or better designed barriers to cut EMF emissions such as used in some of the latest computer chassis.

In houses, certain utility companies recommend placing a loop of electric wire around the eves of the house with an energy level equal to and opposite of the offending field in order to block it out. Metal siding about ¼ inch thick provides some protection but exposed windows and flux around the edges reduce effectiveness. Importantly, the exposure to nearby neighbors may be increased from deflection of the shielded home. A low carbon steel plate placed in the floor blocks out fields. Metal constructed with a material known as *mu* (relating to molecular permeability) will absorb and concentrate flux to a very high degree but is very expensive. The cost to cover an average size house is about $200,000. Also remember that electric lines are grounded by the water pipes running through the house. A diaelectric coupler can reverse or stop the current flow from outside.

Electric utilities are beginning to take some precautions. PEPCO in the Washington, D.C. area, takes into consideration EMF conditions when constructing new lines but offers no mitigation measures for existing lines, reports Keen. Existing lines are primarily bare wires but could be insulated and field protected by "twisted triplex" wiring which is considerably more expensive.

The importance of these findings is that magnetic beds and other magnetic therapy devices do not appear to be influenced by EMF fields, yet these fields may reduce the effectiveness of the body to assimilate the Earth's natural magnetic field. On the other hand, magnetic beds have shown to increase bodily health, strengthen the immune system, raise pH levels, and work at the cellular level to balance the body's magnetic needs. Further study is needed to determine the long-range effects in relation to electromagnetic fields. The possibility exists that magnetotherapy may be one answer to this complex question.

Counter-Attack by Therapy

The question as a nation remains as to what we intend to do. Our highly technological and advanced health care system is having its own problems. Many believe that there isn't any question we need to turn more to prevention and also the therapies that may very well counterbalance the adverse forces of pollution. In the next chapter, we compare similarities and differences between electromagnetic and permanent (natural) magnetotherapies and how these methods can be used to heal or neutralize the adverse effects of man-made radiation. In short, in addition to preventive techniques, there may be a way to counter-attack, even after one is exposed to pollution. At the same time the government is spending $100 million to determine ill effects, it would certainly make sense to assess whether certain magnetic fields applied therapeutically can counteract adverse fields. Let's see if we can convince the NIEHS and others to consider this point.

Chapter 4

Electromagnetic vs. Permanent Magnetic Therapy

The next two chapters (4 and 5) may have more medical and technical terms than the average reader may wish to deal with, so feel free to hit the highlights, move on to the latter chapters and come back later for review or substantiation of information of interest. In any case, the data are vital and reinforce the differences and effectiveness of various methodologies. The mixture of more technical with easier material is almost a necessity when trying to reach both the professional and lay person. Handle these chapters to suit your taste.

Magnetic Energy is Fundamental to Our Health

The application of electromagnetic therapy as a medicine has expanded considerably in the past two decades; however, a clear understanding of its effects is still not widely known. The FDA approved use of various magnetic devices in the early 70's. A number of societies have been formed to support electromagnetic therapy. Thousands of doctors use this therapy and hundreds of thousands of patients have been healed. In this chapter, we explore what electromagnetic therapy is all about and how it relates to solid state or natural magnetic devices and whether their effects are similar or interchangeable. If these two therapies were complementary, even with some modest change in methodology, this would be a breakthrough of sorts for magnetic health.

Manufacturers of magnetotherapeutic devices in Japan, Canada, Germany, and the United States and other countries market a variety of permanent magnets and electromagnetic devices. Permanent magnets can be worn during the day or slept on at night to give the user the maximum exposure he or she may need without detracting from one's normal daily activities. On the other hand, most electromagnetic units require the user to be near an electrical outlet, resulting in less ability to move around freely. Some newer electromagnetic devices are portable.

How Magnets Work

In most cases, a professional provider is needed to treat with electromagnetic devices, while personal or home use is more the case for permanent magnets and after only brief instruction. More serious cases would be first treated in the doctor's office and then a protocol for therapy given for magnetic instruments for a home maintenance program with periodic examination by one's physician. Individuals may also purchase permanent magnets on their own and use them at home with instructions directly from the manufacturer.

Electromagnets are normally made with a solenoid wrapped with wire that emit frequencies and more powerful electrical signals than the permanent magnet. The iron core concentrates and directs the magnetic field produced by the electricity flowing through the coil of wire. Caution must be taken not to burn the skin. The electromagnet can vary in strength by controlling current flow. Normally both polarities enter the body simultaneously which can be a health problem for long-term use. Both permanent magnets and electromagnets can be applied with a single polarity or both polarities simultaneously. Most therapists believe that only trained professionals should treat patients with the more powerful electromagnetic devices. Solid state magnets are usually of sufficiently low gauss strength not to be a problem; even a high strength of 10,000 or 15,000 gauss is not dangerous if used knowledgeably for the proper duration of time and the correct polarity.

Electromagnets can penetrate muscle, bone, marrow and nerves, usually without unpleasant sensation or pain. But if electromagnetic current is too high, it can stimulate constrictions of local muscle groups and cause electrolysis (disintegration of tissue or body chemicals etc.) or other cellular damage. Remember the rule—faster does not necessarily mean better. The slower functioning permanent magnets may be the best course for certain ailments, particularly if a patient is interested in long-term disease prevention or self-administration. Both methodologies can be used for many similar ailments. The application of electromagnetism to acupuncture points for faster and deeper penetration, for example, is used by many therapists. Likewise, the simple solid state, permanent magnet is used for this purpose but normally takes longer for effect. The electromagnet is widely used for bone fusions and major muscle or joint problems that don't seem to cure as fast by natural magnetic fields especially in the quick time-frame that many seek. The risk/benefit factor should always be assessed for each type of therapy. But, importantly, both methodologies are external treatments usually localized at the point of ailment and not nearly as dangerous as consuming a drug or performing surgery.

Systems are Complementary

These two magnetic systems are complementary and can be used together or one after the other. Many practitioners of electromagnetic devices do not recognize this possibility. For example, the appropriate pole of the permanent magnet can be applied to the diseased part of the body and the electromagnet applied nearby or in between two permanent magnets. Since the use of electromagnets usually involves both the negative and positive poles, the permanent magnet can counter possible adverse effects of the positive polarity by applying negative magnetic energy along with the electromagnet bipolar fields. Philpott and others have demonstrated that these two different magnetic systems essentially perform the same healing function, since the end product is magnetic fields. The pulsing effect of electromagnetism, however, if regulated to natural body frequencies can be very effective. And for short-term applications for ununited fractures, pain and similar ailments, the polarity question is not as significant.

Each therapy has its appropriate applications. More severe or immediate problems can be treated first with the electromagnet, followed by continued or periodic use of permanent magnets to relieve pain over the longer-term. The electromagnet, Dr. Bansal reports, has proved successful when placed on the body between two permanent magnets. In this manner, vibrations are created where the permanent magnets are located, resulting in greater efficiency. Bansal states it is simply a matter of placing the permanent magnet where it normally would be best suited for the problem and then applying the electromagnet in close proximity.

Exhibit 7   The Treatment of Fibrous Non-Union of Fractures by Pulsing Electromagnetic Stimulation

---

Sharrard WJ; Sutcliffe ML; Robson MJ; Maceachern AG

Fifty-three ununited fractures with a median time since injury of 28 months were treated by electrical stimulation using pulsing electromagnetic fields. Union was achieved in 38 cases (71.7%) in a median time of six months. For ununited fractures of the tibia the success rate was higher at 86.7%. Previous or active sepsis, the presence of plates or nails, the age of the patient or the time since the injury, did not affect the results. Analysis of the failures suggests that inadequate immobilization, a fracture gap of more than five millimeters or the presence of a screw in the fracture gap were responsible. In four patients no cause of failure could be determined.

Source:*J Bone Joint Surg* [Br] 1982; 64(2): 189-93.

Opening up a New Era

A highly captivating point-of-view concerning magnetotherapy is taken by an experienced practitioner and researcher, R. Lightwood of the Department of Surgery, Clinical Research Unit, Queen Elizabeth Hospital, Edgebaston, Birmingham, UK, who has worked directly with electromagnetotherapy for the past 20 years. He encourages the medical profession to take a closer look and not to be afraid to make the optimum use of magnetotherapy. He says it is long past the point of debate whether anything happens magnetically in sick people. The search, he emphasizes, should move on to discover the best characteristics needed in applying electromagnetic fields, "It is time that we learn to direct and manipulate such benign energy," Lightwood pleads.

Electromagnetotherapy still remains controversial even though the medical community concedes something useful is taking place. The preference in the scientific community, Lightwood says, is to adhere to properly organized trials and well defined theories. He believes that, "If this artificially generated field does nothing more than provide an environment that enhances the recovery of sick and injured cells, then offering it for almost any malady seems no more than common sense."

There appears to be no question of efficacy. Observations over five decades have shown that even with applied energy levels too low to detect a temperature rise, patients have benefitted. It is more than a heating effect as proved early on by A. J. Ginsberg (New York Academy of Medicine, October 1940), who demonstrated other actions were involved. At that time, a unit called "Diapulse" was in common use. Today modern versions are used.

Countless numbers of therapists claim an astonishing variety of ailments are healed or improved by applying magnetic fields. Lightwood first used pulsed energy at 27.12 MHz in 1974 in treatment of facial battlefield injuries. For many ailments, patient hospital stays were reduced by 25 percent, providing Queen Elizabeth Hospital with a very gratifying response. Many of these cases involved wounds that would ordinarily involve long and careful nursing. Wounds that had lain dormant for weeks or were even deteriorating began to dry and close up at a more normal rate. Difficulties with bowel activities (not uncommon with large abdominal wounds) were also resolved. Interestingly, since 1948 Red Army doctors of the former Soviet Union used magnets to reduce pain in limbs after amputations. Research at the Medical Institute of Roslov and Leningrad Military Academy is further confirmation of the effectiveness of magnetotherapy.

Other Uses

All cases of post surgical paralytical ileus (bowel obstruction) are being treated with magnetic fields at Queen Elizabeth Hospital. Surgeons at Queen Elizabeth Hospital consider the application of magnetic fields to be a preferred treatment for ileus, especially after experiencing successful results with hundreds of cases. Magnetic fields are also used on pressure sores, painful or infected amputation stumps, chronic varicose ulcers, sprains, contusions, torn ligaments, fibrositis and tennis elbow, with relief reported usually after only a few hours. For another serious condition, one of the doctors applied magnetic fields on a patient who had suffered a stroke six years previously. After treatment of three weeks of eight hour days and keeping the device under his pillow at night, the patient regained his speech and restored his shuffle to a reasonably normal walk. It is this type of evidence which strongly indicates that both the electromagnet and the permanent magnet function similarly, since the same types of cases have been healed by both methodologies. Nevertheless, each methodology may be more suited for a particular ailment. For some illnesses, permanent magnets appear to work just as fast or faster than the electromagnet, such as in psychosis, epilepsy, and various types of body pain. And, of course, for long-term illness, chronic fatigue syndrome, better sleep, and a host of other complaints, the permanent magnet outshines the electromagnet.

Another area of interest is dental treatment. At Queen Elizabeth Hospital, post surgical dental pain is treated on a casual basis, often showing reduction of both pain and edema. Researchers conducted a six-month double-blind, placebo controlled study of this therapy at a wisdom-tooth extraction clinic. Half of the patients received an hour's post surgical treatment during their bed-rest stage and then were compared to the half that were not treated (using a response on a one to five differential scale of pain, and also visual assessment of the degree of swelling and contusion). The study confirmed that both edema and pain were rapidly reduced in the magnetically treated patients. Similar results of reduction of edema and pain after dental procedures are reported in the U.S. using permanent magnets.

Any individual can carry a permanent magnet with him or apply it at home when a toothache occurs. I have done it successfully myself several times by using a two by one inch, 900 gauss strength, natural magnet. Unable to fall asleep two distinct times during the past year, this simple magnet took the pain away in about 15 to 20 minutes. When I removed the magnet to observe results, the pain consistently reappeared. I, of course, left it on all night to realize a good night's sleep and I have had no need to see a dentist as the pain has never returned after the last ache over eight months ago. The infection has also gone.

Clinical vs. Control Groups

The Queen Elizabeth Treatment Center relies primarily on clinical observations to assess results. They believe it is not wholly ethical to conduct placebo studies for major illnesses because they are dealing with real patients who need treatment and who cannot fairly be denied care while patients around them are being healed. The FDA in the U.S., as well, regards such an understanding as satisfactory for certain critical illnesses. But it seems more appropriate than ever in both Britain and the United States, to conduct controlled, placebo studies on this methodology that reports such a high rate of success and where prominent surgeons have no doubt of its extraordinary effectiveness.

The Science

In explanation of the science, Lightwood believes that accumulated fluids in the cells of ailing tissues are unable to be carried away from the effected site. But when cell membrane potential of a group of sick cells is restored towards normal or full polarization, excess fluid is thrust through the membrane, disbursed, and healing takes place. (This process was explained earlier concerning the opening of cell channels.) In cases of treating the abdomen, as an example, Lightwood explains that a measurable increase in blood flow of the legs occurs where formerly lower limb circulation was non-existent. This presumably works via the sympathetic nervous system, he believes, since patients who have had a double-sympathectomy (resection or interruption of the sympathetic nervous pathway) do not demonstrate it.

In regard to the importance of frequency changes, evidence shows that regeneration of the nerve pathways and regrowth of the central nerve cells take place under the stimulation of magnetic fields whether the fields pulse or not. Pulsing is effective because it sets up resonance in the tissue which results in an energy level many times that of a permanent magnet, yet over time the permanent magnet heals as well. This is verified from thousands of cases of clinical observation and millions of users worldwide.

With respect to polarity, Lightwood states that it does not seem to influence the efficacy of treatment, nor do wave forms. (Of course, treatment can be applied through clothing or dressings.) For brief duration of treatment, where therapy is terminated upon healing—as appears to be the case for the Queen Elizabeth Hospital Center—a noticeable difference in the effect of the two polarities may not be readily evident. It is in long-term exposure where differences may be noted in such things as stress, adverse cell growth, and other consequences. Both the negative and positive polarities can bend and break bicarbonate bonding to produce hydroxide, therefore both are biochemically beneficial. However, Robert Becker's "negative current of injury" stipulates that the body is bathed in electrons (negative energy) when healing.

Functions, Uses, and Cautions

In 1978, the FDA formally approved a number of electromagnetic instruments for healing purposes. This legitimacy of magnetic treatment was primarily sanctioned for healing of human bone fractures that otherwise failed to heal, a prime reason why this therapy has gained general acceptance. Can you imagine if we had to wait for magnetotherapy to be approved for certain diseases only after everything else has failed and there is no risk? This is no way for a sophisticated research system to approve innovation.

Magnetotherapy seems to be effective for a number of diseases, including cancer. Cases are documented involving inoperable brain tumors where the doctors finally relented to permit the use of benign magnetotherapy, safer than any other procedure. Tumors have been reduced, even eliminated. Do we have to treat this discovery as a last resort when it may be a medicine even more valuable as a preventative? Any conspiracy of silence ought to be put to rest by placing all the research and known cases on the table for evaluation and pumping a few dollars into the very double-blind, placebo controlled studies the medical community continues to demand. At least we should have an open mind, even in the review of existing cases. Many practitioners in our health system believe that the FDA should clearly sanction the use of permanent magnets as it has done for electromagnets, particularly since solid state (natural) magnets are likely even safer.

In respect to how electromagnets and permanent magnets function or differ, let's examine a few scientific observations. Research shows that much smaller voltages and currents are actually used by the body's growth-control system to heal than normally assumed. This means smaller values can be used to produce bone healing and other cures without damage to the body system, a more benign approach. In clinical tests, Dr. Becker's technicians were able to show that the same rate of success could be obtained by using silver electrodes with voltages below electrolysis levels and currents a hundred times lower than those in general use. Instead of

10 microamperes, Becker used 0.1 microampere and still caused bone growth and healing of the non-union. Silver electrodes were important because their low resistance permitted the use of low voltages. These researchers turned on the growth-control system in a benign fashion, in contrast to the possibility of stimulating electrolysis from higher currents.

The Importance of Timing

At times, it has been reported that magnetotherapy did not work. Efficacy depends on proper procedure. For example, success rates for fracture healing are quite related to early treatment when cells are still in active growth, not after dormancy has set in or when everything else has failed. (Exhibit 8 explains the use of pulsing electromagnetic fields on 20 patients where early treatment proved more successful than waiting for failure first.) Magnetic fields turn on the system by assisting less active cells to perform. Dr. Becker reports that in 1983, Dr. Abraham Liboff, Professor of Physics at Oakland University, noted that pulsed magnetic fields in normal cells in mitosis (indirect cell division) increased the synthesis of DNA. This was due to the magnetic field not to the induced electrical current. (All electric fields create a magnetic field.) Other laboratory tests have confirmed this synthesis and, most importantly, that it occurs only in cells in active growth. This explains why the success of this technique has varied so greatly, some reporting the usual 70 percent success rate, others reporting almost a zero rate. Success depends on when the therapist declares a fracture non-union. If the therapy begins within three months after a fracture, active cell growth is still occurring and can be stimulated by magnetic fields. The magnetic effect is on cells in active mitosis rather than a formal turning on of the normal D.C. growth-control system. The ongoing process is simply stimulated.

No one argues about the fact that the growth system is energized. Since this is the case, it is apparent that infectious or cancerous cells can be either stimulated or suppressed. Magnetic devices using positive polarity have shown a significant increase in cancer-cell growth and malignant characteristics of cells in mitosis compared to normal cells. This is why a number of doctors believe the dual polarities of the electromagnet need to be neutralized or overcome by infusion of negative magnetic fields at the site location. Negative ions arrest cancer cell growth, according to Becker.

If he is correct, completely new controlled, double-blind studies need to be conducted to verify effects. The entire way these instruments are administered needs to be evaluated. (Another project for FDA's Dr. Kessler.) Nevertheless, sufficient success has been exhibited by magnetotherapy that opposition groups should not be allowed to turn back this medicine simply because all the answers haven't been found or because it has been used in the least effective way. The opportunity exists now to take a remarkable therapy and make it better.

Rules for Application

Safety is paramount and a number of precautions should be taken. Even small electric currents have a variety of major biological effects. Treatment should be conducted at low voltage levels. (A reason permanent magnets are considered safer.) Therapists are either unaware of these concerns or choose to ignore them. These are areas that an active and responsible FDA ought to explore. Dr. Becker lists several rules for the application of electromagnetics:

1. **The rule of thumb for application should be one milliampere per one square centimeter because this is just below the level at which cell damage occurs due to electrolysis.**

2. **The type of electrodes is important. The positive electrode will give off ions of the metal itself, which can be toxic.**

3. **Administer at low voltage. Water within the tissues is subject to electrolysis—a process by which water molecules are broken apart. In biological tissues, electrolysis produces gases, such as hydrogen, which are toxic to cells and are produced proportionately to the level of voltage. At low voltages, the circulation of blood and tissue fluids will carry hydrogen gas away and neutralize it, but at higher levels the gas produced is greater than the ability of our circulation to carry it away. This amounts to an electrolysis level and the death of cells.**

Piezoelectric and Ultrasound Effects

The piezoelectric phenomenon also confirms that electrical, essentially magnetic charges, heal and do so at very low strength. The piezoelectric effect consists of the generation of electrical charges in the body or, in the case of crystalline materials, produced by bending or pressure. A charge is produced instantly which rapidly diminishes to zero. When the pressure or bending is released, the charge turns to the opposite polarity. Working together, Drs. Robert Becker and Andrew Bassett found highly effective results for healing by this method. Many orthopedic surgeons fail to relate the characteristics of this functioning with regular electromagnetic therapy. When Becker and Bassett applied a D.C. current at 1, 10, and 100 microamperes in their experiments, in contrast to using the piezoelectric technique of short, transient pulses, they found no difference in performance. Even at one-quarter microamperes there was not a difference, and pulsing did not appear to make any difference either.

Ultrasound is another variation for treating a variety of ailments by using a different range of frequencies, but accomplishing similar results. These frequencies range to 20,000 Hz which is beyond human hearing. Ultrasound heals fractures with just 20 minutes of therapy daily, reports Thomas Kristiansen, M.D., professor of orthopedic surgery at the University of Vermont College of Medicine. Shin bone fractures treated in 59 patients healed in 92 days compared to a placebo group that took an average of 132 days. "Nothing's ever been shown to accelerate fracture healing before", he says. Apparently he is not familiar with the electromagnetic therapy success rate and healing in one quarter to one-half the usual time frame at Queen Elizabeth Hospital or the numerous controlled studies from many worldwide sources, plus the 100,000 fracture surgeries that take place in the U.S. alone every year.

Lower frequencies are even more effective for treatment as they are able to achieve resonance more easily when interacting with the natural resonance frequency of the body tissues which are under 25 Hz. Furthermore, permanent magnets (without frequency) demonstrate results almost as good as low frequency devices and ultrasound, as long as the correct size (weight) and strength are used for the problem and for the appropriate period of time. Two studies are reported in this chapter—but thousands of experiences exist—where bones and muscles were healed more rapidly and inflammation more quickly reduced for various ailments using permanent magnets.

Treatment Protocol

A variety of important considerations need to be taken into account when treating with pulsed magnetic field (PMF) therapy. A number of treatment sessions are necessary, each usually lasting about 15 to 30 minutes. In most cases, pain relief will last progressively longer as treatments continue to full recovery. Many cases clear up after one session. Increasingly, the negative polarity is used in treatment and at times in conjunction with the positive pole. In a series of clinical cases, it was demonstrated that if the pain had not diminished, the positive polarity was applied with healing results. Some therapists believe that in certain cases the positive polarity is needed to engage the stimulus process, at least for a short period. Then one can switch to the negative field for longer-term treatment.

In electromagnetic application, Buryl Payne, Ph.D , Santa Cruz, California, who has investigated numerous cases, believes that one pole or the other can be used satisfactorily or both poles simultaneously. The positive polarity can be used for certain conditions, particularly if an ailment needs stimulation. Dr. Philpott believes that the positive polarity treatment should be of short duration compared to a much longer, negative magnetic application to follow directly afterwards. Negative magnetic application could further assure reasonable preventive measures against abnormal cell stress or other long-term adverse effects.

Electromagnetic therapy has proved highly successful when one understands its principles. Success has been demonstrated over a long period of time by one of America's most noted researchers who has achieved remarkable results using electric therapy for many types of ailments. He has documented particular success for hip joint injuries and breaks. Dr. Andrew Bassett at Columbia University's Orthopedic Hospital, Presbyterian Medical Center in New York City, on a regular basis has electrically induced magnetic fields to cause the regrowth of tissue, nerve, bone, and blood supply.

Exhibit 8 The Use of Pulsing Electromagnetic Fields to Achieve Arthrodesis of the Knee Following Failed Total Knee Arthroplasty

Bigliani LU; Rosenwasser MP; Caulo N; Schink MM; Bassett CA

Treatment with pulsing electromagnetic fields was used as an adjunct in twenty patients who had a knee arthrodesis after failure of a total joint arthroplasty. Eighteen had an infected arthroplasty; one, mechanical loosening; and one, recurrent dislocation. Arthrodesis had been attempted twenty-five times in these twenty patients prior to application of the coils. These procedures included the use of twenty-two external fixation frames, one compression plate, one intramedullary rod, and one cylinder cast. Two groups of patients were identified: those with non-union and those with delayed union. In seventeen (85 percent) of the twenty patients, bone-bridging was achieved. The average time to union after coil therapy was started was 5.8 months. The patients who started coil treatment earlier after arthrodesis showed a tendency to heal faster. Three patients who had failures were the only ones who did not adhere to the protocol, and all three were in the non-union group. All patients with a solid arthrodesis were free of pain and able to walk at the time of follow-up, none to thirty-one months after the completion of treatment. The use of pulsing electromagnetic fields appears to be a valuable non-invasive adjunct when performing arthrodesis of the knee after failed total joint arthroplasty.

Source: *J Bone Surg* [AM] 1983 Apr.; 65(4): 480-5.

An FDA evaluation shows that approximately 85 percent of treated hip injuries would have required hip replacement without this therapy. The overall success rate of 80 percent compares favorably with the success rate of cortical and cancellous (lattice-like) bone grafting procedures. The success rate of 80 percent from direct current stimulation is verified by Clinton L. Compere, M.D., Northwestern University Medical School, Chicago, Illinois. Tens of thousands of patients have received one form or another of electrical stimulation for non-unions (fracture), delayed unions, pseudoarthroses or failed arthrodeses, each technique with its own advantages and disadvantages.

Electromagnetic therapy methodologies are fairly similar. Normally they require cooperation from the patient to ensure regular treatment over a ten to twelve hour period daily for a number of weeks.

Exhibit 9   Results of Pulsed Electromagnetic Fields (PEMFs) in Ununited Fractures after External Skeletal Fixation

---

Marcer M; Musatti G; Bassett CA

Of 147 patients with fractures of the tibia, femur, and humerus, in whom an average of 3.3 operations had failed to produce union, all were treated with external skeletal fixation in situ and pulsed electromagnetic fields (PEMFs). Of the 147, 107 patients united for an overall success rate of 73%. Union of the femur occurred in 81% and the tibia in 75%. Only five of 13 humeri united. Failure to achieve union with PEMFs was most closely associated with very wide fracture gaps and insecure skeletal fixation devices.

Source: *Clin Orthop* 1984 Nov; (190): 260-5.

This is usually done in the home on an outpatient basis. Some cases of a critical nature may involve surgery to implant devices directly on the non-healing bone. However, Dr. Compere believes surgical methods should not be recommended for routine, primary fracture treatment, only for fractures showing no definite progress toward union after four months.

Dr. Bassett points out that the non-invasive method is of negligible to non-existent risk and produces union with a comparable rate of success as surgically invasive methods. All of these methods are capable of modifying cell behavior so that fibrocartilage in the non-union gap is calcified, vascularized, and replaced by bone (endochondral ossification). Patient self-help, non-surgical processes are not necessarily what surgeons are seeking nor are these methods generally taught in medical schools. Dr. Bassett acknowledges that there is a definite need for surgery in specific cases, but that for the vast majority of problems, non-invasive, including home self-help procedures, are adequate. After a medical examination, the patient can apply and continue a safe maintenance program at home. And we all benefit. As the patient takes greater control of procedures that are in the negligible or non-existent risk category, our national health expenditures may come more in line with our ability to pay. (Exhibit 9 shows that fracture non-unions can occur due to gaps and improper fixations. Exhibits 10 and 11 outline success rates for fracture healing over two periods of time.)

Exhibit 10   **Pulsing Electromagnetic Field Treatment in Ununited Fractures and Failed Arthrodeses**

C. Andrew L. Bassett, MD ScD; Sharon N. Mitchell, RN; Sawnie R. Gaston, MD

Pulsing electromagnetic fields (PEMFs) induce weak electrical currents in bone by external coils on casts of skin. This surgically non-invasive, outpatient method, approved by the Food and Drug Administration in November 1979, produced confirmed end results in 1,007 ununited fractures and 71 failed arthrodeses, worldwide. Overall success at Columbia-Presbyterian Medical Center was 81%; internationally, 79%; and in other patients in the United States, 76%. Treatment with PEMFs was effective in 75% of 332 patients (a subset) with an average 4.7-year disability duration, an average of 3.4 previous operative failures to produce union, and a 35% rate of infection. Eighty-four percent of carpal naviculars and 82% of femoral neck-trochanteric non-unions were united. After attempted arthrodeses could not salvage a failed total-knee prosthesis, PEMFs promoted healing in 85% of patients. When coils were unsuccessful alone, combining them with surgical repair was effective.

Source: *JAMA* 1982; 247: 623-8.

The protocol for treatment and equipment usage, as enumerated by Dr. Bassett and colleagues, for the professional therapist includes the following six steps:

1. **Application of a snug plaster cast to control motion.**
2. **Measurement of the cast diameter at the level of the non-union to establish intercoil distance and an appropriate "driving" voltage for each patient's pulse generator.**
3. **Placement of the parallel coils under roentgenographic control for treatment at home for 10 to 12 hours daily.**
4. **Strict non-weight-bearing during early phases of treatment for unstable lesions in the lower extremities.**
5. **Assessment of the lesion in plaster with standardized roentgenograms at monthly intervals.**
6. **Graded, protected rehabilitation, once roentgenographic in clinical evidence of early union is established.**

Exhibit 11   Effects of Pulsed Electromagnetic Fields on Steinberg Ratings of Femoral Head Osteonecrosis

Bassett CA; Schink-Ascani M; Lewis SM

Between 1979 and 1985, 95 patients with femoral (thigh) head osteonecrosis met the protocol for treatment of 118 hips with selected pulsed electromagnetic fields (PEMFs). Etiologies (causes) included trauma (17), alcohol (9), steroid use (46), sickle cell disease (2), and idiopathy (obscure or unknown) (44). The average age was 38 years, and the average follow-up period since the onset of symptoms was 5.3 years. PEMF treatment had been instituted an average of 4.1 years earlier. By the Steinberg quantitative staging method of roentgenographic analysis, none of the 15 hips in Stage 0 to III showed progression, and grading improved in nine of fifteen. Eighteen of 79 hips (23%) with Stage IV lesions progressed and none improved. In the Stage V category, one of 21 hips (5%) worsened and none improved. Three Stage VI lesions were unchanged. The overall rate of quantified progression for the 118 hips, 87% of which had collapse present when entering the program, was 16 %. This clinical trial shows a significant reversal of disease progression compared to other more conservative treatment methods. PEMF patients also have experienced long-term improvements in symptoms and signs, together with a reduction in the need for early joint arthroplasty.

Source: New York Orthopedic Hospital, Columbia Presbyterian Medical Center, Riverdale, NY 10463; *Clin Orthop* 1989 Sep; (246): 172-85.

Controlled Studies for Various Ailments

Many uses can be made of electromagnetic systems. For example, doctors in both Europe and the United States achieve a high level of success using electromagnetic fields to treat ailments ranging from decubitus ulcers to severe burns. Soft tissue injuries respond as well as those for bone and joint. In the Soviet Union, doctors regularly use magnets to speed wound healing after surgery, also to improve circulation, and to strengthen and mend bones.

At a recent symposium on **Electrically Induced Osteogenesis**, sponsored by the Department of Orthopedic Surgery, University of

Pennsylvania, Philadelphia, Carl T. Brighton, M.D., remarked that orthopedic surgery entered the era of biophysics several decades ago, ever since a Japanese orthopedic surgeon I. Yasuda, in 1953, demonstrated that mechanically stressed bone exhibited electrical potentials. In 1979, the FDA approved three electrical systems for marketing to treat non-unions:

1. The constant direct semi-invasive system developed at the University of Pennsylvania,
2. Constant direct current totally implanted system developed by Dwager and Weckhorn, and
3. The inductive coupling non-invasive system developed by Bassett.

The effects of these procedures are comparable to bone graft surgery. About 30 percent of all non-unions in the United States are being treated with one of these forms of electrical stimulation. It is evident that important progress has been made in the treatment of bone, muscle, joint, and tissue problems, but considerably less understanding for healing disease or preventive medicine, even though there are similar effects on all cells of the body and countless cases to prove it. (Exhibit 12 depicts a double-blind assessment for treating cuff tendinitis, a typical area where progress is evident.)

Perhaps no individual can match the experience of Dr. John F. Connolly, M.D., in applying all three of the above mentioned systems. Dr. Connolly is professor and Chairman of the Department of Orthopedic Surgery and Rehabilitation, University of Nebraska Medical Center, and also Chief of Orthopedic Surgery, Omaha Veteran's Administration Hospital, Omaha, Nebraska. He analyzed 100 consecutive fractures in a period from 1977 to 1982. He says there is no longer any doubt that electrical (magnetic) signals can induce healing of ununited fractures. Clinical application has demonstrated this on many thousands of patients who have benefitted significantly.

Although electric osteogenesis has provided us with a natural way of healing, precautions must be taken. Connolly discusses the need to use plates and fixators to hold the two ends of bones together. The tibia and the femur have become the predominant fracture problems, whereas in the past this was not the case. The shift has resulted from greater use of internal plates and external fixators that seem to help upper limb fractures better than lower. He found that fixation techniques produced fracture distraction or gaps 20 to 25 percent of the time. The key factor contributing to failure of electrical stimulation has been failure to achieve adequate fixation of the non-union, he says.

Exhibit 12   Pulsed Electromagnetic Field Therapy of Persistent Rotator Cuff Tendinitis. A Double-Blind Controlled Assessment.

> The value of pulsed electromagnetic fields (PEMFs) for the treatment of persistent rotator cuff tendinitis was tested in a doubled-blind controlled study in 29 patients whose symptoms were refractory to steroid injection and other conventional conservative measures. The treated group (15 patients) had significant benefit compared with the control group (14 patients) during the first 4 weeks of the study, when the control group received a placebo. In the second 4 weeks, when all patients were on active coils, no significant differences were noted between the groups. This lack of difference persisted over the third phase, when neither group received any treatment for 8 weeks. At the end of the study, 19 (65 percent) of the 29 patients were symptomless and 5 others much improved. PEMF therapy may thus be useful in the treatment of severe and persistent rotator cuff and possibly other chronic tendon lesions.
>
> **Source:** Binder A; Parr G; Hazleman B; Fitton-Jackson S.

In brief, Dr. Connolly states that for most stable non-unions of the tibia, percutaneous D.C. stimulation provides a simple and reliable method for achieving union. Fractures that have been vascularized by injury or previous surgery need additional treatment, such as internal fixation, and bone grafting, supplemented by electromagnetic coil stimulation. Electric stimulation can be abused without adequate fixation. It can be useful as a primary treatment for a variety of fracture problems, particularly in the tibia; but, it should not be oversold as a substitute for adequate fracture management. For fractures and other serious injuries, use of a trained specialist or orthopedic surgeon is advisable to ensure bones are properly placed and held together. One might have to deal with bone fragments. In summary, nature will do most of the healing, magnetic field or electric current will stimulate the process, and a specialist may be *necessary to manage it. (Exhibit 13 describes the result of a recalcitrant non-union, as a case in point.)* *

Therapy for Neck Pain

Let's look at how to eliminate a "pain in the neck," not a laughing matter. Darragh Foley-Nolan, with a group of M.D.s from the Mater Misericordia Hospital in Dublin, Ireland, Department of Rheumatology and Rehabilitation, has used electromagnetic therapy of a pulse frequency (27 MHz) to treat a number of patients for neck pain. Persistent neck pain is a common complaint of middle age and elderly patients, in particular. The two most frequent causes are cervical spondylosis and trauma. Rear end auto collisions that cause soft tissue injuries to the neck, known as "whiplash," constitute about 20 percent of all vehicle accidents. Neck pain after these events tends to be persistent, lasting up to six months in 75 percent of patients and up to two years in 66 percent. One study showed 35 percent of the patients had symptoms after six months and 26 percent at one year.

Important factors in the development of pain are likely encroachment on bodily space and impairment of movement. Compression of spinal tissues at posterior or anterior joints can impinge on local blood supply or spinal nerve routes. Other important factors may be a congenitally narrow spinal canal, inequality of the vertebral arteries, and nerve fibrosis. In a trial using therapies involving soft collars, postural exercise instruction, traction, placebo traction, and placebo medication, no difference in outcome was found between the groups in this double-blind, placebo-controlled study of 20 patients. The treatment had to turn to electromagnetic fields.

The study next evaluated a low energy, portable PEMT (Pulsed Electromagnetic Treatment) to be used at home that allowed minimal supervision because of the lack of side effects or need for prolonged exposure. The researchers point out that short wave diathermy is a well established form of physical therapy in which beneficial effects result from deep heating of the tissues; but, they definitely recognize changes in cell function and oxygen capacity. The time needed to optimize the best effect

---

* The italicized text refers to more complex information.

153

is between five and 30 minutes. Care must be taken against prolonged or excessively intense short wave treatment that causes burning and localized irritation. It is important to note that lenticular and testicular damage have been reported from careless administration. On the other hand, beneficial effects include pain relief, elevation of pain threshold, reduction in spindle excitability, increased collagen, extensibility in tendons, and reduction in muscle spasms and joint stiffness.

**Exhibit 13   Treatment of Recalcitrant Non-Union with a
              Capacitively Coupled Electrical Field**

Twenty-two well established non-unions in twenty patients were treated with a capacitively coupled electrical signal (sine wave, sixty kilohertz, five volts peak to peak) that was applied non-invasively through stainless-steel capacitor plates placed on the skin surface overlying the approximate site of the non-union. The average age of the eleven female and nine male patients in this series was 38.4 years, and the average duration of the twenty-two non-unions was 3.3 years. Seventeen of the non-unions were labeled recalcitrant, meaning that they had failed to heal after either previous bone-grafting or another type of electrical stimulation, or both.   Five of the non-unions had not been previously treated.   Seventeen (77.3 percent) of the non-unions achieved solid osseous union after an average of 22.5 weeks of treatment with capacitive coupling. The results in this small series were not affected by the non-union being recalcitrant, by the fact that one patient bore full weight on the extremity in a cast, by the presence of osteomyelitis, or by the presence of remaining metallic internal-fixation devices in the bone. Since capacitive coupling is non-invasive, involves portable equipment, allows full weight-bearing on the lower extremity in a cast, is easy to apply and does not require precise localization of the capacitor plates, it has distinct advantages over those methods of treating non-unions with electricity.

Source: Brighton CT; Pollack SR; *J Bone Joint Surg* [Am] 1985 Apr; 67 (4):
        577-85.

The study revealed that 75 percent of the patients responded "moderately better" or "much better" and that improvement of movement and relief of pain occurred within three weeks. The researchers concluded that there is a definite role for electromagnetic energy. They also found that three groups of enzymes are sensitive to electromagnetic fields:

1. Membrane bound adenylate cyclase;
2. Cyclic AMP independent protein kinase;
3. Ornithine decarboxylase.

All of these have profound effect on cellular functioning.[*]

(Exhibit 14 shows another successful electromagnet treatment—in this case spinal fusion.)

Facial Nerve Stimulation

Magnetic field applications can be substituted for electric current stimulation, particularly when one wants to cut out pain from the treatment itself. Facial nerve stimulation is just one such example. The use of electrical current is painful and tends to discourage even studying the method. However, transcutaneous (magnetic) stimulation of the facial nerve is painless, easily reproducible, and elicits facial muscle responses identical to electric stimulation, says Dr. Ian M. Windmill, Ph.D, and his colleagues at the Division of Communicative Disorders at the University of Louisville, Kentucky.

Magnetic stimulation of the facial nerve reduces the time necessary to complete procedures and reduces patient discomfort. Electrical stimulation discourages patient cooperation. Magnetic stimulation of peripheral nerves is now the method of choice because it is reliable, painless, and can be performed repeatedly.

The most significant problem with facial electromyography (EMG) is pain caused by electric currents. Typically supramaximal stimulation assures the greatest EMG response; however, these levels may be painful and any reduction to levels below the pain thresholds may yield inconsistent responses. Magnetically induced stimulation of peripheral nerves and cerebral cortex is a non-invasive and painless technique for elevating motor responses. Magnetic signals produce little or no sensation (other then muscle contraction) and are not attenuated by body tissue.

---

[*] The italicized text refers to more complex information.

Exhibit 14   Treatment of Failed Posterior Lumbar Interbody Fusion (PLIF) of the Spine with Pulsing Electromagnetic Fields

Treatment of failed posterior lumbar interbody fusions (PLIFs) of the spine with pulsing electromagnetic fields (PEMFs) has proved successful. Thirteen male patients suffering from failed PLIFs, with an average time of 40 months since the last surgical fusion attempt, were the subjects of this study. PEMFs were applied by the patient according to strict criteria but in the comfort of their home. Initial and subsequent medical evaluations closely monitored the patient's condition and progress. PEMFs promoted a significant increase in bone formation in 85 percent (11 of 13) of the patient pool and achieved body-to-body fusion throughout the intervertebral disc space in 77 percent (10 of 13) over the treatment period. The treatment required no hospitalization, reduced morbidity, and avoided the risks associated with surgical intervention. The results suggest that this surgically non-invasive outpatient therapy may become a successful alternative treatment of failed PLIF.

Source: Simmons JW; *Clin Orthop* 1985 Mar; (193): 127-32.

Of course, as with all cases, when using magnetic fields, caution is needed regarding possible aggravation of seizures in epileptics, short term memory loss, and effects of magnetic fields on pace makers. Importantly, when taking into account proper precautions, magnetic field energy is a highly effective methodology. (see Exhibit 15, **Application of Transcutaneous Stimulation**.)

Periarthritis of the Shoulder

Not all procedures are effective. In one examination that was not successful, Drs. Richard LeClaire, M.D. (Rehabilitation Medicine Service, Notre Dame Hospital), and Jean Vourgouess, M.D. (Department of Pharmacology, University of Montreal), February 1989, presented at the tenth International Congress of Physical Medicine and Rehabilitation, Toronto, Canada, conducted a study called *Electro-Magnetic Treatment of Shoulder Periarthritis: A Randomized Control Trial of the Efficiency and Tolerance of Magnetotherapy*.

Exhibit 15 Use of Transcutaneous Electrical Nerve Stimulation for Postoperative Pain

> This study examined the effects of transcutaneous electrical nerve stimulation (TENS) on incisional pain caused by the procedure of cleaning and packing an abdominal surgical wound. Seventy-five subjects (mean age 56.9 years) were randomly assigned to one of three intervention groups: TENS, placebo-TENS, or no-treatment control. The appropriate experimental treatment was administered during the routine dressing change which took place two mornings after surgery. Using an 11 point, visual analogue pain scale, subjects described pain experienced during the dressing change. Subjects who received either placebo-TENS or no-treatment reported little or no change. Treated subjects reported considerable reduced pain as registered on the visual analogue pain scale. Drug administration variables did not contribute significantly to level of reported pain.
>
> **Source:** Ann Hargreaves; Jance Lander; May/June 1989 Vol 38, No 3.

The study was designed to determine the potential benefit of magnetotherapy on 47 consecutive out-patients with periarthritis of the shoulder. Using a controlled, triple-blind design, one group of patients received hot pack applications and passive manual stretching and pulling exercises; the other group received the same therapy plus magnetotherapy. Treatment was administered three times a week for a maximum of three months. They found no significant improvement in pain reduction or in range of motion with electromagnetic field therapy.

These results are shown because a number of studies indicate little or sometimes zero effectiveness, as mentioned previously. Results are affected by a number of factors: the protocol used; magnetotherapy methodology involving frequencies and strength; the beliefs of participants and observers; duration of illness; whether other methods were used simultaneously on all subjects that could have diminished the single effect of magnetotherapy; plus a variety of other factors. In any case, the zero effect will happen but studies show that in the vast majority of circumstances, significant effectiveness is achieved. A 30 percent failure rate compared to a 70 percent success rate does not mean science should discard the program. The stretching and pulling exercises in the above study would very likely emulate a piezoelectric effect which has a basic magnetic inducement at its source, equalizing all subjects. Reflexology or acupressure might have induced similar results as that of physical exercise, neutralizing the effects of direct magnetic application. And importantly, the hot packs (if strong enough) applied to both groups of subjects could have brought into play the counter-irritant effect (similar to a mustard plaster) which normally rushes negative magnetic fields to the site to counter a build-up of positive ions. Psychosomatically, the brain responds to this irritant by sending signals through the immune system to deliver negative ions to the site.

Treating Abnormal Balance

Electromagnetism also works to balance the body. A study called the **Destabilization of an Abnormal Physiological Balance Situation, Chronic Musculoskeletal Pain**, utilizing a magnetic biological device, conducted by David and Judith Stewart, Department of Biological Research, at the Medi-Electronics Research and Development Corporation in Loretto, Ontario, Canada, in 1989, addressed body balance:

Much of the research in electromagnetism concerns the equipment used for bone non-unions, whereas this study focuses on the destabilization of the abnormal balanced body condition or what happens at the cellular level and pH balance. Most electromagnetic research covers frequency effects on cells in cycles per second. The search in this study is for the effect of pulsing on tissue in a moving field over an area for less than a second, returning over the same area every second for three seconds, then moving away for six or more seconds. Since the falling edge of the poles is in a different orientation to the tissue than the leading edge, the cancellation effect is minimized and a net change takes place. Time away from the affected area seems to be needed to allow tissue an adequate period to respond after each stimulation; therefore, the pulsing effect may play some role, the Stewarts conclude.

Results of electromagnetic therapy are unique, they report, and unquestionably superior to standard therapeutic procedures in the maintenance of chronic musculoskeletal pain, as well as being a nontoxic and non-invasive therapy. These two trials, one short-term, the other longer-term over one year, got superior scoring on the Melzack-McGill *pain questionnaire. Ability to increase the balance of thermal emission was noted. While electromagnetic therapy may interrupt the pain mechanism temporarily or periodically, attainment of physiological balance is longer lasting. They found that hypnosis or distraction averaged a 40 percent reduction in perceived pain while magnetotherapy averaged a consistently 83.3 percent reduction. Their studies show that placebo effect and autosuggestion attain response in less than 40 percent of subjects. Also, they found there are few people on whom magnetotherapy cannot be used or is contraindicated.* *

Permanent Magnets Best over the Long-Haul

Pulsing rates or frequencies for long-term use appear to have a distinct disadvantage. Researchers in various studies have found that using devices with periodic pulse rates can cause the nervous system to adapt to the stimulation over a period of time, lessening efficacy. On the other hand, static-state magnetic system effectiveness appears to be ongoing, as 61 percent of the subjects surveyed remained pain free over the long-term. Temporary pain relief can come about from locally applied, short-term use to attack a singular problem; while, long-term healing is more likely to come about through the attainment of physiological (pH) balance from full body therapy. This, of course, is an important lesson for orthopedic surgeons and thousands of other providers who simply concentrate on solving an immediate problem rather than considering the total body and immune system in order to relieve long-term pain. A surgeon needs to be more than a bone specialist; he very much needs to consider total body health at the same time he is dealing with a localized problem. This might very well include the administration of long-term, permanent magnetotherapy gained from magnetic beds or other daily maintenance devices.

---

* The italicized text refers to more complex information.

Reconstructive Surgery and Permanent Magnets

In the case of the effectiveness of permanent magnets for reconstructive surgery, an interesting study was conducted by G. V. Lud and Professor A. M. Demeckiy, Head of the Department of Surgery at the Vitebsk Medical Institute, Vitebsk (USSR), in 1990, entitled **Use of Permanent Magnetic Fields in Reconstructive Surgery of the Main Artery.** The study used from 10 to 30 mongrel dogs of both sexes for three series of tests involving control, placebo, and experimental groups. Various sizes of elastic magnets were used externally while absorbable magnetic implants were used in the surgical wound.

The experiment was highly successful in demonstrating the following effects: stimulation of the central and peripheral blood flow, hypercoagulation prevention, and reduction of edema and inflammation. It suggests that these magnetic sources and properties should be taken into account during the post-operative period and that permanent magnetic fields can be used for improving the results of reconstructive operations on the main arteries.

The study also showed that permanent magnets had an especially stimulating effect on the extremity haemodynamism. Apart from the direct effect of the central vessel at the surgical site, it was demonstrated that permanent magnets have a reflex effect on vessels by means of cutaneous receptors, which results in a more generalized reaction to the whole organism. Can anyone imagine what benefits might occur if our medical profession would adopt these successful procedures used on animals to humans in our modern medical system in competition with high-tech equipment?

Effects of Permanent Magnets on Skin and Blood

The effects of permanent magnets in healing is being verified by more and more controlled tests. F. Wunsch-Binder of the Department of Radiology, University of Kiel Medical School, Federal Republic of Germany, conducted a study called The Influence of Static Magnetic Fields on Skin Temperature and Blood Flow in Man, using a thermocamera to observe the behavior of the human skin

within a static magnetic field. He found that human skin undergoes temperature change (a similar influence of magnetic fields was found in mice and pigeons). This was conducted on the arms and legs of nine subjects in 39 separate tests, some conducted as blind tests, where the subjects did not know if the magnetic fields were switched on or off. Temperature by variations were from .3 degree centigrade to 5 degrees centigrade. Changes increased with field strength. The critical point for observation of a change was .2 degrees. Four of the experimentees complained of moderate pain, such as aching muscles some twelve hours after the measurements. Assumptions were made that change in temperature was caused by change in blood flow. (Further experiments on the webs of frogs, by J. Grohmann and C. Tesch of the University of Kiel in Arbeit, came to similar conclusions.)

It appears that there are many similarities between pulsing electromagnets and the steady-state permanent magnets. One may work more quickly, the other more safely. But it should be recognized how these two methodologies might work more effectively together at a higher rate of success and comfort for the patient. And it is very possible that permanent negative magnetic fields can offset the possible adverse effects of extended electromagnetic dual polarities, or the effects of incompatible frequencies. The permanent magnet can also extend a pain-free condition for the patient over the long-term by treating the whole body. Perhaps we should ask, is it time to enter these procedures in the medical book of standard operations?

Growth of Societies and Scientific Works

If magnetotherapy can be found to have a significant positive effect on the American populace, a tremendous saving could result in national health care costs. Take for example just one major problem area—back pain. (Exhibit 19 shows estimated costs.) Low back disorders are extremely prevalent in all societies and the rate of disability and costs are increasing. The direct medical and indirect costs are in the range of 50 billion dollars per year and could be as high as one hundred billion dollars. Of these costs, 75 percent can be attributed to 5 percent of the people who become disabled temporarily or permanently—a phenomenon that seems more rooted in psychosocial factors than disease. Spinal surgery plays a relatively small role. The future challenge lies with prevention and optimal management of disability, rather than perpetrating a myth that low back pain is a serious health disorder, say researchers John W. Frymoyer and William L. Catz-Baril.

Exhibit 16   Double-Blind Study Using Permanent Magnetized Foils on Secondary Myotendofasciopathies

This trial examined the clinical effectiveness of localized, alternating polarity permanent magnetic field therapies by comparing magnetized and non-magnetized foils of rectangular size 53x83x0.75 mm and also circular size of 40mm diameter and thickness of 1.5 mm. Treatment was applied for 14 days.

Evaluation revealed that compared to the control groups, significantly higher therapeutic effectiveness was found for all trial groups using magnetized foils. The best results in reducing subjective pain was with the cervical pain syndrome where 80 percent reported pain relief and 60 percent achieved improvement in movement restrictions. Drug consumption was reduced 60 percent for cervical pain syndrome and for periarthropathy humeroscapularis, but somewhat lower at 44 percent for lumbar pain syndrome. The relevant factor for those treated with non-magnetized foils was 25 percent. Results for other symptoms were similar except the population groups were smaller and results more difficult to assess. Study factors embody patients compliance, motivation, how he copes with sickness, duration and intensity of symptoms, and general health conditions.

Source: Dr. Jens Martin, Bioflex, Aug. 4, 1992 from study by
Orthopadisch Neurologisches, Rehabilitations—zentrum, Klinik
Bavaria, 8351 Schaufling, Dr. Thomas Laser, Head Physician,
Medical, Orthopedic-Chrotherupy-Social Medicine Practitioner.

Many of the back "experts" and their societies have given up on even trying to find a solution, preferring to suggest that the pain will go away naturally. Yet it has been shown in case after case that a simple, permanent magnet of the correct strength and depth of penetration will relieve pain in most instances.

The brief sample of studies here verifies the effect on reduction of pain from both permanent and electromagnetic therapies and how these two methods may be used together. Societies have formed to study these phenomena in greater depth and to develop the proper protocol for magnetotherapy.

Progress is being made in the study and use of electromagnetic and permanent magnetic therapies. Nevertheless, two major groups exist with different opinions. Some for example are convinced that electromagnetic fields can alter cell processes and others believe this is pure nonsense. Even with the evidence mounting and the healing that takes place, it is difficult to convince those who have been educated or trained one way to believe something else.

The medical profession has accepted one side of the magnetic issue almost completely, but few understand the other side. They have accepted diagnostic devices without much difficultly even though these magnetic fields are many times the strength of those needed for therapeutic purposes. The medical profession is deathly afraid of side effects and prefers a degree of government regulation to get them "off the hook," so to speak. The risk/benefit trade-off is a difficult equation for physicians, so they prefer to establish treatment regimens that everyone can accept to prevent law suits. With this attitude, the full understanding of magnetotherapy may be many years away.

A good example of sticking to a regimen, cited by Bruce McLeod, is a practice in the United States of continuing the procedure of mutilating radical mastectomy, an operation largely discarded in Europe in preference to simple mastectomy for which the comparative mortality rates are the same. Yet one disfigures and disables and the other does not. Still much of the medical profession clings to the old method, even though it is detrimental to the patient. Fortunately, a good number of doctors are changing their ways for this procedure. But change takes so long and so many are hurt in the meantime.

The FDA is finally taking greater and greater interest in different therapies. They have sponsored a number of conferences on electromagnetism. One held in 1989 at Tulsa University, entitled **Emerging Electromagnetic Medicine**, attracted over one hundred scientific papers and 800 participants. Other joint conferences are planned with other research entities and universities. A number of scientific societies have come into existence to focus on biomagnetism. The Bioelectrical Repair and Growth Society (BRAGS) was formed in 1980 with an emphasis on clinical uses of low frequency fields. The Bioelectro Magnetic Society (BEMS) was formed a year earlier, in 1979, with its emphasis directed more toward high frequency fields and possible health hazards. The Bioelectrical Chemical Society (BECS) was formally incorporated in 1979 and has held regular meetings since 1971. Its emphasis is primarily directed at cellular research, electromagnetic fields and chemical reactions. Another society, The Institute of Electrical and Electronic Engineers (IEEE) formed a special group called Engineering in Medicine and Biology Society (EMBS). This group, as the name implies, is made up primarily of electrical engineers who are interested in how electricity and magnetism can play a role in cell and biological system regulation. We have already mentioned the Bio-Electro-Magnetics Institute (BEMI), Reno, Nevada, that has scientists and practitioners as members who review the whole range of magnetic field effects on the human body. A number of its studies were mentioned earlier. It also sponsors an Institutional Review Board interested in getting physicians and researchers to document a variety of clinical cases in the arena of magnetotherapy to be monitored and evaluated by this board.

Exhibit 17   Studies of Permanent Magnetic Users in Japan

Dr. Nakagawa mailed questionnaires to 11,648 users of magnets 2.5 mm thick x 5mm in diameter with external gauss strength of 590. (Although not mentioned in the study, these magnets were designed with a common procedure in Japan of the positive magnetic side stuck to the plaster and the negative magnetic side for contact with the skin for treatment.) Women made up 57 percent and men 43 percent of the total, with the most represented age group 40 to 49 years.

The magnets were used for the following conditions:

Stiffness of neck and shoulders	45.20%
Lumbago	19.00%
Heuralgia	13.90%
Painful muscles	12.30%
Rheumatism	1.30%
Other	6.30%
No reply	2.00%

Effect usually took place from the second to fourth day. No adverse effects were reported, while over 90 percent of the users classified results as very efficacious, efficacious or fairly efficacious, and 10 percent as ineffective or not very effective.

Three other studies of 400 subjects were conducted in 1976 by professors Akio Yamada and Shuwichs-Hirose of the Faculty of Medicine, University of Tokyo; professor Yamamoto, University Juntendo, Tokyo; and Kyoshi Kurmskima, Kohnodai National Hospital. Some tests were double-blind placebo where both the doctors and the subjects did not know who were or were not using magnetic necklets that delivered 1,300 gauss each. Symptoms were for pains in the back of the neck, and in shoulders, backs, arms, hands and legs. Effectiveness fell in the range of 60 to 80 percent within a time frame of seven to fourteen days. No side-effects were detected.

A double-blind study of 80 subjects to relieve lumbar pain was conducted by Dr. Yoshia Oay using belts containing magnets of 1,500 gauss. Fifty subjects were given strong magnetic belts and 30 received placebos or less powerful belts of 200 gauss magnets. With the full strength belts, almost all showed very marked improvement or marked improvement; while, with the weak magnets or placebos, no subject showed very marked improvement and only 23 percent showed marked or minor improvement.

Source: Dr. E. Helzaptel, P. Crepon, and C.Philippe, **Magnet Therapy**, *Thorsons Publishing Group, Ltd.*, 1986.

Exhibit 18   Therapeutic Effects of the Magnetized Health Mattress in a Double-BlindTest

This double-blind test was conducted on 431 people, approximately 50 percent male and female, 375 with magnetized mattresses and 56 with non-magnetized mattresses. The magnetized mattresses used 104 magnets each of 750 - 950 gauss strength at the surface of the magnet (which translates into approximately 10 - 20 gauss within the body). The testing period ranged from two weeks to six months and was conducted at the San-ikukai Hospital, the Tokyo Communications Hospital and the Kouseikai Suzuki Hospital in Japan. The magnetized mattresses were manufactured by Nippon Athletic Industry Co., Ltd.

Side effects were checked for changes in blood pressure, hemoglobin, number of erythrocytes, and the number of leucocytes before and after using the mattresses. In addition, blood sedimentation, TP, COL, ALP, GOT, GPT, Na, and K were examined at San-ikukai and Tokyo Hospitals. No clinical symptoms were found to suggest abnormal change in the digestive system, circulatory system, neuroperceptive system, cutaneous tissue, or any other side effects in the kidney, liver, pancreas, blood pressure, hemoglobin, urine, and number of erythrocytes and leucocytes.

The following show results for the various ailments treated at the hospitals based on a 99 percent confidence coefficient:

		Effective Rate:
1.	Neck and shoulder pain (stiff shoulder):	56.83 - 85.95%
2.	Back and lower back pain:	68.49 - 92.04%
3.	Back pain:	62.35 - 98.94%
4.	Lower limb pain:	66.76 - 92.06%
5.	Insomnia:	76.82 - 97.47%
6.	Fatigue:	70.64 - 94.98%

More than 70% of subjects realized effect within 5 days, 53.33% within 3 days, for a total effective rate of 48.28 - 58.38%. The conclusion was that the magnetized mattresses proved to be effective in a high percentage of cases and with no adverse side effects as measured within the testing period.

Source: Dr.Kazuo Shimodaira, Tokyo Communications Hospital, Obstetrics and Gynecology, Tokyo, Japan, 1990 (complete study available upon request).

Exhibit 19   The Estimated Direct Costs of Back Pain in the U.S., 1990

Direct Costs

House inpatient	$6,780,462,000
Outpatient & emergency room	$387,980,000
Outpatient diagnostic & therapeutic $2,000,000,000	
Physician inpatient	$1,707,080,000
Physician office outpatient & emergency room $2,411,690,000	
Other practitioner	$3,825,119,000
Drugs	$191,697,000
Nursing Home	$4,952,394,000
Prepayment	$615,080,000
Nonhealth sector goods & services $1,564,651,000	

Total Direct Costs	$24,336,153,000

Total Indirect Costs Range from $50 billion to $75 billion.

Some of the titles of the papers submitted at the 1988 BRAGS Conference included:

1. Ununited Fractures
2. Fresh Fracture Repair
3. Treatment of Osteonecrosis of the Femoral
4. Lumbar Spinal Fusion
5. Enhancement of Bone Maturation
6. Nerve Regeneration
7. The Study of PEMF of Mice Undergoing Bone Marrow Transplantation
8. Wound Healing in Rat Skin Flaps
9. Treatment of Loosened Hip Prosthesis with PEMF
10. Healing of Skin Ulcers of Venous Origin in Humans

The annual meeting of the Bioelectric Magnetic Society, Frederick, Maryland, held in Salt Lake City, Utah, in June 1991, included over one hundred papers such as the following:

1. Effect of Static Magnetic Fields on Neurotransmitter Relief
2. Leukemia in Telephone Lineman
3. Reduction of Electric and Magnetic Field Emissions from Electric Blankets
4. Effect of 60 Hertz Magnetic Fields on Human Cancer Cells
5. Undersensitivity of Cells and Tissues to Electromagnetic Fields
6. Reduction of Magnetic Fields from Video Display Terminals
7. Functional Condition of the Health of Populations Living Within the Places of Radar Location
8. Methodological Approaches to Hygienic Standard Setting for Populations
   Exposed to Electromagnetic Fields
9. The Effects of Growth of Hela Cells Due to Strong Exposure to Constant Magnetic Fields
10. Lay Peoples Preference for Alternative Strategies for Limiting Exposure to 60 Hertz Fields

As an example of the activities of these groups, BEMS was founded in 1978 to promote research on the interaction of electromagnetic fields with biological systems, including the response of living organisms to electric and magnetic fields at frequencies from D.C. to visible light, mechanisms and models of interaction, absorption and distribution of electromagnetic energy, and diagnostic and therapeutic uses of electromagnetic energy. Each year its eight hundred members meet and 180 or more scientific papers are presented.

The first world conference for Electricity and Magnetism in Biology and Medicine was held in Buena Vista Palace, Orlando, Florida, in June 1992. This brought together those interested in the beneficial purposes of bioelectromagnetism as well as those concerned with potential adverse health effects. It looks like the future is here.

Chapter 5

Important Differences of the Negative and Positive Polarities

Exploring the Mysteries of Life

How Long Must We Wait?

Biomagnetic therapy is at an important cross-roads for use as a medicine. Biophysicists, doctors, nurses, and therapists are seeking additional studies and information in the field of magnetic energy. A conventional methodology needs to be developed so that this basic life force receives the critical consideration and evaluation it deserves. Although much has been written on the subject, it is difficult to draw absolute conclusions in several controversial areas, even though the evidence appears to rest more logically in one direction than the other. In any case, we are forced to make judgments from the existing reports, studies, and expert opinions. In the end, both lay persons and professionals must draw the most rational conclusions from this information. If the medical community does not act in some sensible and humane fashion early, this natural phenomenon may not ever become available on a large scale for the improvement of the nation's and the world's health.

In this chapter, we discuss several important theories as well as the safest and most beneficial use of magnetic fields. First, we must learn how to identify correctly the two different polarities.

Identifying the Negative and Positive Poles

It is important for everybody who uses magnetotherapy to understand that there are two opposite conventions for identifying north and south poles. If one is engaged in magnetotherapy, he should know the wisest and safest polarity use.

The two conventions for designating polarities are: the industrial and the scientific. These are discussed in a Bio-Electric-Magnetics Institute journal. In the industrial and engineering world, as well as in the geological sciences, the designations of magnetic polarities is made by suspending a bar magnet balanced on a string and free to rotate within the Earth's magnetic field. When it stops, one end will point north, the other south, and the poles are so designated. This incorrect designation is made even though we know opposite poles attract. The end of the magnet pointing north is actually south, or the positive polarity being attracted by the north pole.

Apparently it would be too unrewarding and costly to make changes now for all of the erroneous designations made over many decades. The engineers get around this convention by stipulating incorrectly that the Northern Hemisphere contains the south magnetic pole. Most technical journals and encyclopedias and other sources of information have named the magnetic poles opposite, as well. Many people and industries do not recognize a difference in the negative and positive polarities or do not understand which is which. For instance, several corporations that sell magnetic beds and devices for many years told their customers that the north pole was properly designated the negative polarity in its mattresses when it actually was the south pole. Only recently have some recognized the difference and made the modification; others believe it is of no consequence.

Dr. Bansal too has accepted the industrial designation as legitimate, stating the Earth's north pole is really magnetic south. Yet clearly the suspended magnet test, as well as scientific instruments such as the magnetometer, specify the Earth's Northern hemisphere as the negative magnetic field. The north pole is both geographic north as well as magnetic north, as it spins on its axis. The north pole of a magnet, by the scientific convention, will attract the arrow head of a compass which actually is a south polarity attracted by the true magnetic north pole. A magnet's polarity can be tested by aligning one end with the north pointer of a compass. If it attracts, that end of the magnet is geographic, magnetic south pole, but negative polarity since the tip of the compass pointer is both the geographic and magnetic north, but of positive polarity; if it repels, that end of the magnet is south or positive polarity. A magnetometer, which can be purchased from manufacturers of magnetic products, can also readily verify correct designation.

Importance of North vs. South Polarity

One of the most important questions for the application of magnetic energy is which polarity is most beneficial and to what extent both or either energy poles are therapeutic or troublesome. It may be beneficial to list the different effects between north and south as enumerated by some experts. Exhibit 29 (Negative and Positive Polarity Differences) shows the negative field as the healer; the positive field—when overused or incorrectly used—an adverse factor. The positive polarity can be beneficial for certain applications and ailments when used under proper time limitations. Both poles together are beneficial under various circumstances. The negative polarity can be used to help balance the effects of bipolar use. The positive fields, as reported by Davis and Rawls, are beneficial for a number of purposes: to stimulate waking up; for biofeedback central nervous system response testing; for stimulation of specific organs and glands to evoke production of hormones or enzymes; to evoke production of endorphins; and for use as an irritant to evoke the body's own counter-irritant or negative magnetic healing energy.

As explained earlier, the counter-irritant effect takes place, for instance, when the positive (south) magnetic fields are placed on an inflammation, or sore joint or other painful spot. Negative (north) energy rushes to the area causing the body's own energy system to fight the pain. It is similar to placing a mustard plaster on the sore area to effect relief. This irritant causes the body's energy system to awaken and attack the alien site as a counter-irritant.

Differences between north and south polarities continue to mount. Indirect evidence from various sources indicates that negative (north) energy increases cellular oxygen while positive (south) energy decreases it. Philpott has documented evidence that negative magnetic fields encourage deep restorative sleep, fight infection, support biological healing, normalize acid-base balance, and relieve pain. On the other hand, he has found that positive energy does just the opposite—stimulates wakefulness, inhibits biological healing, anlling. Philpott believes that d increases acidic levels. The negative polarity works to reduce inflammation while the positive field tends to increase swelling if placed directly on the inflamed site; but it can help reduce edema if the magnet is placed several inches to the side in order to pull fluids toward the positive field and away from the site of the swethis is true of fatty deposits as well, where negative fields help to dissolve fat and positive fields encourage deposits.

Can Magnetic Fields Benefit Arteries?

It would appear nothing short of miraculous if it could be shown that magnetic fields over time remove fatty materials from arteries, as some believe. This would be significant for a number of disorders. Consider a 1991 study funded by the National Institute of Neurological Disorder and Stroke involving 669 high risk patients in the surgical removal of plats of fatty plaques from inside the carotid arteries (which carry blood through the neck to the brain). This review showed a 17 percent reduction in the risk of stroke for up to two years. The number of patients nationwide undergoing this procedure rose from 15,000 in 1971 to 107,000 in 1985. The New England Journal of Medicine stated that this surgery is a stunning affirmation of a safe and effective treatment for stroke prevention. Yet many referring physicians have shown a declining interest in the procedure, lacking more evidence of lasting effect because the procedure usually has to be repeated a number of times. Normally the surgery is not conducted until the patients are quite ill, such as after having experienced neurological dysfunction or blindness in one eye or at the point the blood flow is reduced 30 to 99 percent through these arteries. Certainly early treatment as well as therapy after surgery to extend curative time, either from proper diet, exercise, or the possible application of magnetic fields, would be good preventive medicine and call for further prudent investigation.

Dr. Philpott says preventative negative magnetic field therapy should be examined for the possible cleaning of arteries in general, including those to the heart and brain. Magnetotherapists believe that the process of reducing fatty substances in arteries takes place but only with long-term application over a number of months or years. But they report it

172

is effective, is of no risk, and that it is sound medical practice to use the technique.

Metabolic Disorders

The reported effects between the poles tends to reinforce their differences. Negative magnetic application promotes restorative sleep, while the positive polarity stimulates over-activity. Under certain circumstances, in cases of depression or lack of desire to sleep or eat, the therapists use positive polarity for a limited time to arouse senses and stimulate activity, but are cautioned by Philpott and some others to follow with negative pole application to bring the system into balance. Every human body and condition is different. No one can tell what is best in every case without some trial and error. A major desire of many physicians is that they be enabled to diagnose and treat instantly without much time spent recognizing differences in individuals. But much of what is good procedure requires testing and trials that may have to be done over a number of weeks or months. In the case of magnetotherapy, results may be obtained in matter of minutes or it may take weeks or months. One can only imagine, not only the patient's surprise but the doctor's bewilderment when pain is relieved in short order with magnetotherapy, yet patients need to be prepared for long-term therapy as well. In about one-third of the cases, results may not be dramatic or noticed at all for a variety of reasons already discussed. Certain healthy individuals with high pH levels who have engaged in penetrating exercise or good nutrition may not notice a difference for some problems. But it appears that all persons will evidence improvement over the long-haul in such things as better rest and reduced stress.

The healing process, whether a cut, burn, blood clot, allergic reaction, addictive state, infection, toxic state, emotional or mental reaction, or any metabolic disorder, is capable of responding to methodically produced magnetic energy. Dr. Philpott says that this will almost always be externally applied negative magnetic energy. The brain and spinal cord are positive relative to peripheral body tissues, while most human illnesses (emotional disorders, seizures, infections, toxic and acidic states) are of positive polarity in the body. It has been observed clinically that many of these diseases have been corrected by local application of negative energy of sufficient intensity and duration to counteract any abnormal positive polarity.

Negative Polarity Fights Pollution and Misapplication

Prolonged, simultaneous, high gauss exposure to both magnetic fields is capable of producing the positive polarity effects of lethargy, fatigue, and various other illnesses. Also, we may involuntarily experience these effects as explained earlier from electromagnetic pollution all around us. According to Dr. Philpott, electromagnetic pollution and improper application of positive or bipolar polarities may be counteracted to various degrees by the use of the negative polarity. This application not only is a wise health measure when ill but should be part of a regular daily regimen in the battle of diverse energies, he says. Are there adverse effects from negative fields? Researcher Richard Broeringmeyer, in his **Energy Therapy Training Manual** (1987), states that negative magnetic field energy is alkalinizing but, with extended use, can become over-alkalinizing, producing symptoms by interfering with cellular and organ system functions. In contrast, Dr. Philpott, who has gone beyond theoretical speculation, cites from his practice on thousands of patients that no matter how strong the gauss strength or how prolonged, no alkalinization illness develops from application of negative field exposure. A sluggish organ is not evidence of alkalosis, says Philpott, but rather evidence of a chronic state of fatigue from prolonged stress from positive magnetism. The answer is to apply negative fields so that the organ can recover and heal its disordered biological state.

Stimulation vs. Production of Energy

The biological response to a positive magnetic field is acidifying—the central problem in degenerative disease. Philpott has observed this effect in thousands of acute reactions involving allergies, addictions, intolerance to certain foods, chemicals and inhalants. Correction is by negative field application. Formation of insoluble

174

products from amino acids and minerals is caused by acidification and does not occur with alkalinization or normal biological pH, according to Philpott. Philpott has relied on both the original research of others and verification of results by treating his own patients clinically with the observation of conditions from before treatment to a reasonable period afterward.

Broeringmeyer says positive magnetic fields increase energy by raising the hydrogen ion. Philpott disagrees, pointing out that positive fields only stimulate use of energy but do not produce energy, and in fact, if continued into a chronic state, cause fatigue and energy collapse. Positive fields raise hydrogen concentration, but this is a rearrangement of stored chemical energy rather than the production of new energy, Barefoot testifies. This is certainly an important observation, particularly for athletes, some of whom may be sleeping on positive oriented magnetic beds. Observe the case study of Mr. Canada of 1990, cited previously, who increased leg extensions 47 percent and also bodily strength over the long-term by sleeping on a negative magnetic pad. Athletes or anyone else sleeping on positive magnetic beds receive temporary stimulation (from the alkalinization of body fluid) and then eventually fatigue, Philpott believes.

Negative magnetic fields increase energy by conserving oxygen. Energy is a restorative process from negative fields, not a stimulation process from positive fields (Bradford, R.W. 1989; Semm, P. 1980). And oxygen can only be present in an alkaline state. While certain non-oxygen respiratory plants and microorganisms grow in a positive field, this is not true in the human system that functions best in the alkaline state.

Philpott believes that long-term use, day and night, of magnetic beds for the full body reduces adrenal and gonadal hormone functions temporarily but these functions, almost immediately, return to normal levels. Treating the adrenals relieves stress which they are often under, while the function returns normally. Selective treatment at the crown of the head makes corrections in both the adrenals and gonads, Philpott says. Treatment of the pineal glands can erase menstrual problems, whereas treatment of the ovaries directly with negative fields can completely stop menstruation, he observes.

Generalizations cannot be made of the influence of magnetic fields on microorganisms in the laboratory compared to what occurs in the human body because of the antibiotic response of the body that makes it *impossible to replicate results. Philpott has observed that bacteria, fungi and viruses all die out in the human body with adequate negative magnetic application. A prolonged application of these same fields oxygenates cancer tissues as well, he notes. Cancer results from an initial acidification that produces a loss of oxygen and further cancer growth; and cancer can only grow in oxygen deficient tissue.* [*]

Philpott produces abundant evidence that negative magnetic fields are effective against scar tissues and also can resolve atheromatous plaques and other hard fibrous tissues. If treatment is extended long enough, scars disappear. Of course, low level gauss bipolar magnets will attract the negative polarity to the scarred area and also heal; consequently, both the negative and bipolar magnets are useful.

The Range of Human Adaptation

Interestingly, simultaneous magnetic pole exposure, at low gauss power, has been observed to evoke anti-stress response much as the negative pole exposure does alone. Positive fields stimulate cells, push fluids and gases and can activate the human system. If the gauss strength is within the range of the body's human adaptation, any ill effects from a positive magnetic orientation or a simultaneous negative-positive application will not likely occur.

Worldwide users of magnetic devices provide different international experiences and range of choices for adaptation. The Germans are said to believe the combined negative-positive anti-stress point is up to about 200 gauss, the French believe it to be up to 450 gauss, and the Japanese 850 gauss. Some researchers speculate that anti-stress may only be within the range of human adaptation to the Earth's known magnetic field of only 50 micro-tesla (0.5 gauss). The most predictable symptom relieving effect appears to be about 450 gauss. However, much of this is inaccurate and misleading at best, since effective gauss strength depends on a lot more than surface measurements or manufacturer's ratings. Only a fraction of the specified gauss enters the body.

Importantly, chronic, high gauss exposure to simultaneous both negative and positive, magnetic fields can introduce the same adverse effect

---

[*] The italicized text refers to more complex information.

of stress as the positive alone. Regardless of the accepted range of adaptation for each of the methodologies mentioned, stress occurs at some point from positive magnetic application. When it happens, it is closely related to gauss strength, duration of treatment, where applied, and importantly the volume of tissue exposed.

The feeling of stress also occurs with the application of negative polarity under certain circumstances. Stress has been noted to occur in about one-third of cases on high gauss strength, negative magnetic beds after one or several nights of use. This stress is due to the discharge of toxins and passes usually in a few nights, but in some cases may last several weeks or longer depending on the seriousness of one's preceding condition. Once the body is relieved of toxins, symptoms disappear and the system feels greatly improved—so its worth the limited stress. It is more likely to occur on extra-strength magnetic beds or beds with considerably more magnets than the average. Philpott says he has not experienced it with the beds with which he is familiar, whereas Canadian companies with more powerful and quickly performing mattresses indicate that it occurs in about 30 percent of the cases. Presumably, these beds are more effective, at least over the short-term. In the long-haul, the lower strength beds may prove just as effective as the body gradually builds up its energy level without experiencing sudden stress symptoms. Also some people experience stress even with lower gauss strength pads. Regardless of the strength of pads, one should gradually ease into their use until all toxins are expelled.

Standards of Use Set

The Japanese Ministry of Health and Welfare, which must approve all magnetotherapy healing and pain relieving devices in Japan, has set standards for use for magnetic devices at a minimum of 500 gauss which they believe is necessary to reach reasonable effectiveness. This is for single polarity application. There is little discussion concerning simultaneous magnetic field utilization, although they condone dual-pole therapy. In simultaneous application, one pole will diminish the strength of the other pole, weakening the combined magnetic effect. The Japanese Ministry does not relate to this problem. It appears, the lower the gauss strength, the safer when using positive exposure or simultaneous positive-negative exposure. Of course, if results are not achieved, a higher gauss strength may become necessary. Importantly, many experts believe that there will never be damage from use of the negative polarity alone regardless of duration of use.

For centuries, the simultaneous application of both polarities was used for healing in jewelry, necklaces, wrist bands, and all sorts of devices, with reportedly effective results. Massage therapists and chiropractors use both poles in relaxation grids to facilitate their work. Miniature (one-eighth inch diameter) magnets are used over specific acupuncture points to energize them to greater potency, either with both polarities or unipolar. We have witnessed and gathered information where countless patients have experienced either pain relief or healing benefits from using simultaneous applications of positive-negative magnetotherapy. We can cite examples from personal observations where people have been almost instantly relieved of pain and suffering from simultaneous pole exposure for such conditions as painful shoulders, sprains, tennis elbows, headaches, gout and various other ailments. When this type of application is limited to the point where healing occurs, then withdrawn, stress is avoided. Low strengths under 100 gauss, usually found in jewelry and similar devices, will likely avoid stressful symptoms.

Balancing the Poles

After initial success is obtained, a maintenance regimen of one-half hour to one hour per day is recommended using negative magnetic application. One may apply a magnetic device to various parts of the body or sleep on a magnetic bed. None of the experts or the literature challenge the benefit of negative magnetic therapy, with the single possibility that prolonged use of the north pole may lower adrenal production over the long-term. Too much of anything, whether water, drugs or vitamins is not good. Everything must be taken in correct proportion to the need and the proper balancing of the body.

Researchers confirm the differences between the polarities. Albert R. Davis cautioned about overexposure to the positive polarity which could cause overstimulation, particularly harmful if any type of infection or cancerous cells were present. Davis indicates that positive polarity over-stimulation can accelerate the aging process or aggravate disease, which the opposite, negative pole has been found to cure. Caution must be taken that emerging symptoms from the positive fields are not scoffed off as simply "allergic reactions" or "healing crises." Contact with the true positive pole may have energized a deep-seated infection or overenergized an acupuncture point. Dr. Nakagawa, from his experience in Japan, states that most of these symptoms can be improved within a week or so by simply staying off the magnetic device. Continuous usage over several months may cause symptoms to return in what he calls a "habituation effect." Applying more can become a stress factor rather than relief. He does not relate to the ability to counteract adverse effects of the positive polarity by using the opposite or negative field.

As previously mentioned, in order to offset adverse effects of the positive pole, Philpott maintains the application of the negative magnetic fields will cancel out symptoms and protect against overstimulation. The negative, he says, will not drain the body. Once the magnet is removed, the body resumes an equal balance between the poles, becoming bipolar at a higher level of balanced magnetic energy. The north pole normalizes the alkaline state of the body but does not produce an over alkalinized condition. It oxygenates the body, Philpott says, but never produces oxidized free radicals. A lengthy exposure to the positive pole can block the detoxifying process and disorganize the central nervous system. On the other hand, the positive energy can help when applied to chakras and glands that require stimulation, and it can also drive calcium to broken bones to accelerate the healing process. In any case, both forces are necessary to maintain life, while the key is balance.

Positive magnetic energy has a number of useful functions, such as exciting the return of response capacity of neurons that have undergone an extinction of disuse, and nerve response testing or facilitation of responses for testing purposes. Theoretically, Philpott states, applying a 2,000 gauss positive magnetic field (3 inch wide, 1/8 inch thick plastiform magnet) on the forehead for three minutes upon awakening and a 12 inch to 24 inch positive magnet on the spine for three minutes could replace bright light therapy—to be followed at bedtime with a negative magnetic application for 30 to 60 minutes. Response of the central nervous system can occur in three minutes.

Effects of Bipolar Magnets

Magnetic Fields Versus the Body's
Alkaline and Acidic Base

It is common knowledge that a number of health therapies have an element of reflexology at their base structures, which causes interaction with the magnetic forces of light. Reflexology invokes magnetic field switching that occurs when the energy applied exceeds the point of fatigue, turning to stress rather than healing. Eventually, the brain sends negative ions to the source of the problem to effect pain relief and healing. Homeopathy is another example that even its founder Hahnemann understood worked by magnetic forces. Shaking (or seccusion) the homeopathic remedies agitates these substances in the Earth's magnetic field. These dilutions, as explained earlier, get so minute that they are undetectable, yet sufficient energy is created to elicit response from the brain.

The negative polarity, used in alternative therapies or as a conventional medical application, has an alkalinizing and oxidizing effect which can be a large part of the answer for cures for many human illnesses. Allergies, intolerance, chemical hypersensitivities, pollution of various sorts, insect stings and most toxins are acid or biologically acid evoking and hypoxic producing. In a test of the concentric magnet, the Massachusetts Institute of Technology demonstrated that this magnet causes some degree of vasodilatation (widening of blood vessels). Dr. Ted Zablotsky speculates that vasodilatation from the bipolar magnet increases oxygen to tissues and therefore is effective in relieving pain. On the other hand, Philpott states that predominantly positive magnetic circles are acid producing therefore symptom producing as well, particularly when these magnetic fields are applied beyond the human level of adaptation. When both magnetic fields are used simultaneously but are overwhelmingly high gauss positive, therapy is acidifying to the tissues, therefore less oxygen is carried in the blood rather than more, according to Philpott.

Barefoot believes that the production of hydroxides occurs with both poles which raises the extracellular pH, but that the positive pole suppresses normal biochemical activity and so has a countering (acidifying) effect. Dr. Zablotsky instructs patients to use a weaker concentric magnet if pain is experienced or use a concentric magnet with the outer pole negative which provides a largely negative field, and not to use a dual polarity on acute swollen areas or where bleeding occurs because vessel dilation might increase bleeding or swelling. Dr. Philpott says use of the negative polarity alone would solve the problem and allow immediate therapy on both swollen and bleeding parts, since the negative fields are alkalinizing—normalizing the pH of the blood and tissues. Philpott also believes that negative magnetic fields aid in reducing fat and calcium deposits in the circulatory system by normalizing the acid-base balance (pH) of undesirable cholesterol and triglycerides that adhere and build inside artery walls.

In further understanding of the role of negative magnetic energy, Robert Becker points out that large amounts of bone growth accumulate around negative electrodes, as well as the resorption of bone at the negative pole and at bone unions and where there is bone growth. Although these data were accepted in the United States originally in the 1960s, the scientific profession has been slow to discern a difference in north-south polarities except to indicate direction.

Differing Theories

Different schools of thought persist around the world as to which polarity works best. It seems because of long tradition, in nations such as Japan, India, and Germany, bipolar application is acceptable for treatment. Dr. Bansal confirms that the most favored practice in India is the bipolar method. Nevertheless, many who subscribe to dual pole treatment generally follow its use by applying the opposite pole shortly after the other to achieve balance. Although Bansal uses both poles and believes he gets better results from this methodology, he states that he has no basis for favoring one method over the other. He places one pole to the side that is to be healed and the opposite pole in another location nearby to either push or pull nutrients. Philpott says it is unnecessary to use both poles, that the negative is sufficient and preferred. The positive pole, when located at any substantial distance from the negative pole is unlikely to have any noticeable effect in any case, he believes. More than six or eight inches of separation would not have measurable effect at the injured site.

There is a disagreement by many American and foreign doctors and therapists as to how magnetic fields function. Bansal is challenged in one of his main reasons for using the bipolar method. He believes that it is technically necessary to use two poles in order to complete the magnetic current circuit which would not be achieved with a single pole. However, science shows this to be incorrect. It is unnecessary to complete a circuit in dealing with magnetic fields. The magnetic field performs whether or not there is a ground at the other end, since we are dealing with body cells that are bipolar in nature and are influenced by either external negative or positive magnetic fields alone or together.

Bansal also diminishes the force of his bipolar argument when he refers to his own experiment with magnetized water of north polarity which he demonstrates neutralizes bacteria while south pole magnetized water hastens production of bacteria. North pole, he says, is very effective against diseases caused by bacterial infection such as arthritis, boils, burns, eczema, ear and tooth aches, goiter and kidney infections, tumors, ulcers, wounds and even cancers; however, he believes the south pole works better on neuralgia, stiffness, swellings, poor digestion and gas formation. As already stated, for certain types of ailments some initial stimulation may be necessary in order to turn on the system or hasten results.

Bansal and other Eastern therapists, in particular, talk about north and south rather than negative and positive. Direction in itself is of no consequence. What is significant is whether a particular side of the magnet is negative or positive and that the therapist knows it. Furthermore, the direction of the Earth's poles is not significant in treatment because the entire surface of the Earth is negative poled as described in Chapter 2.

Negatively Charged Curative Instruments

The successful use of various magnetic devices reinforces the beneficial use of the negative polarity. A variety of therapeutic instruments utilizing negative polarity, as opposed to the positive magnetic field, are being used with considerable effectiveness in both the Unites States and around the world:

A study by Professor Caomin Sun of Beijing Institute of Technology and Dr. W. D. Stanish and J. W. Kozey, Orthopedic and Sports Medicine Clinic of Novia Scotia, tested 50 people with a control group using a therapeutic device for a period of 14 days. Conclusions were that the treatment did not materially reduce pain compared to a placebo group but that it did reduce swelling and also increased mobility as early as seven days after surgery, a much quicker recovery time than normal. The unit used is called Therapeutic Electro Membrane and is fabricated from a non-woven, non-allergenic and sterile high electron density polymer, designed to form a closed circuit but placed tightly against the skin to emit low electric current and promote healing and relieve pain. It is effective for temporary relief of minor arthritis, bursitis, muscle spasm, sports and soft tissue injuries associated with whiplash, low back pain, sprains, strains, inflammations and swelling.

Another study of the therapeutic membrane involving 251 treated patients, conducted by the Orthopedics Departments of Beijing Union Medical College Hospital and Beijing Red Cross Yang Hospital and Jishutan Hospital, showed a highly effective success rate of 86 percent. The lowest success rate of 50 percent was for protrusion of an inter-vertebral disk; while 100 percent success rates were indicated for sprains, tenosynovitis, neck and shank pains, backaches, tennis elbow, bursitis, among other ailments.

The significance of the electro-membrane is that it has a negative charge which tends to support the findings that the negative polarity neutralizes histamine which causes pain.

In other cases using the negative oriented membrane, a 90 percent effectiveness response was reported by Dr. Winston Green of Texas who treated many popular sports figures, such as Bernie Kosar, quarterback of the Cleveland Browns, and Evander Holyfield, professional heavyweight boxer, and others. About 25 percent faster healing rates were reported. The device has been approved for the federal Medicare and Medicaid insurance programs and for most private insurance reimbursement. It has a Current Procedural Terminology (CPT) code for reimbursement. A large number of physicians and therapists are using it regularly. However, bipolar magnets are also effective (see exhibit 20 **The use of Alternate Magnetic Foils**). The question always arises which is the most effective and safest. Low gauss, bipolar magnets could very well function more quickly and be just as safe as negative foil alone at a particular site for brief periods of time when adaptation has not yet occurred. Both negative pole and bipolar magnets are safe and effective as demonstrated in numerous studies and thousands of patients.

Exhibit 20   The Use of Alternate Magnetic Foils In the Treatment of Chronic Lumbago

The Oberarzt of the Neurosurgical Clinic, Vienna, Austria, conducted a blind test on 40 patients with similar complaints of severe Lumbago three months after a disk operation without surgical complications. Twenty were treated with alternate poled magnetic foil and twenty with a non-magnetized foil. Conclusions reached were that magnetic foil had a strong effect on pain, specially in the first weeks of use. While four patients were free from complaints over the same period who were not treated with magnetic foil but with physiotherapy, 13 patients were free from pain after four weeks of therapy with the alternate magnetic foil—more than three times as many. The study demonstrated that in the case of long-term pain, effects—from substantial improvement of pain symptoms to practically complete freedom from pain—could be observed in about two-thirds of all patients investigated.

Source: Kletter, Dr. Gerhard, Oberarzt of the Neurosurgical Clinic, Vienna, Austria, Zehenthofgasse 37, A, 1990.

Evidence for the Negative Healing Polarity

Comparing device effectiveness is important. For example, the TENS (transcutaneous electrical nerve stimulation) units and ultrasound units have some benefits and some problems. These particular devices, claims Dr. Rer Nat, retard the healing process and only mask the pain. T.E.N.S. treatment up to 500 volts at one second intervals, he explains, traumatizes the tissues and causes the release of endorphin in the brain which blocks pain. The high current reduces ATP (Adenosine Triphosphate) production in the cells, retarding the healing process.

Ultrasound soothes pain by causing blood to flow to the area, but it also reduces ATP. On the other hand, the bio-analgesic membrane described above provides an electron transfer, exchanging the positive polarity of the injured tissue for the healing negative polarity. It also produces ATP which increases protein synthesis, ion transfer through cell membrane and other chemical reactions as well.

Information Brief

Bioflex Concentric Bipolar Magnets

Junella Robb has been under the care of Dr. Eddie G. Benge, M.D., New Mexico Arthritis Clinic, Albuquerque, N.M., since July 28, 1983 for diffuse musculoskeletal pain. The clearest diagnosis he and his colleagues, Dr. Erik E. Carlson, M.D., and Dr. Douglas E. Roberts, M.D., have been able to make is fibromyalgia syndrome (fibrositis), although she does have mechanical problems in the cervical spine that may be symptom producing. She has tried a number of therapeutic modalities, including most of the available nonsteroidal, anti-inflammatory agents and has been forced to take Fioricet on a regular basis. She also takes Ludiomil at bedtime. She has used different narcotic analgesics and has been evaluated by the St. Joseph Hospital Chronic Pain Program by Dr. Brian Delahaussage, participating in their pool program. Extensive physical therapy plus other modalities were unsuccessful.

In the first month of using bipolar magnetic devices, improvement for Ms. Robb was 75 - 80 percent and today she is much better and is more functional in doing daily activities. Dr. Benge states physical examination shows that she exhibits much less tenderness than in any of her prior visits. Other cases are also documented.

Low ampere power should also be the mode of use. High power devices cannot only create damage, says Dr. Becker, but can also cause cell death. As early as 1971, Dr. Zachery Friedenberg, University of Pennsylvania, reported the first successful electric treatment of non-unions in a human being using a low 10 micro-ampere D.C. current. Low voltage micro-amp stimulators (10-60 volts) can overcome tissue resistance because they are sensitive to the impedance properties of the tissues being treated; whereas, high volt stimulators that drive currents in large quantities do not readily adapt to tissue resistance because impedance increases with higher voltage. Small micro-amp currents more *closely approximate naturally occurring bioelectric currents in the body and therefore more effectively assist tissue healing and repair.**

The user needs to be cautious of the kinds of devices and the claims made for them. Some of these devices, as they became popular, where pushed by unscrupulous suppliers as performing cures were absolutely no evidence existed. For example, when the TENS unit first appeared, the FDA warned the public that there was no evidence that these devices were good for weight loss, body shaping or muscle building, breast development, or non-surgical facelift, among other claims. It seems so often that things worthwhile are misused by profit seekers against the public interest. So much good can come out of the proper use of magnetotherapy that suppliers should not oversell or abuse its value.

No question exists that the simple, permanent magnet relieves symptoms and heals certain ailments. Numerous double-blind, placebo controlled studies show effectiveness on healing fractures, sprains and all sorts of pain. Since magnetic fields do not recognize a difference between cells involved in bone-fusions or any other type of body cells, it appears logical they heal or influence all cells. Because a difference exists in the understanding about the effects of the various polarities, science ought to immediately set out to find the answer for the benefit of mankind. This could be done in short order, if we set our research minds to it. Lay aside competitive arguments and proceed to conduct practical controlled clinical tests to confirm conclusions. We owe that much to the public (see appendix I Areas for Possible Research).

---

* The italicized text refers to more complex information.

Effects of Bipolar Magnets

Swiss scientist Arno Latske in 1981 introduced an alternating polarity magnet, observing that when applied over areas of pain, a healing effect occurred from the charged particles (such as electrolytes in the blood) that passed through the magnetic field in a perpendicular direction to that field, in accordance with the principle of physics known as the Hall Effect. Theoretically, the alternating polarity magnet generates an alternating current in the blood. Furthermore, the poles of the magnet (as shown in Figure 5-1 below) are arranged in parallel strips so that the

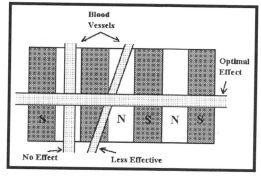

Figure 5-1 Healing effects from applying bipolar magnets

perpendicular therapeutic effect is limited to blood vessels that run across alternating poles.

German scientist Horst Baermann developed a concentric magnet that was designed to improve performance under the Hall Effect. However, a certain amount of blood vessels still were not affected. If they did not cross at or near the center of the pattern, the alternating current effect was minimal.

Trying to improve on these designs, American engineer Vincent Ardizzone, of Nu-Magnetics, Inc., N.Y., developed a design that takes into greater account the random angles of blood vessels by utilizing a checkerboard pattern. The previously mentioned designs have two sides per pole adjacent to

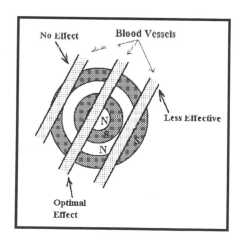

Figure 5-2 Parallel arrangement of the poles of the magnet

opposite poles, while the four-sided checkerboard configuration (shown in Figure 5-2) mathematically increases the probability that a blood vessel will cross alternating poles. This design is also more versatile because it can be cut into any shape or size without creating gaps in the pattern.

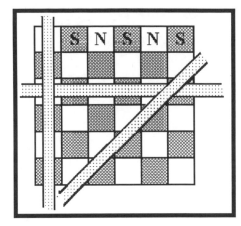

Figure 5-3 Checkerboard pattern increases chance that blood vessels receive optimum effect

The checkerboard pattern results in more alternating pole sequences. Ardizzone's device also utilizes a steel foil backing that he says causes the pad's fields to reflect back onto itself to enhance field strength and penetration, while making the product more durable as well.

Magnets generally have a long life, particularly if they are not exposed to another source that might drain energy or disrupt internal alignment. The energy product or stability of a permanent magnet is a measure of the inherent field strength of the material multiplied by the magnetic force required to neutralize that field. Concentric pads generally have been tested to have an energy product of 0.9 MGOs (mega gauss-oversteads). Checkerboard pads have an energy product of 1.4 MGOs which means they retain magnetic strength considerably longer because of increased energy intensity.

Latzke's tests showed that effective therapeutic results are obtained when poles are from 4 to 10 mm wide. He also argues that to obtain the alternating therapeutic effect, the minimum number of pole changes is three. For the concentric and checkerboard patterns, Ardizzone has mathematically calculated the probability of blood vessels crossing with fewer than three pole changes and/or less than 4 mm or greater than 10 mm between alternations. His data show the probability of effectiveness for the concentric type magnet at 64.3 percent and for the checkerboard magnet 93.8 percent or about a 30 percent difference. Nevertheless, the *makers of the concentric magnet say it is mathematically impossible to design a configuration more efficient than the circular magnet.* *

Remember that effectiveness is related not only to the assembly of blood vessels, but quite explicitly to gauss strength, penetration depth, and the volume of tissue covered. Larger and heavier magnets affect more tissue and cells deeper in the body. So to get around the varied configurations, other researchers say to simple apply larger and/or stronger magnets. But the convenience of application and flexibility of wrapping around a body part is also very important; therefore, thin, ceramic or foil magnets may be most appropriate for specific treatments.

Deeper disorders may require a heavier and stronger magnet. A steel backing can provide increased strength and penetration by reflecting the magnetic field. However, penetration is primarily related to weight. The greater the weight, the deeper the penetration. A thin magnet of extra, high gauss strength will not penetrate as deeply as a thick, lower strength magnet, although the thin bipolar magnet will most likely turn on the biofeedback effect more quickly because the body is dealing with a smaller irritant factor (less tissue volume) that negative fields need to overcome at the site. In a thin bipolar magnet, lines of flux are drawn horizontally to each other across the face of the magnet rather than inward toward the body tissue, resulting in diminished penetration.

The Hall Effect states that magnetic fields will only influence another property when angles of force are perpendicular to each other. Since the body has over 60,000 miles of blood vessels that flow in many directions, magnets whose lines of force are at right angles to the vessels would logically affect more blood vessels, so magnets that are mathematically superior in design should be more effective than those not so configured. Arteries flow linearly, straight, and parallel to the longitudinal axes of the body; however, if a magnet penetrates deeply enough the fields will be perpendicular to most of the large arteries, which are deep. One must take into account all the factors as described above. Importantly, all configurations have varying degrees of healing effect.

---

* The italicized text refers to more complex information.

Various Configurations of Magnets
Have Therapeutic Effect

Concentric and checkerboard magnets, as well as a variety of other bipolar configurations offer effective therapy, depending on the type and severity of disorder. If results are not forthcoming, stronger or heavier magnets, or an extended period of use may be in order. Dual polarity magnets that emit less than 200 gauss at their surface (one-third of the internal manufacturer's rating) are deemed perfectly safe, especially for local application or for brief periods of time. It appears that the north-south pulsing effect (more accurately the drawing of ions and repulsing of ions in spatial frequencies or cycles per unit of area or polarity change per foot) of a bipolar magnet may perform more quickly than a single pole magnet of the same gauss strength and thickness. Some experts believe that there is no pulsing effect at all, simply the response of the predominant polarity of the particular magnet. A negative oriented magnet of higher gauss strength can equal or better the performance of a lower strength bipolar magnet.

In brief, bipolar and single pole magnets can be used safely and effectively when applied locally with the proper gauss strength; but, a much higher gauss strength can be used safely with the negative polarity.

For long-term application, negative magnetic fields are considered safest, as described earlier. Nevertheless, sleeping or sitting on a positive or bipolar field pad with magnets of 850 gauss or less each is acceptable and safe according to many experts. These magnets emit about one-third strength or 283 gauss at their surface and normally from 10 - 20 gauss on body tissue, depending on the distance from the body. The farther the magnets are imbedded within the mattress or pad, the less the gauss strength to the body tissue.

Stress may occur with the positive field after a few months or sooner. Stress does not appear to occur with the negative field, regardless of gauss strength, except initially when the body releases toxins. Stress is limited according to Philpott and Bonlie, since the counter-irritant reflexology is not being used, rather the body directly receives the negative energy that controls the metabiology of healing. With both bipolar and positive magnetic fields, the body acts in a counter-irritant function by signaling the brain to send negative magnetic energy (similar to the response to a liniment or other medication) to the injured site to relieve symptoms. Importantly, the body is limited as to how long it can keep up this reflex response, usually for about eight weeks when the counter-irritant effect wears off and symptoms return. The subject then needs to go off the therapy to rest the body.

Pulsations that parallel human organ systems can be used to facilitate a magnetic field. It is assumed that the effectiveness of smaller gauss permanent magnets is increased by the so-called pulsing effect of such bipolar magnets as the concentric or checkerboard. The negative poled magnet can produce a similar effect but at a higher manufacturer's rating in the range of 1000 to 4000 gauss in the "closed system." In the "open system," or that which is released against the body, only about one-third of the magnetic field is available therapeutically. This means that a manufacturer's rating of 3,950 gauss renders about 1,200 gauss to the subject, while a rating of 12,300 renders 4,000 gauss to the body, and considerably less internally to the tissue.

Neither the negative or positive pole evokes any type of radiation injury to cells; therefore, brief exposure, even to the positive field, is not harmful. However, prolonged exposure to positive magnetic fields can disorder metabolic functions by producing acidity, reducing cellular oxygen supply, or encouraging replication of latent microorganisms, pointed out earlier. The positive field also evokes the production of endorphins, as all stressors do and can become addictive when applied to the head. (Rosenblatt, Michael, **The Endogenous Opiate Peptides**, pp.378-382, **Harrison's Principles of Internal Medicine**, McGraw-Hill Book Co., 1987.)

Electrically Negative or Magnetically Negative

Robert O. Becker demonstrated, by use of a magnetometer, that a broken bone initially registers electrically positive for about three hours, then becomes electrically negative. He has shown that the negative field is indeed the field which governs the healing process. Although Dr. Zablotsky agrees with the different biological effects of the negative and positive poles, he states that this is the effect of electric current, not magnetics. Dr. Becker states that any magnetic effect would be minor. On the other side, Dr. Philpott and Dr. Bonlie among others say electric and magnetic effects "go hand-in-hand" and you cannot have one without the other.   Robert Barefoot says, "they are indivisible, magnetics create electricity to cause and stimulate biological activity. One need only ask the question whether Becker's electricity was devoid of a magnetic field—which is impossible."

To demonstrate that increased negative magnetic fields are relayed to the site of injury, Dr. Dean Bonlie offers a test that anyone can conduct. First, he measured the palm of the subject's hand and the wrist with a magnetometer (measures magnetic field strength), which indicated a negative field of 210 milligauss. He then pinched the palm with a toothed clamp that immediately changed the milligauss to 40.00 positive field at the point of injury. After removal of the clamp in 20 minutes, the wrist was measured and found to have increased its negative field from 210 to 400 milligauss, which would indicate a biofeedback effect from the brain sending increased negative field currents toward the injured site. In short, the brain sends electromagnetic negative currents to the site, increasing the negative magnetic field as measured by a magnetometer. In approximately one hour the palm (point of injury) had returned to a normal magnetic field reading again.   Becker's and Bonlie's experiments indicate that both electrical and magnetic fields are at work in the healing process.

This procedure can be repeated using a 1" diameter x ¼" thick neodymium disc placed in the palm of the hand with the positive side to the skin to stimulate an injury. The magnet needs to be left in the palm for at least 20 minutes. When the magnet is removed, there is a 52 percent (150 milligauss) increase in the negative magnetic field at the wrist.   This increase gradually declines over a period of three hours from a 20-minute exposure.

Further indication of differences in polarity effects is that certain therapists recommend not putting a bipolar magnet on a swelling or bleeding area for a day or two, rather first applying an ice pack. On the other hand, Dr. Philpott states that the patient may immediately apply negative fields on an injured site to reduce swelling and bleeding. This oxidizes the histamine in the region, he says, which reduces swelling and pain. A positive oriented or alternate poled magnet can be placed about six inches to the side of the injury, he points out, which will increase pulsed magnetic energy from the brain to the site. Philpott believes that bleeding does not appear to be a contrary factor because as swelling is reduced, blood flow subsides. Zablotsky and some others believe magnetic fields dredge swamps, creating channels, and therefore fluid flows more easily.

Oxygen is the strongest of the paramagnetic gases. It is assumed that the oxygen in the air is carrying the Earth's magnetic field and if it is magnetized to a greater degree, it will impart this increased charge to the DNA—an additional source of human energy beyond nutrition. Negative magnetic fields have been observed to reduce cellular edema rapidly, most likely by activating the sodium pump, according to Philpott, that more readily diffuses oxygen into the cells when the site is not swollen. Philpott has used hyperbaric oxygen and ozone to ozonide the blood. This clinical experience permitted the assessment of several procedures: the significance of oxygenation caused by pressure, ozone by ozoniding the blood, and negative magnetic field therapy. Philpott draws the conclusion that negative magnetic fields are more oxygenating or oxidating to human cells than either hyperbaric oxygen or ozone therapy.

Energy or Simply Force

Zablotsky argues that magnetism is not energy, only force, and that there is absolutely no transfer of energy from a permanent magnet to a person. Robert Barefoot says that we are really quibbling over the definition. Magnetism is force that can be readily converted into energy. The production of hydroxides by magnetism generates heat from the energy released by the breakdown of molecules. Energy is not transferred but it is released.

Energy involves movement. A static magnetic field produces energy. Movement through a friction field to convert to energy. Vibration of live cells in a magnetic field produces energy. Blood flowing through the friction of a magnetic field produces energy.

A magnetic field itself is not energy, however, a static magnetic field moves electrons in the magnetic field to produce energy. The principle of magnetic resonance is further evidence that a static magnetic field energizes charged particles in the biological system as demonstrated in the technique of magnetic resonance imagery. Furthermore, positive and negative electromagnetic direct current poles and solid state poles have 180° oppositeness in physical fact and predictably in human systems. Negative magnetic-electric energy response in humans is oxidative and functions like that of adequate oxygen, low hydrogen ions, and maintenance of a biologically normal alkaline state. The positive energy behaves oppositely—oxygen deficit, increased hydrogen ions and acidity.

Different Biological Effects

Clinical observations show that negative fields are a universal antibiotic, such as in bacterial, fungal and viral infections. Most microorganisms have a low tolerance for oxygen and some no tolerance. Human cells require high oxygen tension, thus the process of oxidation to the human is the breath of life and to microorganisms is the kiss of death.

A vector potential is associated with a fixed magnetic field (Aharonov-Bohn effect that a solid state magnet moves electrons in the magnetic field) and therefore it becomes easier to explain how magnetic fields from a permanent magnet may influence the motion of static charged particles and accounts for some of the biological effects observed, confirming empirical observations of biomagnetic effects associated with opposite poles. (Bradford, Robert W. Rodriquez, Rodrigom Garcia, Jorge and Allenm Henry, The Effect of Magnetic Poles on Accelerated Charge Neutralization of Malignant Tumors in Vivo, Robert W. Bradford Research Institute, presented at the International Symposium on Biomagnetology, Magnetotherapy and Posturography Salve Regina College, Newport, R.I., May 29-June 1, 1989 Aharabiv, Y. and Bohm, d., Significance of Electromagnetic Potentials in Quantum Theory. The Physical Review, 115, 485 (1959).)

General malaise and soreness of muscles are associated with numerous types of acids produced by bacteria as the end product of metabolism. These include lactic acid, acetic acid, propionic acid, gluconic acid, and kojic acid. Ethyl and butyl alcohol, acetone, and 2,3-butylene glycol are also produced as end products. Ammonia is a byproduct of some bacteria metabolism. Fatty acids, antibiotics, pigments, and certain toxins are produced. Also exotoxins are circulated in the blood and endotoxins are found in the bacteria itself.*

A negative magnetic field is known to cancel out acids, as well as oxidate exotoxins and endotoxins, and inhibit bacterial replication by interfering with bacterial metabolism and production of enzymes used by

---

*   The italicized text refers to more complex information.

bacteria to break down human cellular structure. The positive magnetic field increases microorganism replication, for example, as observed by microorganism epidemics following sunflares which are known to be a positive magnetic field.

The effect of magnetic fields are related to multiple factors working at the same time, such as interference with nutrition of bacteria, interference with microorganism replication, the pH factor of the human host, and the oxidation and oxygenation factor.

In further discussion of the differences in poles, some argue that it is impossible to separate one pole from another on any magnet and that the lines of flow are really abstract lines to aid us in visualizing direction of force. However, it is a fact of physics, says Barefoot, that the north pole is negative and the south pole positive, and although they cannot be separated, they are diametrically different.

Supportive paraneural cells and Schwann cells concentrate negative energy at the site of injury. From this knowledge, it has been determined that magnetic fields can be used not only for symptom relief but also to promote healing by application over an extended period of time. And this works both for the negative and positive fields or both fields applied simultaneously as long as the anti-stress gauss level is maintained. But the negative magnetic fields appear to have a more predictable response. They also produce melatonin, the central governing neurohormone over all energy functions that has been documented to be anti-stressful, anti-aging, anti-infectious, anti-cancerous, and also to exert control over free radicals and respiration. (Semm, P. Nature 228 (1980): 206 Magnetic Sensitivity of Pineal Gland; and Fontenot, J. and Jevine, S.A., Melatonin Deficiency: Its Role in Oncogenesis and Age-Relative Pathology, Journal of Orthomolecular Medicine, 1st quarter, 1990, Vol.5, No.1).

Magnetic fields also help to produce the growth hormone (an anabolic hormone) primarily at night when asleep, which controls the thickness of skin, muscle mass, growth of hair and nails, and also effects healing by turning amino-acids into proteins. (Daniels, G.H. and Martin, J.B. **Harrison's Principles of Internal Medicine**, 11th Edition, 1987, *McGraw-Hill Book Co.*, pp.1701-5.)

SCIENTIFIC DIGEST

Effect of Negative and Positive Polarities on
Tumors, Cancers, and Pain

For over 18 years, Davis and Rawls experimented with the effects of magnetic fields on the development of tumors and cancers. This mainly involved the transplanting of cancerous cells into healthy rats, rabbits, mice and other animals. Results showed that when the north (negative) pole was applied, the pathological conditions improved and development of tumors and cancers slowed down or were stopped in over 90 percent of the cases, depending on the stage of the disease and age and physical condition of the animal. When the south (positive) was applied, the invariable result was an aggravation of the pathological condition and a more rapid development of the tumors.

In addition, where healthy animal tissue was exposed to negative energy before transplantation of cancerous cells, animals treated with these cells displaced a remarkable increase in resistance to the cancerous graft and further development.

In regard to injuries, in every case where internal repair is occurring, whether animal or human, an increase in negative bioelectric potential takes place on the external surface of the affected region. Upon recovery, the negative potential drops and returns to normal. When nerve terminals are affected by pressure, infection, burns, etc., they inform the brain of danger and send negative energy to the site. If negative magnetic energy is applied directly on the pain, a reduction in the external positive potential on the outer envelope of the nerve fibre occurs creating a sedative effect produced by the diminution in the sensitivity potential of the positive ions.

In reinforcement of this understanding, Dr. Bhattacharia and Dr. Sierra have demonstrated that in different parts of the body, the skin has an electric charge that is positive, negative or zero. The highest positive voltage in the front of the body is around the heart with a value of about 70 microvolts. Voltages vary a great deal from person to person and type of disease. Appropriate magnetotherapy can restore the correct potential.

Source: Davis, A.R., and Rawls, W., **Magnetic Blueprint of Life**, 1979, and Dr. Bhattacharia and Dr. Sierra, **Power in the Magnet to Heal**.

Chapter 6

How to Apply Magnetotherapy

Controlled Studies and Clinical Experiences

Doctors and therapists around the world have known for centuries that magnetic energy assists the body with its healing and pain relief mechanisms. They have used this energy to cure every disease imaginable. Almost no illness is omitted from their list of therapeutic attempts. Every claim known has probably been made for magnetotherapy. The Far Eastern nations in particular have used these healing powers in almost every way possible. Eastern Europe has been quite vigorous in its pursuit as well, much ahead of the United States where greater proof of success is demanded. The U.S. insists more on double-blind placebo controlled studies. Already hundreds of controlled studies and scientific reports exist (over a dozen cited in this book) for the healing of fractures and sprains and bodily pains, but few controlled studies are available on the effects for most other ailments, although some are cited here. Mainly the evidence involves less sophisticated clinical experiences or anecdotal evidence.

Although prevention of disease is one of societies main goals, the efficacy of it is more difficult to prove. Certainly one of the main purposes of good nutrition, exercise, yoga, magnetotherapy and other natural systems is prevention, where controlled studies would take years to conclude. Nevertheless, they should be done. But the sick and weak should not be expected to wait. Providers from all over the world have observed improved well-being, cleansing of the body and new vigor and energy in their clients. When someone feels below standard, one of the options certainly is to consider magnetic energy to spare the consequences of more serious problems.

Additional Studies Needed

If physicians do not choose to use magnetotherapy, society will be the loser. However, we know that thousands of doctors are using electromagnets and permanent magnets all over the world, with an increasing number in the United States. Canada seems to be one step ahead of the U.S. in the use of magnetic devices, where one can purchase magnetic bed pads and seats and simple magnets over-the-counter and other outlets. In the U.S., the FDA approved the use of electromagnetic devices in 1978 but has said little about the safer, permanent magnet. However, American physicians are using analgesic membranes and similar electric/magnetic devices which emit negative polarized currents to relieve pain and heal many types of ailments. M.D.s and licensed therapists can charge these treatments to approved medical plans. If the use of permanent magnetic devices would receive official sanction for reimbursement from government and private insurers, their use would escalate. It has already been done for similar devices.

Fortunately, at least a few small studies on the efficacy of permanent magnets are in progress by such interested groups as the Muscular Dystrophy Society and the World Health Research Foundation. Dr. Philpott and Dr. Zimmerman are undertaking part of this work. Zimmerman is also conducting a preliminary pilot study of how a magnetic mattress pad affects subjectively perceived sleep and the effects of magnets upon implanted cancer in nude mice. These few studies will answer only some questions. Yet the most fundamental research may not be able to show what truly happens to human cells and their membranes. This should not stop the medical community from testing and using magnetotherapy as long as successful end results can be demonstrated, especially in cases where all else has failed.

Inexpensive Therapy

Magnetotherapy is widely used, yet in many cases with too little knowledge of the safest way. In the United States alone, it is estimated that hundreds of thousands of people are using self-help permanent magnetic devices. As a matter of fact, if one chose he could buy a simple magnet at a Radio Shack outlet or one of a hundred other manufacturers or retailers of magnets designed for use in toys or motors or dozens of other appliances. Results from these magnets would be similar to the magnets promoted by the health care companies, if one can identify correct polarity and strength for the particular ailment. Magnets are relatively inexpensive, but their correct use is very important.

The appropriate size magnet for the particular ailment and, of course, the proper polarity and time-frame must be observed for best results. This information should be given by the manufacturers who should have knowledge of how magnets function. Merely buying a magnet off a retail shelf is not going to do the trick. It may work, however, because one magnet of similar size and strength is essentially the same as another. But proper understanding is necessary, otherwise one may or may not get successful results or he may receive adverse side effects.

Magnets are probably the least expensive medicine that anyone can purchase. And a magnet can be used almost indefinitely. It won't change it's power unless it is exposed to some other very intense magnetic fields or subjected to excessive heat or mechanical shock such as pounding it with a hammer. In short, once purchased, a magnet can last for ten or twenty years or even a lifetime. Can you imagine what this could do for our costly health care system where people could self-medicate for simple ailments ! We have already been told that a large percentage of people who seek out doctors do so unnecessarily. A number of studies show about one-third of all tests and procedures done by doctors are unnecessary and simply add to the gigantic cost of the system. Magnetotherapy might solve many temporary pains, saving the most severe ills for professional analysis. With appropriate education from our school systems and family doctors, we could learn to use magnetic devices as preventive medicine. From this, a great deal of good could come, while people learn to take control of their bodies.

The Mechanics of Magnets and Equipment

The average person does not have to become familiar with the following technical information, but providers will have an interest. For example, we may ask what gauss means. The term denotes the electromagnetic unit of magnetic flux density equal to one maxwell per square centimeter, or the number of magnetic force lines through a unit of area. Magnetic flux is the number of lines of magnetic force that flow from one pole of the magnet to the other. For example, 500 gauss is equivalent to 500 lines of magnetic force passing through an area of one square centimeter.

The power of a magnet is very important. The strength of a magnet is measured by a gauss meter in gauss units (oersted) or by the iron-weight it can lift, which is more approximate.

IRON WEIGHT LIFT	GAUSS POWER
2 Pounds	500 - 600
5 Pounds	900 - 1250
25 Pounds	2500
50 Pounds	3500 - 4500

Magnets used in therapy are usually imprinted with north and south polarity labels and protected by a transparent top coating to help prevent chipping and breaking. The strength of a magnet is dependent on size, weight and the kind of material used. Iron lift is measured by the manufacturer using an electronic gauss meter or magnetometer (see Figure 6-1).

Therapists generally agree that magnets between 1000 to 3000 gauss surface power should be applied to large muscles or severe ailments, such as hands, back, shoulders, abdomen, arthritis, backache, paralysis, hips, knees, legs, feet or chronic diseases like rheumatism. The power of 500 gauss would more likely be used on more delicate parts like eyes, ears, nose, throat, etc., although relief from aching large muscles comes at lower power levels, as well. In the case of children, weaker magnets are usually recommended but it very much depends on the nature of the ailment.

Depth of magnetic field penetration is in direct relationship to the physical size (mass) of the magnet as well as gauss power—the larger the size the deeper the penetration. A small round neodymium magnet, even though 12,300 gauss, penetrates only two to three inches into the body; whereas, a 4"x6"x½" magnet of 1,000 gauss penetrates completely through the body or about 17 inches. Of course, the most appropriate magnet for

Figure 6-1   Gauss Ratings

Magnet Size	Manufacturer's Rating	Electronic Magnetometer Rating	
	(Interior gauss strength)	(gauss strength at surface of magnet)	(gauss strength at distance in inches)
4" x 6" x (1/2)" ceramic magnet	3950	900-1000	20 at 5.5"
2" x 5" x (1/2)" ceramic magnet	3950	900-1000	20 at 5.5"
2" x 1" x (3/8)" ceramic magnet	150	1250-1350	10 at 4.25"
2" plastic	2200 - 2450	250-275	10 at 2"
3" plastic	2200 - 2450	250-275	10 at 2-2.25"
Neodymium Super Magnet (small 1")	12300	3500	10 at 2.5

the particular illness should be used; on the other hand, almost any gauss strength utilizing negative polarity can be applied without fear of harm, according to Dr. Philpott. Some trial-and-error is necessary. One of the reasons some physicians may not appreciate magnetotherapy is because it is difficult to predict precisely when symptom relief might take place—in a matter of minutes, days or months. It depends very much on the patient's individual constitution, overall state of health, and, of course, the type and extent of illness. Practical experience provides a reasonable scale for healing periods. But even if it takes trial-and-error and time, as long as it is safe and patients get cured when they otherwise might not, the therapy seems appropriate.

A magnet can lose magnetism if subjected to repeated impact or heat at higher than 400 degrees centigrade, yet it is impervious to cold or boiling water. Magnetic devices should be removed when bathing to avoid the accumulation of perspiration or oil residues under the magnet that could develop rashes.

The greater the number of magnets, size and strength in a mattress, the more efficient the therapeutic effect. Covering material is also important. Wool has about 2 times the hydroscopic (water absorption) ability as that of cotton and 37 times that of polyester. Urethane is not fibriform and is without hydroscopic properties. So wool is most comfortable, followed by cotton. Humans emit about a glass of perspiration per night's sleep to maintain constant body temperature, but if sweating does not occur, the body warms and may prevent sound sleep. It is difficult to prove that magnetism can keep the body warm, but evidence indicates that energy levels increase which stimulate the body. Magnetic insoles, for example, in Eastern medicine are called the "second heart" because so many key acupuncture points are located in the soles of the feet that are able to stimulate the entire body.

Methodologies Differ Worldwide

It would be extremely beneficial if we could trade information between countries more easily and frequently. In this regard, the Japanese Ministry of Health and Welfare regulates magnetic devices. They specify that the strength of a magnetic curing device shall not be less than 500 gauss in flux density; some are 1600 gauss. Their clinical tests indicate that 500 gauss is the minimum for significant effect. Normally, they report that the higher the magnetic force, the better the results; but this is not always the case. Magnetic treatments are therapeutic in nature, and therefore can take longer for effect in contrast to a quick fix. The best advice, the Ministry states, is to be patient and to continue application until it has produced the desired effect without excessive concern for intensity. In most cases, an effect will be felt within a few days or a week. They say minimum of seven hours per day is advisable during the first stages, in the daytime or while sleeping. Dr. Bansal of India, on the other hand, elects to treat for much shorter durations but recommends sleeping on a pad the entire evening, which would be in line with the Japanese point-of-view. Differences may simply be in the strength and size of the magnets. The more powerful magnets may be used for much shorter duration.

In Japan, magnetic cure devices must be submitted—with clinical data—to the ministry for approval before being put on the market. The Japanese report that prolonged use, two or three months after a successful recovery, may cause symptoms to reappear in some cases. Resistance to magnetic stimulation may develop, an adaptation phenomenon observable with drug users as they adapt to certain levels of drug use. If one does become accustomed to magnetic treatment, he should discontinue use for a period of time or until symptoms of stress disappear or the original complaint recurs. Dr. Bansal, reports that in his practice the habituation factor involving stress may come about in a few weeks or months. This condition is reported to occur in users around the world when using simultaneous or south exposure in order to give the body time to balance its forces. A stressful condition can occur with the negative field as well for some people, at least initially until all toxins are thrown off. Barefoot believes that this is partly caused by the "sex without love" syndrome, meaning that magnetotherapy should be accompanied by nutritional love, in order to alleviate stressful symptoms and to achieve long-term success.

We know that as early as 1936, Davis and Rawls and, again, in 1938, Dr. Hansen, found in their investigations that magnets relieved sciatica, lower back pain, and joint and other bodily pains. Significantly, at that early date they found different effects for the north and south poles when applied to plants and animals. This was followed by additional research during the 1950's and 1970's, which demonstrated that the negative polarity was the healer and that which arrests infectious growth.

Purpose: To Eradicate Ignorance

The treatment protocols described here and used by many leaders in the field give the average user and the professional the most acceptable alternatives of how to apply this medicine. The purpose is to erase as much ignorance as possible and to demonstrate the safest methods for the benefit of new users and also for all those who continue to use magnetic fields.

This chapter describes how several of the long-term successful providers of permanent magnetic therapy practice this medicine and what the best methodologies might be. Everybody who uses magnets for health purposes ought to know at least these basic differences. Without further study, particularly long-range effects of various kinds of devices, definitive answers can not be given. We must draw conclusions from the knowledge of the most expert in the field at this time. It is too late to turn back. It is here. The federal government and the medical community have a responsibility to provide definitive answers now.

Explanation of Treatment Methods

The Simultaneous Polarity Methodology

$\mathbf{D}$r. H. L. Bansal, who has practiced magnetotherapy extensively in India, cites case studies along with the conditions and treatment methods that he recommends. His therapeutic methodology consists primarily of using both polarities (negative and positive) simultaneously, which is different from most American and Canadian usage. (A sampling of his methodology is shown in Exhibit 21 to give an idea of his approach)

Dr. Bansal claims success for many diseases and problems, including asthma and bronchitis, colic, constipation, corns, coughing, diabetes, diarrhea and dysentery, ear troubles, eczema, herpes and ringworm, epilepsy, epistaxis (nose bleeds), eye diseases, fissure and piles, flatulence, giddiness (vertigo), goiter, heart diseases, insect bite, jaundice, kidney infections, leucoderma, liver enlargement, lumbago, memory loss, mumps, migraine, nervousness, oralogy, orchitis, paralysis, pneumonia, polypus, psoriasis, sciatica, sinusitis, spondylitis, stones, swelling of feet, tonsillitis, tooth ache, tuberculosis, tumors, ulcer, urticaria, vomiting, and many specialized diseases of women and children. As you can see, this list covers just about everything. The whole Eastern philosophy is that magnetotherapy offers relief, if nothing else, for most diseases. Some of it may be psychosomatic or a combination of other medicines. Such vast claims question the credibility of this approach but Dr. Bansal insists that magnetotherapy strengthens the immune system and raises energy levels which allow the human body to fight off most diseases in a more efficient fashion.

Exhibit 21   Dr. H. L. Bansal Treatment Methodology

BACKACHE:
Lumbago, rheumatic pain, spondylitis, and slipped disk.
TREATMENT:
Pain in upper and lower back, apply north pole on upper portion, south pole on lower. Pain in right and left side, apply north pole on right and south pole on left.

HIGH OR LOW BLOOD PRESSURE:
Common symptoms are severe headache, vertigo, blurred vision, disturbed sleep.
TREATMENT:
For high blood pressure place high powered magnets on both palms of hands 5 - 6 minutes or medium power on for 10 minutes. For low blood pressure, same treatment for 15 - 20 minutes for high power and up to 30 minutes for medium power.

FRACTURES:
Pain and swelling.
TREATMENT:
Apply north pole to upper part of crack to soften and release calcium from the main bone; place south pole of a similar magnet on the lower part to draw fluid and calcium. Apply several times daily for 15 minutes or longer.

GOUT:
Excess uric acid in the blood is deposited as urates in the joints with swelling especially of the big toe. May be caused by chemical changes in the body during assimilation of proteins. It may be hereditary or occur from excess eating or drinking. Temper, fever, or headache may result.
TREATMENT:
A balanced diet, and avoid the use of alcohol and salt. Apply the north pole of the magnet over the top of the painful toe and the south pole below the toe.

HEADACHE:
Simple or bilious, hemicrania, migraine or neuralgia.
TREATMENT:
Trace the cause first if possible, advise rest and check blood pressure. Apply magnets on forehead or on both temples. A magnetic headbelt may be tied on for 15 - 20 minutes once or twice daily. High powered magnets may also be placed under the soles. (Note: Bansal does not specify polarity which can be extremely important when applying magnets to the head.)   *(Cont'd)*

Exhibit 21   Dr. H. L. Bansal Treatment Methodology (cont'd)

KNEE PAINS:
The most common sites for joint pain, feelings of heaviness, fatigue, stiffness, and swelling.
TREATMENT:
North pole of high powered magnet over the effected side of the right knee and the south pole on the left knee for 10-15 minutes or longer as needed.

PROSTATE ENLARGEMENT:
Prostate gland is sometimes enlarged in males usually over 50 years of age. Patient experiences pain in lower abdomen, restlessness, difficulty in passing urine or retention of urine. The gland lies at the neck of the bladder and may increase in size or shape to cause an obstruction of the urethra.
TREATMENT:
In some cases a catheter may have to be used to draw blood or an operation may be necessary. High powered magnets should be applied on both ends of the enlarged gland two or three times daily.

RHEUMATISM:
Inflammatory or degenerative infections of the fibrous textures of joints, muscles and other parts. May be accompanied by fever and pain.
TREATMENT:
Apply high powered magnets under palms if the upper part of the body is effected more, and under the soles if the lower part of the body is effected more.

SLEEPLESSNESS (INSOMNIA):
Most causes are anxiety, brooding, disturbance in the digestive or circulatory systems, excitement, anger, fear, strong stimulants, headaches, or the stress of family or work life.
TREATMENT:
Apply the south pole on the forehead for 10 to 15 minutes before bed for a week or so (magnetic mattresses and pillows are also effective).

Source: Dr. H. L. Bansal, RHMP, Homeopath and Magneto-therapist, President, All India Magnetotherapy Association, Director Indian Institute of Magnetotherapy. New Delhi, India 1990.

Duration of treatment and the period of relief varies from case to case and disease to disease. It depends, Dr. Bansal says, on such factors as

1) nature of the disease, 2) length of the illness, 3) age, 4) climatic conditions, 5) eating habits, 6) constitution 7) and response of the body. He says certain diseases like arthritis, spondylitis, sciatica, polio, paralysis, etc. do not yield to any system of treatment quickly and are often incurable; but, magnetic treatment does offer relief, usually in quicker fashion than most other therapies.

Bansal says that the more powerful magnets, in particular, should not be applied for more than five minutes at a time, with a gradual increase after susceptibility of the patient has been studied. Treatment beyond 10 minutes a day should only be extended upon expert advice, he advises. Some persons may feel a slight tingling sensation, others feel warmth or heaviness of head, dryness of tongue or throat, or an urge for passing urine, and some a slight giddiness or a degree of perspiration.

Certain other practitioners believe that if symptoms appear in a large number of persons, especially under short duration of treatment, the incorrect polarity is being used. In light of the adverse effects Bansal experiences with use of mixed polarities or south exposure and for such short intervals, it seems to reinforce further the differences of magnetic fields. And with magnetic negative field application also, toxins must be driven from the body; therefore, some of these same symptoms will occur initially until the system is cleaned out and balanced. Magnetic-X Corp., Canada, for example, that uses negative field application reports detoxification occurs in about one-third of cases, lasting hours or weeks and includes symptoms involving lack of energy, tingling, soreness, and sciatic nerve sensitivity. Some therapists recommend supplements such as 500 mg of calcium, halibut liver oil capsules, 400 i.u. vitamin D and 5000 i.u. of vitamin A daily to reduce symptoms by neutralizing toxin release. In order to ease the onset of symptoms, it is recommended to gradually increase the length of time one applies magnetotherapy from one or two hours per day up to a full night's application, plus supplements.

Single pole polarity as a methodology

Let us turn now to what Dr. Philpott prescribes. First, he wants us to take some precautions:

- Do not use magnets on abdomen during pregnancy or on a chest with a pacemaker or defibrillator.

- Do not use a magnetic bed 24 hours daily if ill because the adrenal function may be suppressed causing slow energy recovery.

- Do not use on abdomen 60 to 90 minutes following meals in order to allow peristalsis (digestive process) to take place.

- Do not use positive energy unless under medical supervision because the positive fields can overstimulate brain activity, producing seizures, insomnia, addiction, hyperactivity, and hallucinations and also promote growth of tumors and micro-organisms.

Routine Preventive Care

Total body treatment is preferable. Otherwise, 30 to 60 minutes before retiring, apply the negative polarity to the back of the head at the base of the skull; at the spleen to the left side low back junction of the rib cage and abdomen; to the thymus-anterior mid chest; to the neck lymph nodes at the upper and anterior of neck under the chin. Upon retiring apply to crown of head all night.

Philpott also recommends drinking a minimum of two eight ounce glasses of magnetic water daily. During a flu epidemic, drink magnetic water every four hours for prevention and relief.

Exhibit 22 presents a sampling of Philpott's approach. The methodology essentially consists of 15 to 30 minute applications for most ailments and sleeping on a magnetic pad for several hours or more each night. All applications are of the negative polarity. For any serious matter, people should consult their own doctor and also examine Dr. Philpott's manual directly and in detail.

Dr. Philpott says that there are several valuable applications in regard to the positive polarity, but that one should always apply the negative polarity afterward to counter any potential for addiction, seizures, micro-organisms and parasite activity, inflammation, tissue oxygen deficit, and other side effects already enumerated. Drug consumption can become more potent or effective with the use of the negative polarity so that there is a need to reduce or discontinue the use of medication after a period.

Exhibit 22   Dr. Philpott's Protocol for Magnetotherapy

The following is a summary description and sampling of the types of ailments treated by Dr. Philpott. All applications are of the negative (north) magnetic polarity:

ACNE
> Apply directly to the area and check for food allergies, especially dairy products

ALCOHOLISM
> Apply to liver, pancreas, diaphragm

ALLERGIC REACTIONS
> Nasal and sinus, place above, below or the side of the area to pull fluid

GASTROINTESTINAL
> Preferable to wait one or two hours after eating because the motility of the stomach and intestine is reduced while exposed to north pole magnetic fields

EYE REACTIONS
> Fifteen to 30 minutes two or more times daily placed directly over eyes with the exception of glaucoma where magnets are placed several inches to the side of the eye to draw fluid away to relieve pressure

ARTHRITIS
> If inflamed, apply directly, otherwise treat two to three inches to the side to avoid drawing additional fluid to the area which can possibly add pain

ASTHMA
> Treatment is mildly constricting so may increase acute bronchospasm. Apply to tolerable limits, remove and reapply frequently to relieve edema

ATHEROSCLEROSIS (hardening of arteries)
> Cells and walls are normally negative poled. All blood elements are of the same polarity to prevent sticking and clumping. When pH drops lower than normal (7.4 pH), fatty acids (positive) begin to stick to the walls of arteries (negative) to reduce blood vessel elasticity and to narrow passageways.

(Cont'd)

Exhibit 22   Dr. Philpott's Protocol for Magnetotherapy (cont'd)

BACKACHE
>   Apply directly to area and sleep on a magnetic pad. If discomfort continues, bladder or kidney infections should be considered.

BED WETTING, BLADDER PROBLEMS, INSECT BITES
>   Use recommended maintenance program applied directly to part of body affected.

BRAIN ALLERGIES
>   Caused by hypersensitivity to food, chemicals, etc. can produce swelling in brain resulting   in fatigue, poor concentration, head ache, depression, lethargy, and hyperactivity. Apply to CNS, forehead, temporal areas and the spine.

BREASTS (LUMPS)
>   Apply negative fields directly across lymph system.

BRONCHITIS
>   Apply to chest.

BURNS
>   Apply negative fields as soon as possible before tissue deterioration occurs. Can resolve blisters. In stove burns, apply quickly and normal pink color will return.

CATARACTS
>   30 - 60 minutes three times daily application of negative polarity.

CEREBELLAR VESTIBULAR SYSTEM (CVS)
>   Apply to low occipital area at upper neck.

CHRONIC FATIGUE SYNDROME (CFS)
>   Total body treatment.

CONJUNCTIVITIS
>   Place directly on eye.

CONSTIPATION
>   Apply to liver, gall bladder, and colon areas.

CRAMPS, MENSTRUAL
>   Apply directly to cramped areas.

DEPRESSION, ANXIETY
>   Can be helped by raising melatonin from magnetic fields. A therapeutic bright light to the eyes at the beginning of each day may also help.

DIABETES
>   Refer to, **Victory over Diabetes: A Bio-ecologic Triumph** by W. H. Philpott, M.D. Magnetic bed plus food testing medically supervised are recommended.

DIARRHEA, DIZZINESS
>   Can be helped by negative polarity application.

Exhibit 22   Dr. Philpott's Protocol for Magnetotherapy (cont'd)

DRY EYE
   30 minutes daily or several times daily as needed.
EAR ACHE
   Apply to ear, throat, neck, forehead.
ELECTROMAGNETIC INTERFERENCE
   Apply negative to offset disordering influence.
FRACTURE
   When bone is broken it becomes two separate magnets which repel each other. Application of a strong field overrides the weaker of the bones and healing takes place.
GOUT
   Same as for arthritis.
PMS (PREMENSTRUAL SYNDROME)
   Whole body application is recommended.
SCAR TISSUE, SORE THROATS, SPRAINS OR STRAINS, URINARY PROBLEMS, WARTS, MOLES, SKIN LESIONS, ETC.
   Apply directly to problem area, or if internal, use total body treatment.

(Dozens of other ailments and treatments are described in the manual.)

Source: Biomagnetic Handbook: A Guide to Medical Magnets, The Energy Medicine of Tomorrow, William H. Philpott, M.D. and Sharon Taplin, Enviro-Tech Products, Choctaw, OK, 73020

Symptoms of over-medication are more likely to appear when magnetotherapy is applied to the overall body because toxins are released and metabolism improves. The need for medication will be reduced by using either polarity. A case with which I am familiar that occurred just a few months ago illustrates this phenomenon. The person slept on a magnetic pad for two weeks and was able to cut his medication in half in that short period and felt considerably better. However, he developed stress symptoms so he discontinued use. He has been instructed to use to use the pad only an hour or two each night until his toxicity has cleared so that he will not only feel better but will be able to eliminate stress symptoms gradually and will also be able to reduce or possibly cut out the need for pain killing medication. A number of body builders, weightlifters and Olympic contenders, who are sleeping on magnetic pads, have completely eliminated the need to take aspirin and more potent drugs to relieve pain due to strenuous muscle strain. They have also increased energy levels and body strength.

Research Implications and Clinical Observations for Magneto-Electric Energy Therapy

Dr. William H. Philpott points out the great need for studies in many areas using controls to test efficacy of the negative magneto-electric fields (technical terminology for permanent magnetic fields.) Some of these are listed below with a sampling of clinical observations. Testing of positive magneto-electric fields consistently showed a pattern of acidosis compared to a relief of acidosis and symptoms with the negative fields. More comparative tests are advised. Controlled tests using permanent magnets for these chronic ailments could readily answer the question of magnetic field effectiveness in fairly short order. Tests could include the following areas already observed by Philpott as worthy of consideration (See Appendix I for additional Research Needs):

1. Degree of growth hormone use during sleep. (Fingernail and hair growth increased considerably.)
2. Degree of intactness of the pH buffer system during exposure separately to the negative and positive magneto-electric fields. (Negative observed to relieve acidosis and no evidence of over-alkalinization.)
3. Degree of reversibility of fibrous organized material in arteries and veins after a blood clot. (Post-birth blood clot in groin completely disappeared.)
4. Degree of reversibility of insoluble gels when exposed to a negative magneto-electric field. (Symptoms of cardiac and brain atherosclerosis have been observed to disappear after six to eight weeks of nightly exposure.)
5. Degree of resolubility of kidney stones with a negative magneto-electric field. (Kidney stones have been observed to disappear.)

6.	Degree of resolution of calcium deposits in inflamed tissues. (Deposits around joints observed to be dissolved. Question of what degree of resolution and length of time it takes to occur.)

7.	Degree of antibiotic effect of microorganism infection. (Relief from toothache and periodontal abscess exuding puss within 10 minutes and no infection after four days. Relief from candidiasis of the vagina and fungal infection remission.)

8.	Degree of oxygenation and oxidation metabolism of tissues. (Patient diagnosed with arteriosclerosis of the heart was given EDTA chelation and eventually cardiac bypass surgery. In spite of this, he continued to have severe heart pain, mental dysfunction and difficulty walking. With magnetotherapy, the heart pain was relieved in 20 minutes, and within a month other symptoms improved, most likely explained by oxygenation.)

9.	Degree of control of brain exposure (psychotic condition from pesticides and petro-chemicals alleviated, and person returned to same condition by placing negative magneto-electric field of magnets bitemporally. Person depressed and socially withdrawn from eating wheat relieved of symptoms. Person with post-brain injury grand mal seizures became seizure free. Also temporal lobe confusion type seizures eliminated).

10.	Degree of melatonin production by the pineal gland during sleep with the crown of the head exposed (patients observed to sleep more soundly and ceased having sleep apnea, considered a melatonin deficiency).

Miracle of Magnetic Water

Both Dr. Bansal and Dr. Philpott are advocates for the use of magnetic water. Bansal says magnetic water reduces excess acidity and bile in the digestive system and regulates movement of the bowels, expelling all accumulation of poisonous matter; it soothes the nerves and helps clear arteries. Magnetic water can be used for washing swollen or sore eyes, wounds, and for eczema. Bansal says the north pole is excellent for the eyes and that "there is nothing like daily washing with magnetized water." Barefoot states that the hydroxylation of water by magnetism creates a digestive environment that stimulates the absorption of minerals.

In a typical case, Mary Louise J., Washington, D.C., (Jan 1992) complained of problems of indigestion and extreme nervous condition and stress that plagued her for many months while her doctor was unable to bring relief. A user of magnetic water suggested she try drinking four ounces of negative magnetic water twice daily—prepared from placing a plain glass of water over a negative oriented 900 gauss magnet for at least 30 minutes. After several days, she reported that her digestive tract felt marvelous, she slept better, and felt much calmer. She asked her husband who also had sleeping and stress problems to try it. As a true skeptic he was reluctant, joking as he drank the magnetized water, "Here goes, my whole life is going to change!" Surprisingly, for everybody involved, in short order his symptoms also were eliminated. Hundreds of anecdotal case histories may not change minds or prove anything, yet all anybody has to do is to try this almost cost-free treatment and appraise it themselves. There are just too many people who experience results for there not to be an effect, and, of course, results well beyond placebo.

Magnetic water can be made by simply placing a glass or plastic container over a magnet of your choice (negative or positive or both polarities) for at least five minutes, preferably longer. Bansal uses 3000 gauss strength for 12 - 24 hours for a quart of water. But 500 or 800 gauss strength can also be used. He prescribes three doses daily—two ounces for adults and one ounce for adolescents. Philpott says it only takes 15 minutes to magnetize water and he recommends drinking two, eight ounce glasses daily. Other liquids can also be magnetized the same way—milk, fruit juices, beer, and body oils. Magnetized olive oil is reported excellent for treating gout and rheumatism.

You may have heard of the phenomenon where hundreds of thousands of men, women and children line up daily, sometimes in lines as long as a mile to fill plastic containers with a miracle water from the Jesus Chahin's well in Tlacote, Mexico to cure or relieve everything from AIDS and cancer to obesity and high cholesterol. For some reason, the curative power requires "movements" of the water from one metal tank to another. Chahin says that this is light water that weighs less than H_2O, and "scientists can study it all they want but they'll never find the secret." The local bishop is recovering from cancer by using it, and some of the staff of President Carlos Salinas Gortari reportedly use it. Magic Johnson, the famous U.S. basketball star with AIDS arrived with a dozen local boys to help him cart off 150 gallons of water to his plane.

We know of the healing power of baths at such famous places as Lourdes, France, and Sedona, Arizona, and other locales around the world where magnetic energy is reportedly at higher levels. Could the Tlocote water simply be magnetized? Water running over the Niagara Falls is magnetized. One of the best ways to magnetize water naturally is to let it run through about 30 feet of sand where it will come out negatively poled from the quartz crystals in the sand and become loaded with oxygen that will kill germs, build body strength, and improve the immune system. Structured (light or magnetized) water changes its properties of temperature, density, surface tension, viscosity, and electrical conductivity. Any physics student knows that chemicals change weight under the influence of magnetic fields. So does water. More hydroxyl (OH^-) ions are created to form calcium bicarbonate and other alkaline molecules. Perhaps all Magic Johnson had to do was place a pitcher of plain water over a strong negatively oriented magnet in his kitchen to get similar, perhaps better results. The water he carried back begins to lose strength in several days (if refrigerated somewhat longer), dissipated naturally by the oxygenation of the air around it. In short, its a waste to carry that much water back home and unnecessarily costly.

Bob Barefoot reports that cancer is virtually unknown to the Hopi Indians of Arizona and the Hunza of Northern Pakistan, as long as they drink from their local water supply which is rich in rubidium and potassium in the case of the Hopi water and rich in caesium and potassium for the Hunza. The salts of rubidium and caesium have extremely alkaline metal ions that can enter cells through large nutrient channels, raising body pH and killing cancer cells under rich oxygen conditions. The decomposing dead cells provide nutrients for renewed health and normal DNA replication, Barefoot informs us. Magnetized water can have similar effects. Normal water has a pH level of about 7, while magnetized water can reach 9.2 pH after exposure to a 7000 gauss strength magnet, enough to kill cancer cells. (Barefoot and Reich)

Magnetized water has many uses not only for our bodies but for solving a variety of mechanical problems which tend to reinforce its effectiveness. Water pipes, for example, need to be scrubbed periodically to clean the inner walls of salt deposits that restrict the flow of liquid. Magnetized water causes such hard deposits to fall off, dissolving in the water, and either lessening further concentrations of deposits or arresting them completely. Similar results have been obtained in keeping automobile radiators and other types of equipment and devices clean. Several companies promote magnetic kits that improve automobile performance and gas mileage when placed on gas lines and other specified points to enhance gas burning efficiency. People using these kits express how much more smoothly their autos function.

Enviro-Tech Products, Choctaw, Oklahoma, manufactures different kits called fuel energizers that clamp to auto fuel lines to change the molecular structure of the negatively charged fuel and oxygen so that these naturally opposing molecules attract each other for combustion efficiency. The fuel energizer puts a strong positive charge into the fuel which attracts the negative oxygen which they claim can improve gas mileage 10 to 20 percent. Certainly, the auto industry and environmentalists ought to explore this in greater detail.

The National Safety Association (NSA), among other companies promote products made of magnetic substances that eliminate deposits in pipes and other mechanical vessels. Magnetic water assists in dissolving pipe line debris in tubes and machinery, as well as enhancing the growth rate of agricultural products. (U.S. Dept. of Energy; Busch; Collins)

Technically, magnetism works because it increases the speed of sedimentation of suspended particles in water (and other liquids) and enhances conductivity and the process of ionization or dissociation of atoms and molecules into electrically charged particles. (*New Scientist*, June 1992)

Japanese Treatment Philosophy

The Japanese are in agreement with the U.S. on the overuse of drugs in both societies. They too say that the over-dependance on chemicals has contributed to ill health and to the extensive flood of processed foods on our tables. The time has changed since chemicals were considered the cure for everything. The Japanese believe that the secret of good health very much revolves around good blood circulation, therefore their deep concern for magnetotherapy.

The Japanese experience a longer life span than Americans and statistically fewer problems of overall health, even though they live in a highly stressed work environment of strict work hours, compressed transportation and housing, and strong allegiance to rules. Their good health is not simply due to diets of less fat or sound nutrition, but a culture of positive mental attitudes, a variety of exercises, including yoga and magnetotherapy. Ten percent (about 10 million) of Japanese sleep or sit on magnetic pads and another 20 million treat their bodies with magnets of many sorts. Perhaps the world has something to learn from them about the benefits of magnetotherapy, and they from researchers in the U.S. on how to use magnetism more effectively and more safely. We can all benefit from such mutual experiences.

The Japanese realize that many ailments are an absolute mystery as to cause, yet magnetotherapy plays a major role in relief. Chronic fibrositis of the shoulder is one example. This is an enduring stiffness or pain in the shoulder muscles, more common among women, with no apparent etiological cause, such as a local infection of the cervical vertebrae or shoulder joints or a disorder in the integral organs (stomach, intestines, liver, lungs), but magnetic fields have proved quite effective in relieving symptoms. Key punchers and factory workers and other persons in occupations doing routine work are the primary victims. Repetitious labor creates the bulk of victims. The U.S. and other nations have hundreds of thousands of cases of stiffness of body parts and ailments such as rheumatism, uncus rheumatic pain in the chest, backache, recurring headaches, dulling of senses, casual dizziness, insomnia, chronic constipation, and weariness. These are all disorders that the Japanese treat with magnetism.

Chronicity of pain (continually re-occurring over the long-term), another serious problem that has alternating periods of remission and relapse, is of such an elusive nature for symptoms that it defies detection by clinical tests, but is precisely a candidate for magnetotherapy. Doctors may not be able to help or even diagnose the problem; on the other hand, medical checks cannot diagnose magnetic deficiency either. And it is not simply a matter of trial-and-error because with proper training it is possible to identify otherwise elusive disorders. Physicians seem to hate trial-and-error treatments because they are time-consuming and make them look like they don't know what they're doing. Yet doctors should be able to identify problems readily without a lot of trial-and-error, if they are well grounded in these diseases and the cures that apply. Trying to find out a particular patient's constitution, the relative strength of his immune system, and generally what makes him tick is part of successful treatment, yet it has been too long neglected in America because prevention has not been one of our chief priorities or money-makers.

People are healthy, unhealthy or ill. Unhealthy people are the most likely candidates for magnetotherapy because the doctor can readily identify such things as—headache, lassitude, and constipation—and therefore can prescribe specific treatments. But some patients go from better to worse without apparent cause. It takes a knowledgeable, caring doctor to be able to recognize that there is a striking relationship between magnetic deficiency syndrome, for example, and so called autonomic ataxic imbalance or general malaise complaint syndrome, among other elusive ailments.

Autonomic ataxic syndrome occurs when the autonomic nervous system—that governs the internal organs—fails. The human body has two main nervous systems called central and autonomic. We are less familiar with the autonomic nervous system which is especially responsible for the automatic, unconscious regulation of bodily functions and internal organs. It functions in the sympathetic and the parasympathetic modes. The sympathetic system enhances physiological activity, while the parasympathetic generally has the opposite or different effect. One stimulates the heart, the other suppresses it. Acute stress can cause the system to fail, resulting in autonomic ataxic imbalance. Magnetic deficiency syndrome, the Japanese believe overlaps with these symptoms. The doctor or patient is encouraged to try magnetism and observe results.

Another ailment with which Japanese health authorities have found excellent results from applying magnetotherapy is chronic constipation relief. It occurs in either of two opposite bowel conditions: atonic and spastic. In atonic, food residuals are carried down the digestive tract too slowly, and so are excessively deprived of water due to slackened vermicular motion of the bowel. This causes the feces to become hardened. In the spastic condition, bowel contractions are excessive, so that food residuals cannot move smoothly, thus remaining too long in the intestines, becoming dehydrated, and resulting in blockage of the large intestine. A magnetic belt corrects the condition time-after-time, involving a series of magnets with gauss strength in the range 550 - 850. A mixture of polarities has been used, positive and bipolar. The Japanese claim a very high success rate (in the 70 percent range), much better than drug therapy. Furthermore, this is not trial-and-error. They know the symptoms and they know the cure. American physicians could very well benefit from this experience. Again we are experiencing the effect of hydroxylation from the magnetic belt that assists the intestine to absorb minerals, such as magnesium—"Mother Natures" laxative.

Magnetic treatment works very well for backaches. It is not, however, recommended for ruptured disc or conditions inherent in the internal organs. If one has chronic stiffness or pain of fibrositis of no apparent cause, then magnetotherapy is advisable. The Japanese inform us not to rely solely on magnetic treatment. Exercise, hot bath, and good nutrition should always supplement magnetotherapy.

Another ailment—sciatica neuralgia—has eluded our medical profession as to where and how it originates in the organism. Also trigeminal neuralgia—sharp piercing pain that runs through the cheek or jaw and most common in women in their 40's and 50's—has been found elusive to cause. Not only the Japanese, but also American doctors have experienced remarkable relief from symptoms with magnetotherapy. On the other hand, gastritis or gastric ulcer is not helped very much, but relief does occur. Dr. Pawluk states he has had success on gastritis with small magnets over acupuncture points.

A number of research studies have been conducted by the Japanese which certainly should have some validity with the American medical community and the NIH and FDA. One, reported by the Ministry of Health and Welfare, involved 116 patients with severe fibrositis of the shoulders. Subjects wore 700 gauss magnetic (bipolar) necklaces for a specified period and their self-reported relief from chronic pain was graded according to the following scale:

1. *Outstanding*
2. *Greatly satisfactory*
3. *Satisfactory*
4. *Slightly satisfactory*
5. *No improvement*

*After 10 days, 51 answered outstanding, 67 greatly
satisfactory, 38 satisfactory, 10 slightly satisfactory, and 0
no improvement. The satisfactory or better answers
amounted to 94 percent.*

*Another study of 212 patients with backache, but
without discovery of problems in the lumbar vertebrae,
were asked to wear magnetic belts consisting of 24 magnets
of 800 gauss each. In this case, 62.7 percent to 72.1
percent were in the success range of outstanding and
greatly satisfactory, with a 95 percent confidence ratio.
Additional studies showed that for most ailments involving
pain relief, the favorable response rates averaged around
70 percent or proven success in 7 out of 10 cases.**

In general, many Japanese doctors are not much different than their
American counterparts who ridicule magnetotherapy or simply walk away
from it with a wry smile, mostly because they have never understood it or
tried it. This attitude or "conspiracy of silence" then translates over to the
general population. They fail to connect or have no desire to associate
conventional medical knowledge to magnetotherapy. Ostentation and
complacency still prevail on the assumption that it is just a lot of folk
therapy without acceptable principles on which a doctor can prescribe
treatment. Yet the science here is that each patient's constitution and state
of health is different and so requires some trial-and-error and deep concern
with his or her problem that may involve much more than a physical disease
easily identified. Magnetotherapy treats the total human immune system,
undeniably raises the pH, and accelerates the cells and body energy better
and more safely than any host of drugs (Barefoot and Reich; Philpott). It
lets the body heal itself.

Some still attribute the high success rate to psychological effects.
Yet, as the studies have shown, the placebo effect occurs in less than 17
percent of cases. A series of Japanese studies, as reported earlier, show
that psychosomatic conditions occur in only the small percentage range of
6.3%, 11.9%, 17%, 20%, 23%, and an average of 15 percent.
Furthermore, based on controlled studies published in Japan and the U.S.,
FDA analysis sets the value of psychological effect at 13 percent. The 70

---

* The italicized text refers to more complex information.

percent to 90 percent therapeutic effect is extraordinarily high compared to other medicines and better than the greater majority of drugs and chemicals when safety is taken into account.

The Japanese report no evidence of any side effects from magnetotherapy outside the habituation factor. Workers in a magnetic manufacturing factory were surveyed and medically checked, finding no significant abnormalities—subjective or objective—attributable to the magnetic environment. Blood tests and urinalysis fell within the normal statistical range. However, the effect of different polarities and long-term implications of infectious cell growth were not thoroughly investigated.

From the Japanese experience, two of 100 persons may experience a dullness or slight dizziness after using magnetotherapy the first few days. Intermittent use, until one becomes adapted to magnetism, is recommended. Adverse symptoms will gradually disappear and a therapeutic effect will come about.

Most therapists suggest that infants and pregnant women should avoid exposure to magnetic fields to be on the safe side; however, there are no reports of ill effects. For any medicine, the prevailing rationale is that extreme care should be taken with infants and embryos and that it is better to refrain from using anything not necessary, regardless of how safe it might be.

We have a lot to learn from the Japanese and other nations and they from us. We have begun to share and honor each other's knowledge. For society's benefit, we need to gather more and newer research to find definitive answers on which we can agree and improve each nation's health. The protocol for treatment within these pages and the American and Canadian knowledge of the effect of different polarities will certainly benefit the Japanese. On the other hand, their wide acceptance of the therapy may encourage greater use in the U.S. After all it is difficult to believe that 30 million users have been duped into feeling good.

Chapter 7

Nutrition, Drugs and Magnetotherapy

The Question of Choice

Choice and You

Treatment for most diseases and ailments as prescribed by professional and licensed magnetotherapists involves common methodologies of little mystery or complexity. Too many doctors hide diagnoses and treatments in complex language and drug prescriptions. In magnetotherapy, very fundamental procedures emerge that all of us can understand. Importantly, however, for any serious illness the patient should see a medical doctor and evaluate the advice given very carefully, perhaps with a second opinion. But, the ailing individual should not be afraid to consider additional methods of treatment.

As a matter of course, if your doctor does not provide choice of options and alternatives, he has failed to do his job in the best possible fashion. It is his responsibility to become knowledgeable with all types of successful treatments and it is important that you also become familiar with as many of them as possible. Your life may depend on it.

The case histories described in the next couple of chapters cover only a limited number of ailments and treatments but represent a fair sampling so that one can understand the scope of this medicine. If the ailment is not mentioned, procedures for magnetotherapy are sufficiently common to fit most problems. It may be scorned by some because it so simple.

"All disease is biochemical," says Dr. Derrick Lonsdale, a former Cleveland clinical pediatrician. "The trick is to find the biochemical that fits the lock." However, chemical change can come from many sources including magnetic application. Magnetic fields enhance body chemistry in one respect by providing increased energy by means of cyclotronic resonance. Magnetotherapy improves the ability of the body's immune system to generate defensive cells to fight off disease. Better than any pharmacist, the body's own system can find the cure or "magic bullet" when strong and healthy. Why do some people in the same household, same environment and diet, get sick and others do not? One answer is a more viable immune system, made stronger by higher energy levels from various sources. The body then becomes its own pharmacist.

Threat of Invasive Procedures

Surely the public needs to be cautious of dangerous drugs, invasive chemotherapy and radiation treatments, as well as unnecessary tests. The American Cancer Society found that "the side effects of cancer chemotherapy can cause more anxiety and distress than the disease itself", as described by Jean Heimlich (wife of the famous physician of the "Heimlich method") in her fascinating book **What Your Doctor Won't Tell You**. Long-term effects include damage to the heart, loss of fertility and increased risk of developing a second cancer. A surgical biopsy—a procedure to detect cancer in its earliest stages—may contribute to the spread of cancer. She informs us that when one patient asked his doctor what chemotherapy would do for him, the blunt answer was,"It will either cure you or kill you." One in three Americans gets cancer and only 50 percent live as long as five years after these so-called conventional treatments. That record is dismal and we ought to be ashamed of it.

Of the more than one million new cases of cancer each year, only about eleven thousand infected with advanced disease can be cured. If this improbable choice for curing were routinely offered in the doctor's office, the $100 billion a year cancer industry would be out of business, says Heimlich. Those who work in the industry—a greater number than those who have cancer—would lose their jobs. But economics is just one factor. Your doctor doesn't tell you the alternatives because he either doesn't know or he doesn't want to know. When you call the NCI Hotline, they will tell you alternative treatments have been tested in the laboratory and have been found to have no tumor-inhibiting effect. Case closed.

Information Brief

Causes of Cancer

According to the National Cancer Institute, 30 percent of cancers are due to tobacco, 35 percent to diet, and most of the rest to radiation, chemical exposure, alcohol, and other factors mostly preventable. But we push roughly equivalent amounts of money into tobacco advertizing and cancer research and also believe we can't influence proper diet, says Neal D. Barnard, M.D. president of the Physicians Committee for Responsible Medicine. Only one in five women knows that breast cancer is linked to fatty diets. Personal stories of heroism against cancer and high-tech research efforts cloud the central issue that cancer is preventable, says Barnard.

Source: **Physicians Committee for Responsible Medicine**, Neal D. Barnard, M.D., *Journal Health, Washington Post,* January 14, 1992.

Jean Heimlich says that the American Cancer Society, the world's richest private charity with an annual budget of $150 million, is aligned with the AMA, Cancer Inc., and pharmaceutical and insurance company lobbyists who say that the proponents of unproven methods deceive patients and their families with false promises and exaggerated claims. For this reason, they respond, consumer protection laws are necessary to restrict sale of "worthless health products" to the vulnerable public. And they maintain a blacklist. But let us recall, Heimlich says, that the Supreme Court in 1914 stated that every human being of adult and sound mind has the right to determine what shall be done with his own body, embedded in the "right to privacy" clause of the Constitution.

Heimlich recounts a case of a woman who had enough of drugs. "When they started to draw black marks on my ribs," the woman said, "to radiate them, I said that I had enough as a guinea pig and insisted on going home." She returned for treatment at the Miami hospital where she first started her examination, but they gave her stronger chemotherapy drugs and Valium and Compazine to counteract nausea and vomiting. Her body couldn't take it any longer. She developed pneumonia, her lungs collapsed and they sent her home to die. But like Dr. Bernie Siegal's "exceptional patients who refuse to be victims," whom physicians consider "difficult or uncooperative," she said she wasn't ready to die and wished to try some alternatives. Learning that Laetrile was not a drug but a food substance made from apricot seeds that could be purchased at a health food store, she incorporated the Laetrile diet of fresh fruits and vegetables and raw vegetable juices into her routine. She is now also receiving chelation therapy—a slow drip that includes Laetrile, Vitamin C, calcium, magnesium, zinc, and live-cell therapy. With this combination, she now feels healthier than she did before she had cancer.

Magnetotherapy is even more effective than chelation therapy, according to Dr. Philpott who has eliminated a variety of skin cancers. Dr. Harry Park cites a case of a man from Iowa whose doctors said had about three months to live. He was diagnosed with a large tumor about one-half the size of a fist on his right liver lobe due to spreading carcinoma. His visit to the Mayo Clinic stipulated that nothing further could be done. He was then referred to Dr. Park in January of 1993. Dr. Park instructed him to rest on a 12 inch solid negative magnetic oriented bed for eight hours per day for one week, then sleep with his head between a negative magnetic board.

After three months when further X-rays were taken, the tumor had been eliminated and there were no signs of carcinoma. This case was confirmed by both radiologists and a neurologist before and after. It was not spontaneous remission. Other cases are cited by Dr. Park.

In respect to radiation therapy and chemotherapy, these methods are also used on children. Because of such treatments, those with leukemia have a chance at a longer life yet a greater chance of developing bone cancer later. Dr. Orlando J. Martelo, hematologist/oncologist of the University of Cincinnati Medical Center, calls the results of cures with present chemotherapy drugs "unacceptably low." Nevertheless, in breast cancer, he says, "We cannot cure patients with metastatic cancer, but with chemotherapy we can extend their lives three or four years." But six British cancer researchers dispute the claim that chemotherapy prolongs survival, contending that "survival may even have been shortened in some patients given chemotherapy."

In regards to radiation therapy, a 1993 study found that patients in 28 percent of the cases were never told of improper amounts, according to the Nuclear Regulatory Commission. "People should not relinquish the basic right to know if unnecessary harm has been done to them," remarked Senator John Glenn of Ohio. Widespread misuse of radiation therapy, including cases involving serious injury and death have been reported. Over 20 million radiation therapy procedures are conducted in the U.S. every year, while 1.1 million new cases of cancer are reported annually and about half treated by radiation. In 23 states, operators of radiation equipment are not required to be certified. Government regulation is inadequate and almost unenforceable behind the closed doors of medical offices. Greater emphasis should be placed on the patient and his family taking charge of their own health and lives.

Allen Oseroff, Associate Professor of Dermatology at the New England Medical Center in Boston, reported in Science News, January 19, 1989, that existing cancer treatments "are all different and they are all lousy, so you pick the one with the least side effects." Which would you choose, chemotherapy that takes months, even a year or more, during which you can expect to lose your hair or become debilitated—or a Vitamin-C "drip," Laetrile, chelation "drip," or magnetotherapy whose only side effects are an energy boost? With only partially effective alkaloid pharmaceuticals, Oseroff says, we are poisoning our systems.

Exhibit 23   Erratic Drug Testing

Since the late 1960's, the Church of Scientology has waged a war on psychiatrists and drug medications—early targets included Valium (diazepam), an anti-anxiety drug, and Ritalin (methylphenidate), a stimulant used to treat hyperactivity in children. Now they have petitioned the FDA to remove Prozac from the market but without result. Yet the FDA may be more receptive to a petition filed by Public Citizen (a Ralph Nader consumer group) to require Eli Lily to beef up its suicide warnings on Prozac's label. When a powerful drug that affects the mind becomes popular, its heyday is followed by "the appreciation that there is no free lunch," Public Citizen says.

The Journal of Clinical Psychopharmacology in 1988 reported suicidal thoughts with other drugs as well, including Desipramine, Norpramine, and Pertofrane. Of course, suicidal thoughts and deeds are more common in depressed people than in the general population, but the rate with these drugs is exceptionally high.

The world's most widely prescribed sleeping pill (seven million Americans take it) Halcion was banned by the British government in October 1991, after it was shown to cause a much higher incidence of depression and memory loss than expected. The Upjohn Co. did not make all the data available when it received FDA approval in the early 70's. Ian Oswald, professor of psychiatry at Edinburgh University, Scotland, states that Halcion has an entirely unorthodox range of actions on the brain that Upjohn never admitted.

A problem exists with generic drugs as well. In 1992, twenty generic drug company executives and five FDA employees were convicted or pleaded guilty to charges of fraud and racketeering, obstruction of justice, receiving illegal gratuities, and speeding approval of new drugs and improper testing of drugs. Judge John R. Hargrove said, "cutting corners is ... tremendously dangerous. There is virtually no testing of some products ... and they are thrown out on the market." And now we also see illegal and unsafe herbal drugs from Mexico entering the U.S. to be used mostly by poor Americans who can't afford regular health care.

Drugs affect young children and damage our pocket books as well. Congressmen Ted Weiss, of New Jersey, recently lashed out at the FDA for allowing the billion dollar drug industry to market antihistimines for colds when all the studies show that they are not effective for this purpose. These products have been marketed since the early 70's without any positive effect on the nation's health—a national disgrace of a system primarily seeking profit that has gone awry. These are just some of the ways to cut health care costs by billions of dollars and improve health at the same time.

Source: *The Harvard Health Letter*, October 1991, Vol. 16; *Washington Post*, October 3, 1991; author.

New things are happening in the science of magnetic fields that may allow us to cut down on dangerous radiation treatment. Experiments show that cancer cells can be picked out of bone marrow with magnetic beads, as one example. Engineers at Dartmouth University have developed a new technique for magnetically stripping cancer cells out of bone marrow by using upwards of a million tiny magnetic beads, each coated with a monoclonal antibody that binds to cell surface antigens typical of tumor cells but not of normal cells. When the marrow is passed through a series of powerful magnets, the beads are pulled out and cancer cells with them. The success of this procedure could save one from the agony of having bone marrow stripped, cancer cells then irradiated in the bone and, finally, cancer-free marrow replaced, as in the case of former Senator Paul Tsongas. Several medical centers are working on the new technique. In other experiments, at least two centers have been successful in using magnetic separation to treat childhood neuroblastoma.

Science also may be closer to proving that unwanted cancer cells can be destroyed by negative magnetic fields, rather than the need to strip cells. If magnets can pull unwanted cells out, they can change cell composition. Dr. Robert O. Becker's studies show that the permanent (steady state) magnet is strong enough to halt mitosis in malignant cells. Walter Rawls, in the July, 1989, National Medical Association Journal, reported how magnets can kill cancer cells in 96 hours. Dr. Philpott verifies how the negative fields restore proper balance of acid/alkaline pH in the body to arrest cancer growth. The health of the colon, for example, depends on proper pH. Good and bad bacteria flourish in alkaline colon, but if too acidic, the bad bacteria outnumber the good. Magnetotherapy raises the pH; good nutrition keeps it there. They work hand-in-hand, used together or before or after one another.

Diets, Supplements and the Mind

Diet and Change

Most cures for serious disease must involve the whole body. This is the prevalent point of view for long-term healing. A healthy body has an immune system that can destroy cancer cells and prevent their multiplication. Compare this to the standard treatment and belief that cancer starts as a localized tumor and, if not detected in time, will spread throughout the body so that the physician must eradicate the tumor by cutting, burning or loading the body with poisonous chemicals.
Good nutrition is an alternative that affects the entire body. But the AMA says that we don't know enough about diets yet, maybe in another 10 or 15 years. But everybody agrees that a full, nourishing and balanced diet is a must. If we have that, few vitamins, if any, and only some mineral supplements are needed. Nevertheless, for specific illnesses, such as lung cancer, vitamin C drips and fresh carrot juice and Beta-carotene have proved successful, reports Heimlich. She also speaks about the Hoxsey treatment that is mainly an herbal tonic for internal and external use; the Burton treatment involving administration of four blood proteins that are deficient in cancer patients; and the Livingston treatment, which combines diet and psychotherapy. Then there is electic therapy that involves a variety of immune system-enhancing techniques, including nutrition, psychotherapy and magnetotherapy. Dr. Bonlie, among others, says that

all nutritional reactions are bioelectrical, such that these reactions are accompanied by the flow of electrons which must have an associated magnetic field.

We must be careful that too much nutrition talk does not create a backlash against doing anything. An American Dietetic Association survey found more than a third of Americans do not consider nutrition important and are not interested in changing their eating habits; and another 38 percent know that they should be eating better but aren't. Too many people will not change their eating habits until threatened with a health crisis. But that is human nature. I recall when my brother would not stop smoking and drinking to excess until the doctor told him he would die in a few years. He hasn't touched the stuff now in ten years. But eating less fat and more fiber might seem inconsequential to most people, especially those seeking a drug or magic pill to make it easy. If you are worried about your job or income investments, nutrition is less important.

People are still confused about what is good, but for certain kinds of cases some diets are clear. Dr. Dean Ornish believes that we know enough about diet and nutrition that most of us could go on a healthy regimen right now. He has studied nutrition for the past fifteen years and is in the last year of a five year control study involving 48 treated patients and a similar size control group. He says that there isn't any question that those on this diet have improved their health. Those who had serious arterial blockage actually reversed their condition to regain normal health, regardless of age. Even those in the 60 and 70 age group improved, compared to the control group who consumed their regular, higher fat diets.

The Ornish diet is strictly vegetarian without fish or poultry. For the average person, the American Heart Association recommends a thirty percent or less fat intake, perhaps knowing that it will be difficult for the average American to cut out all meat, fish and poultry. For those who need to reverse serious conditions, Ornish recommends no more than 10 percent fat intake, and for those in better health who wish to maintain their condition, he approves a 20 percent fat intake, a diet he believes most people can continue and enjoy satisfactorily.

Doctors should know that certain diets work and that they don't have to hesitate to recommend them. The unexpected result of the Ornish diet is that it actually reverses disease. Patients in emergency conditions, of course, still have to rely on the best available medicine of the moment; yet, doctors need to recognize that preventative techniques must be included. If we were sensible —which we are not—we could cut the nearly $1 trillion national health bill in half with prevention alone. For every dollar in preventive care, we could save ten times that down-the-road.

We know more about nutrition than medical professionals want to admit. One diet we could easily fathom is a one ounce fiber intake daily to cut breast cancer significantly. A four-year study, involving 451 women who were diagnosed with breast cancer and 451 with no history of cancer, found fiber was the dietary component with the greatest role in preventing breast cancer. Peter Baghurst, of Australia's Commonwealth Scientific and Industrial Research Organization, states that some women could reduce the risk of developing breast cancer by as much as 50 percent by increasing intake of fiber-rich food. Fiber is more strongly related for some women than other factors, such as fat and total calories. Women with the least risk ate about an ounce of fiber a day; those with the greatest risk ate about half an ounce a day. Understanding this, it needs to be pointed out that nations and cultures vary in their fiber intake. Britain has the highest death rate from breast cancer at 36 per year per 100,000 population, with much of Europe close behind; the lowest is in Peru at 5.6, with Ecuador, Japan and Mauritius close behind; and the U.S. at the high end at 27 deaths per 100,000.

Diet, Cholesterol and Heart Disease

When we consider diet, we must relate to the most popular discussion of all—cholesterol. Yet the effects of cholesterol remain controversial. Various studies show that for two-thirds of Americans, lowering dietary cholesterol will not effect plasma cholesterol levels.
Incorrect assumptions cost the nation dearly. The price of comprehensive cholesterol-screening programs, for example, could cost the U.S. over $50 billion a year that might benefit one percent of the population. One of the largest studies found that 973 of 1000 men treated with cholesterol-lowering drugs survived five years without a heart attack. Of a similar group given a placebo, 959 remained healthy for five years. So to prevent 14 heart attacks, we would have to put 959 people under continuous

---

* The italicized text refers to more complex information.

treatment with powerful, costly drugs that would give no benefit. And the long-term risk of these drugs are unknown, although short-term evaluation of the drug takers show inexplicably higher rates of violent death and death by other diseases.

Information Brief

Heimlich recalls the work of Ross Hume Hall, professor at McMaster University. His study of the consumption of egg yolks is a case in point. Fifteen egg yolks were fed daily to 13 subjects and only two showed marked blood cholesterol elevation, while a greater majority showed absolutely no change.

Nutritionists say that it is regrettable that we have learned to exclude the wondrous, healthy egg from our diet. Recently the American Heart Association increased its recommended allowance of eggs to four, up from three. Cholesterol in diet is only dangerous when exposed to air or it oxidizes, reports Dr. Allan Goby, authority on Vitamin B_6. If you break the yoke, oxidation takes place more rapidly when exposed to air, he says, therefore, poached, boiled or sunny-side up are the best, while, scrambled eggs, omelets, and egg custard should be avoided. A scientific diet study by the NIH or Office of Technology Assessment could readily confirm this in order to improve our health and the proper consumption of eggs so that there is no mystery about it. Eggs are too nutritious to waste.

A Finnish study, published in October 1991, in the Journal of the American Medical Association, found that 10 years after the end of a five-year intervention, a group of middle-aged men who had their cholesterol lowered actually had higher overall mortality rates than a similar group without treatment. Consider that psychologically telling people they have troublesome cholesterol levels or high blood pressure creates higher rates of absenteeism and impaired outlooks compared to those unaware of any problem. Analysis of any health care system should take this into account.

The National Cholesterol Education Program in the U.S. recommends drug therapy for people with LDL levels in the top 25 percent of that population, while Canadian standards call for treating the top 10 percent. The life expectancy difference over the next 30 years in the U.S. is 26.29 years and for the same group treated in Canada 26.24. So for twice the cost and number, life span would be increased 18 days.

Another study reported in JAMA, June 1991, stated that lowering the amount of fat intake to 30 percent of total calories consumed from the average of 37 percent would increase life expectancy only three to four months. Importantly, stable weight means less stress to the body compared to constantly losing and gaining weight and, consequently, a marked decrease in heart disease. Furthermore, Dr. Ornish's studies show that cutting fat intake down to the 10 or 20 percent level has a significant effect on clearing arteries and actually reversing disease. So it appears that if you have serious problems, go on as low a fat diet as possible, then gradually ease up to a level you can maintain over the long-haul.

Robert Barefoot tells us that cholesterol is not the instigator of atherosclerosis but rather a last stage participant of a process that is started by the cellular breakdown of the arterial muscle. Heart disease is not a function of the chemistry of the heart muscle but rather the chemistry of the blood. The process is explained in the digest on the following page.

Magnetotherapy, as described by Barefoot and Reich and others, opens up the ion channels to allow the nutrients access to the cell and the pH to rise to repair and prevent further cell breakdown. Negative magnetic field treatment plus calcium and other nutrients work together as a team, both as a cure and a preventive measure. The intake of drugs is highly questionable. For preventive health, proper diet and nourishment are recommended, as are a variety of alternative, non-invasive therapies, including adequate exercise and a good mental attitude.

Vitamins and Minerals

Questions still remain as to how much vitamins we need. Some say the equivalent of a thimble full is all the supplements we need for a year. Several decades ago, Dr. Reich called the government's Recommended Daily Allowance (RDA), "legislated deficiency." Some promoters have recommended massive amounts to cure our ills, which most experts agree is unwarranted. Megadoses cause headaches, dryness of the mucous membranes, liver problems, and if taken for a very long time, Barefoot explains, even death. But if you take too much of anything, even water, it can lead to death, and has. The correct amounts are what good medicine seeks.

SCIENTIFIC DIGEST

Cholesterol Not the Instigator of Atherosclerosis

The arteries which deliver blood to the heart build up with plaque, composed of collagen, phospholipids, fibrin, triglycerides, mucopolysaccharides, cholesterol, heavy metals, protein, muscle tissue and debris—all bonded with calcium. Plaque does not build up in the much thinner walled veins that return blood to the heart. It is the arteries that have inner circling muscular layers that allow for expansion and contraction in order to regulate blood pressure and delivery of blood and nutrients to all organs. Acidic cells result in the breakdown of the inner coat of the muscle to be replaced by an immobile collagen that causes inflammatory degeneration rupture of the lining and a harming patch of repairs. Polar (electrically charged oppositely at each end of the molecule) fats begin to stack on calcium in the arteries, with cholesterol only one of them. (Dr. Robert O. Becker also says that cholesterol is not the cause of heart disease, only one of many participants.)

Cholesterol is a vital component of the body, found in every cell and crucial to the production of Vitamin D. But 80 percent of all body cholesterol is manufactured by the body, not ingested in the diet. Dozens of controlled studies have shown that low cholesterol diets do not reduce heart disease. Consumption of food with cholesterol is only poorly correlated to heart disease. This is controversial mostly because it is difficult for the medical community to believe that there is only a minimal problem when cholesterol is found in the arteries as an end product. All the attention tends to mask the more important factor of calcium deficiency associated with polar stacking in the arterial walls. Deficiency of various nutrients causes the organs to become more vulnerable to disease.

Source: **The Calcium Factor**, Robert R. Barefoot and Carl J. Reich, M.D., Bakar Consultants, Wikenburg, Az, 1992.

Barefoot and Reich permit us to understand vitamins better. They report that the recommended amount of Vitamin A is 5,000 I.U. (International Units), yet eating a modest meal of carrots and liver is about 100,000 I.U. Spinach, sweet potatoes, red peppers and dried apricots would be disallowed under the recommended limits. The RDA for Vitamin D has been 400 I.U., yet the human body can generate 10,000 I.U. on a good sunny day at the beach. Only 1,200 I.U. (60 milligrams) of Vitamin C are recommended, yet we exceed this in the first glass of orange juice. Nobel Prize winner Dr. Linus Pauling recommends up to 100,000 I.U. daily (5,000 milligrams) of Vitamin C. In the early 1970's, the FDA tried unsuccessfully to make a drug prescription necessary to purchase over one and half times the RDA, but public outcry was too much. This single mandate, if successful, would have increased our trips to the doctor's office and pushed up, even further, the national health bill.

Larger than normal amounts of vitamins and minerals are recommended for a limited time only or until a desired result has been achieved. For large amounts, the patient's blood, urine and medical symptoms should be monitored by doctors. Depending upon a person's weight and other factors, Dr. Reich recommends vitamin A up to 54,000 I.U., vitamin D up to 7,200 I.U. and calcium up to 1,250 milligrams. He believes that effective doses can correct both immune and adaptive deficiency syndromes and significantly help asthmatic sufferers and attack a host of other diseases. But the general medical community seems to prefer vaccines and anti-viral drugs to vitamins. Nevertheless, much of the public has taken to greater use of vitamins and minerals on its own initiative. *

A close associate of mine cleared up his young daughter's prolonged bout with asthma by daily intake of vitamin D, B6, and calcium. This in only a few weeks and after many visits to physicians who did not consider vitamin deficiency as a factor, particularly at a young age. This asthma case can be multiplied thousands of times over by the experiences of Dr. Reich and Barefoot. Barefoot recognized that, as a young man, his asthma attacks were inversely proportional to his exposure to getting a good sun tan which gave him plenty of vitamin D, resulting in more effective processing of calcium.

The proper intake of all minerals is important, but calcium appears to have been particularly neglected in the RDA. Calcium can relax the muscles surrounding the bronchial tubes and alter permeability of the cell walls to allow nutrients to get in. Recently the RDA for calcium was increased to 1,200 mg. Importantly, the National Research Council says that because of Western diets and lifestyles even that "may not be optimal." Studies show that high calcium intake reduces hip fracture rates by as much as 60 percent. Certainly now doctors can recommend high calcium intake for their patients as preventive health. *

---

* The italicized text refers to more complex information.

The importance of the consumption of large doses of vitamins is still unclear but certain studies point to its increased value. Vitamin A, C, and E are part of a large family of chemical compounds known as anti-oxidants that are believed to have a protective effect on organs. A study in the Journal of Epidemiology describes the experience of 11,348 men and women who were interviewed about their diets in the early 1970's and observed for 10 years. Men whose vitamin C intake was the highest—equivalent of two oranges plus a 150 milligram Vitamin C pill a day—had a 42 percent lower risk of death from heart disease and a 35 percent lower risk of death from any cause compared to the population of white men as a whole. For women, the risk was 25 percent lower for heart disease but no significant change in total death rates for any cause.

Reduction in mortality held up in this study even when adjusting for age, sex, race, disease, history, education and other variables, including cigarette smoking. This relationship to vitamin C "is stronger and more consistent in this population than the relation of total mortality to serum cholesterol and dietary fat intake, two variables for which strong public health guidelines have been issued over the years," say researchers from the School of Public Health, University of California, Los Angeles.

Source: David Brown, School of Public Health, University of California, Los Angeles, Ca.; *Journal of Epidemiology; Washington Post*, May 11, 1992.

Mineral Supplements and Cancer

Both deficiency or excess intake of certain minerals and vitamins can cause health problems. For example, a common denominator exists between calcium deficiency and diseases of aging, allergy, stress and cancer. A link is apparent, reports Barefoot, with Duchenenne's muscular dystrophy and lack of dystrophin protein in the cells. A calcium regulation problem is evident in this case, for the calcium concentration within the cells is twice as high as normal.

Let us be mindful of osteoporosis which affects most older Americans and also Alzheimer's which affects 10 to 50 percent (relevant to age) of older people. Calcium deposits in the tissues and joints are a sign of calcium deficiency. These bony deposits are created to bolster skeletal structural strength resulting from the osteoporosis or decalcification of the bones. They also create fear in us that we may be consuming too much calcium, which is precisely the opposite case, says Barefoot. This author was told a number of times by physicians that my system was over-calcified after several accidents, including a fall on the ski slopes which left my arm in a 90° angle for six months. Recently while jogging, I stepped off a six inch curb, twisting my leg, causing a bony deposit to appear. My first thought was the usual, "I am over calcified," but now I believe I know better.

This last resort removal of calcium from the bones, Barefoot explains, leads to such diseases as osteoporosis, arthritis, rheumatism, sclerosis and periodontal disease. Also, he says, Alzheimer's disease has been associated with aluminum accumulation in the body which is associated with the overproduction of parathyroid hormones that stimulate removal of calcium from the bones. *

In regard to the second biggest killer, frightening cancer, we must look at alternatives and gain a better understanding of how cancer functions. Cancer can be defined as a malignant tumor eating away and spreading indefinitely while tending to recur when removed. It occurs when the DNA (deoxyribose nucleic acid) is chemically altered, producing mutant cells that multiply without restraint, spreading to distant sites and into the blood stream. Most scientists agree that a relationship exists between the food we eat, the air we breathe and certain chemicals and carcinogens that can, in massive amounts, trigger cancer. Also specific ultra violet radiation and various adverse and unacceptable electromagnetic frequencies can incite cancer.

With the advent of chemotherapy and radiation, the nation is winning many minor battles but losing the war on cancer. Greater understanding is necessary about the chemistry of carcinogens and how these cancers are energized to be able to interact chemically with the DNA. We need to incorporate this knowledge into an appreciation of the electron physics of the cell membrane and to the fact that all carcinogens are highly electrophilic (electron loving) reactants. These powerful electron acceptors are free radicals, says Barefoot, eager to gain electrons that can enter the body through such elements as unsaturated oils, food additives,

---

* The italicized text refers to more complex information.

238

nitrites, inhalation, and skin absorption of toxic chemicals from such elements as benzene and the tar of cigarette smoke.

Information Brief

Fake Advertising

Secretaries of agriculture seem to put citizens last. The latest USDA's food pyramid is little more than a side dish of information. Advertising remains the most popular medium for influencing our dietary choices, yet much of it is deceitful. It is up to the public to figure out that General Mill's Honey Nut Cheerios has less honey and nuts in each box than it has sugar and salt. Prego Spaghetti sauce is "made with fresh mushrooms"—a half mushroom per serving. Pillsbury Hungry Jack Buttermilk Pancakes have less than 160th of a cup of buttermilk per three pancakes. The seven ounces of Banquet Vegetable Pie With Chicken has 10 peas, 120th of a carrot and a 19th of a potato. All this and more compiled by the Center for Science in the Public Interest. Will President Clinton's new Agriculture Secretary do better!

Source: **Center for Science in the Public Interest,** *Washington Post,* May 1992, Colmon McCarthy.

A 1990 study, conducted by the Office of Technology Assessment with an eminent panel, concluded that more study needs to be done concerning alternative therapies and that there should be a "mandated responsibility of NCI to pursue information and facilitate examination of widely used unconventional cancer treatments for therapeutic potential." Unfortunately, this report did not give much encouragement to alternative health procedures. NCI has not formally sought out alternative medicine, usually reacting only to reported problems or Congressional pressure. The Natural Products Branch, OTA suggests, might examine herbal treatments, for example. The panel confirmed the difficulty of obtaining accurate information from clinical tests because of wide variables in procedure and also in human condition. Better examination results might be obtained, they suggest, by visiting the facilities where alternatives take place and make evaluations. They say that this could be a revolution of sorts and might be the best way to test validity of patient cures. The question is whether the scientific community has sufficient innovative spirit to do this or the stamina to overcome political and corporate adversity. Yet it may be the most practical way to determine effectiveness. NIH's new Office of Alternative Medicine is preceding in this direction but with very limited resources for such important questions.

Surgery and Alternatives

Data on the health care system should awaken our senses and cause us to look more to prevention and alternatives. Heimlich reveals that uncontrolled hypertension is a leading cause of 500,000 strokes each year and a major contributor to the one and one quarter million heart attacks. Bypass surgery has increased from 175,000 operations in 1982 to 332,000 in 1987. Depending on the surgeon, from three percent to 23 percent die from bypass surgery, one in five incur mental impairment, and most of the others experience trouble remembering, depression, and lassitude. The surgeon earns from $20,000 to $40,000 per operation and the hospital gets a substantial slice. The average surgeon generates $1 million in revenue for the hospital every year, while over $5 billion is spent on this surgery nationally. It would be difficult to turn off this industry.

An August, 1991 study reports that balloon angioplasties have jumped from 32,000 in 1983 to over 200,000 in 1988. Still, 10 percent of this group suffer heart attacks or need emergency surgery shortly thereafter; while, for a third the vessels become blocked again in a few months and need to be cleared. For most of the others they become blocked again within a few years. Here is a group of people that could benefit from something approaching the Ornish diet. The question is how many M.D.s recommend a strict diet and what is the responsibility of the AMA to inform their membership and the public about what is truly effective!

Heimlich further stirs our senses by describing a number of procedures, such as live-cell therapy and oxidative techniques like hydrogen peroxide (5,000 articles have been written about its beneficial effects) and DMSO (dimethyl sulfoxide) treatment, involving an inexpensive industrial solvent used as medicine in 55 countries but only permitted for a rare bladder inflammation in the United States (6,000 articles have been written on its effectiveness). Apparently, the number of articles and studies is not enough to overcome the objections of the medical community.

Compare the unfortunate statistics of failed or blundered surgeries to the 400,000 people who have experienced successful results, just over the past decade, from chelation therapy without any deaths attributed to the treatment. The opposition to this and similar alternatives by much of the medical profession is that these treatments are unproven. Without FDA approval, health insurers won't cover the costs. Yet cites Heimlich, chelation therapy (as do some other alternative methodologies including magnetotherapy) improves blood flow naturally throughout the body, reverses arteriosclerosis, reduces blood pressure, forestalls heart attacks and strokes, relieves angina pains, and improves sexual stamina and vision. Patients may also experience reduced symptoms of arthritis, multiple sclerosis, Parkinson's disease, psoriasis, and some relief from Alzheimer's disease, of which there are 337,000 people afflicted.

Furthering the reinforcement of the positive effects of chelation therapy, Heimlich cites a 1988 study in Brazil of 2,870 patients with various chronic degenerative diseases. It showed that 90 percent of the subjects with peripheral vascular disease and blocked arteries of the legs, and 76.9 percent with ischemic heart disease, showed marked improvement. In a 1985 Cypher study at the Great Lakes Association of Clinical Medicine, Inc. involving 25,000 patients and 300 controls, results showed a significant improvement in 79 percent of the cases. These studies aren't even available in the computer search INDEX MEDICUS, so doctors know nothing about them. Surely the AMA and data information sources have some responsibility in reporting these findings to let the membership and other practitioners draw their own conclusions.

Last year, I had the unique experience of attending a two-day conference in Gettysburg, Pa., conducted by Golden Pride Raleigh, which markets health products. Raleigh was founded in the last century and was bought out by Golden Pride about eight years ago. They market eight formulas in tablet form for daily consumption of vitamins and minerals, stating that 99 percent of all Americans are deficient in minerals in particular and that being insufficient in any one of these can cause disease. The natural formulas consist of such substances as honey bee pollen (the only food that contains all the nutrients needed by the body), proplis (an antibiotic), fiber caps, and green barley juice.

SCIENCE DIGEST

Pollution and Nutritional Supplements

If you lived a Tarzan lifestyle of clean nutrient-rich foods, exercised to a lean body, avoided pollution and drugs and stress, supplements would not be necessary, says Patrick Quillin. RDA is designed for "normal" people like the average American who gets six colds per year, wears glasses, is overweight, wears dentures by age 45, is plagued with lethargy, constipation, depression, and gets sick in the 60's and dies in the 70's of heart disease or cancer. The RDA is the governments' "yardstick" for the poverty line of enough groceries for a family of four. If it were elevated, the number of Americans living below the poverty line would triple, a calamitous event for politicians in office. Yet a couple hundred dollars of supplements could prevent $100,000 worth of long-term illness that would cut the comprehensive, national health bill way down, but somewhere in the future.

However, professional schizophrenia among health care professionals, registered dietitians, the American Dietetic Association, and a lot of physicians seems to prevail. Yet 60 percent of dietitians (Journal of the American Dietetic Association vol. 84, P. 795, 1984) and 71 percent of vegetarians and 57 percent of non-vegetarians in the U.S. take supplements anyway (Draper, H.H. and Bird, Free Radical Biology and Medicine, vol 3, p. 203, 1987) and their use is higher among the well-educated. About 98 percent of older adults and 30 percent of children are on prescription drugs at any given time. What have we come to? Dr. Jeffrey Blumberg, Tufts University, Boston, finds drug-induced malnutrition in the elderly a serious problem and typical poor immune response.

The Oregon Medical Priority Setting Project (Bioethics Consultation Group, Inc, Berkeley, CA, Mar 1989), whose program was recently approved by President Clinton's new Secretary of Health and Human Resources, Donna Shalala, endorses nutrition supplements (food and pills) as a top priority to prevent long-term health problems. Dr. John Kitzhaber, physician and president of Oregon's Senate, and an elite panel of experts believe in a broad-spectrum of vitamin and mineral supplements. Kitzhaber says if they were passed out in school each morning there would be "less cancer and other health woes."

(Cont'd)

242

SCIENCE DIGEST

Pollution and Nutritional Supplements

(Cont'd)

Cancer, especially in these heavily polluted times (electro and chemical) may be a deficiency condition of vitamins E and C, says Dr. William Pryor, Louisiana State University. Evidence warrants doubling the RDA for vitamins C, three to five fold increase for vitamin E, and a separate beta-carotene requirement, according to Dr. Anthony Diplock, London Hospital. And Dr. John Bieri of the National Institute of Diabetes, Digestive and Kidney Diseases, in Maryland, is convinced of the need for higher intakes of vitamins A, C and E and carotenoids. And the list of believers goes on as noted in Free Radical Biology and Medicine (vol 3, 1987). Swedish, Japanese, Finish and Australian studies (controlled and large based samples) all show substantial reduction of cancer under various nutrition supplement programs including national efforts to supply whole populations (Lancet, Jan 24, 1987; Science, vol 233, July 1986; Nutrition and Cancer, vol 9, 1987).

Experts have argued that since most of our morbidity and mortality in the U.S. comes from degenerated diseases (heart, cancer, emphysema) and most degenerative disease are caused by free-radical damage, and free-radicals can be slowed down with supplemental antioxidant nutrients, it is foolish to neglect these valuable protectors in our polluted times, as reported by Machlin and Bendich (Federation of American Society for Experimental Biologists vol 1, 1987). Hillary Clinton's health plan needs to take the idea of supplements and pollution seriously. Quillin reinforces a quote about a wealthy America, "May you make lots of money and spend it all on doctor bills."

Source: Quillin, Patrick, PhD, RD., Safe Eating, M. Evans and Co., Inc, NY, 1990, Vice President for Nutrition Services at the Cancer Treatment Centers of America, Tulsa, Oklahoma.

Their prime mission, however, appears to be a chelated, formulated capsule hailed as the health product of the decade. They have the patent on a formula that they say no other company has been able to reproduce. After taking the capsule, a simple blood test for EDTA could verify results. It uniquely combines royal jelly, honey bee pollen and EDTA (synthetic amino acid with chelating properties). Golden Pride says it does the same thing as chelation therapy performed by M.D.s that requires a series of injections over a six week period. It takes more time to have an effect but some users report improved health in a matter of weeks, as it removes accumulated toxins and other harmful substances from the cardiovascular system. Numerous testimonials at the conference ranged from better vision and reduced body pain to improved memory. One employee of IBM reported walking away from his wheel chair after just a few months of treatment. Reportedly, it has an effect on hypertension, clogged arteries, varicose veins, strokes, arthritis, diabetes, gout, kidney stones, cataracts, Alzheimer's, senility, and the list goes on. You could not convince its 25,000 distributors and many times that number of users that this product is any thing but effective from their own personal experiences. The question arises, can a couple of hundred thousand users be bluffed or does this stuff work!

Harry Hersey, president of Golden Pride Raleigh, has proved the effectiveness of his chelator in laboratory tests over several years. In his book **New Answers to Old Questions**, he defines a free radical as a reactive, oxygen-derived substance that fulfills a certain necessary physiological function, but is also capable of causing great harm when in excess or in the wrong place. A chelation substance binds naturally to minerals and specific free radicals to help them work normally or assist in their discharge from the body. Aspirin, for example, is a copper chelator that behaves like the anti-oxidant enzyme SOD (superoxide dismutase) that rids the body of harmful free radicals implicated in heart disease, arthritis, aging and other diseases. Aspirin inhibits platelet stickiness which improves circulation. The requirements are less than a quarter of an aspirin daily. In conversation with Hersey, he concurs that there is a basic magnetic reaction to chelation therapy, which again reinforces the significance of magnetotherapy.

Certainly, the NIH ought to explore just how effective these therapies are. Considering the thousands of doctors who inject chelation treatments annually, the more simple procedure of taking capsules or applying magnetotherapy could improve the nation's health bill substantially. Does this capsule perform as well as injections? Should chelation therapy or special diets be recommended after or before heart surgery? What is the role of magnetotherapy? Since President Bill Clinton and Vice-President Albert Gore are looking for answers to the ineffective and costly health system, this should be one of the prime areas for review.

Exhibit 24   Health Evaluation

A computer program, the APACHE (Acute Physiology and Chronic Health Evaluation), invented by William A. Knows, physician at George Washington University, predicts a patient's chances of dying in the hospital from various ailments using an 18,000 person data base and treatment methods at 40 hospitals. It shows that medicines straddle science and art and that uncertainty is respected. It doesn't direct the decisions of doctors but lets them know how they are doing in comparison to other doctors. It remembers far more than what is in one physician's experience, demonstrating prognostic powers about equal to the country's best-trained academic, intensive-care physicians.

A data base such as this could be very useful in predicting possible cures and healing rates for ailments treated by a variety of alternative therapies and could alert doctors to a wider scope of medicine and preventive remedies. Doctors don't have the time to read everything available and many are afraid to make a mistake recommending something unusual. A good data base could take some liability away from them which could be quite welcome. It would make them think more about each individual case and the wide range of opportunities available for the practice of the art of medicine. If a patient has a 50 percent chance of living five years from a certain cancer but has odds of living 10 years with a change in lifestyle or an alternative therapy, the patient ought to know this from a data base that may be more convincing than the doctor's dictum. The patient should at least be able to make a choice from state-of-the-art information. An intelligent data base could cut the costs of liability insurance and national health expenditures.

Source: William A. Knows, M.D., George Washington University,
Washington D.C., *Washington Post*, January 1st 1992,
David Brown; author.

The Mind

We cannot forget mental conditioning as an alternative cure. Earlier, the psychosomatic or placebo effect was discussed. Mental conditioning is much more proactive and will ordinarily have a higher success rate than control subjects who passively believe that they are receiving treatment. I like to refer to a course I took some years ago given by an authority on human effectiveness, Louis Tice, The Pacific Institute, Seattle, Washington, who lectures on the powers of the subconscious mind to visualize events and desires. The mind, he says, can visualize or believe something is real many times more powerfully than reality itself. In other words, we can fool the mind. Through strong, daily and repetitious visualization of what one wishes to accomplish by setting goals, the mind actually believes it is happening and therefore it is much more likely to occur. A real event would not necessarily be as strong.

Our creative subconscious is a magnificent storehouse of solutions to solve any problem necessary to reach a goal we have set. "Many creations are in the process and each will have its moment." Do not wait for the exact, right moment or method to achieve an objective. Set the goal first, follow with visualization and desire, and the means and solutions will come.

Members of the Olympic team and other sports figures use goals and visualization to improve their abilities. Eastern European and Russian teams used these methods long before we decided on their viability. Chief executives, police officers, productivity experts, and persons in almost every walk of life have been trained to use these techniques successfully. Numerous investigations and studies have demonstrated that mind manipulation may also be why one believes he or she is floating over his own body in an "out-of-body experience" or why some people truly believe that they have visited with creatures from outer space. We can train or reinforce our thinking process to believe or visualize almost anything as vividly as we desire—even greater than reality though that may not seem possible.

People can make heart rates go up or down with will power. Hypnotized subjects show a variety of metabolic responses, including heart rate increases of 25 beats per minute simply by visualizing exercise. While exercising, for example, those who simply think highly of themselves as top performers show lower levels of exertion at equal levels of effort than those who don't. In other words, macho or self-confident minds make lighter work for their bodies. Those who think that they are straining, actually are. These tests have great implications for the elevation of stress. Think "cool" and your stress level will be lower. The highly excitable are more likely to develop high blood pressure or heart disease.

The significance about the practice of visualization is that the patients can picture cancer cells or some other ailments dissipating or curing in the system at any given time. Whether he believes that there be spiritual assistance or simply a pure scientific desire to effect mind-over-matter, the process has been proven to help in many cases and is used as part of many doctor's armenatarium to good health. Little doubt exists that one must think positively to get the best results.

Numerous cases can be cited where a physician has told his patient that he has a specific time to live and, unwittingly, to the day the patient succumbs. In one interesting case, the doctor told the patient he had six weeks to live. The patient visited another physician who prescribed medication that appeared to arrest the cancerous condition. The patient was fine for a year or so until he visited his original doctor again to tell him the good news. This first doctor told him the drug he was taking was worthless and he would soon be ill again. Indeed, it happened. The patient fell ill at the command of the doctor who felt he should be honest with his patient about the efficacy of a particular drug, combined with the idea as to how long one has to live in the judgment of the doctors so the patient could make proper burial preparations. Until he was able to believe again that the drug was working, the patient remained sick. Convinced by the second therapist that the drug was working, the patient returned to normal health again.

This is an example as to how our minds can turn on bodily energy and the immune system for the production of certain hormones and enzymes. For many people, a positive effect will occur but also for many it may not be enough. No doubt positive thinking helps, yet the vast majority require some therapy to turn the system on. The right combination can be most beneficial.

Richard L. Weaver II, in a speech, "Developing Self Esteem," asks if you like yourself. If you don't like yourself, nothing you do will be successful for long (not even your health). He lectures for you to associate with groups that are friendly and understanding and helpful. But you must be constructive, accepted, and appreciated, in order to improve your own condition. Think happy and healthy. Weaver enumerates four ideas:

1. People are illogical, unreasonable, self-centered: love them anyway.
2. If you do good, people will accuse you of selfish ulterior motives. Do good anyway.
3. The good you do today will be forgotten tomorrow. Do good anyway.
4. People need help but may attack if you do help. Help them anyway.

And we add, you may have been told you are sick and your chances of survival are slim. Seek out a reliable therapy that makes you feel good and inspires you and makes you an active participant in your recovery, and you will heal anyway. Even if you have surgery, you must think positively. Since the more passive, placebo effect functions in only a small percentage of cases and more aggressive mind control works on only a slightly higher number, most patients still need a substance, or a therapy such as acupuncture, magnetotherapy or some additional treatment to effect better health. The combination of a strong mind and alternative treatments is the best procedure.

Chapter 8

The People Discover Magnetotherapy

Relevance of Studies

Thousands, and if we could take the time and expend the resources to examine them, we would find millions of successful cases of treatment or satisfaction with magnetotherapy reported around the world. A sampling of cases are reported here from personal experiences of individuals and from medical professionals, noting that only a limited number of controlled tests are available mostly because of lack of funding. For these real experiences, called anecdotal, there are no control patients on the opposite side with the exact condition and age and temperament and immune system to play the placebo role. Controlled studies are desirable but they should not rule everything else out. Many of these cases have been evaluated individually with the same care and depth of analysis as tests involving a control group. People were healed in these cases where they were not before, whether or not a control group existed. Most clinical tests do not involve control groups yet results can be valid. A major reason for controlled testing is to determine psychosomatic response; but, as we have reported, the placebo effect involves only about 15 to 17 percent of subjects in most cases, substantially defusing the absolute necessity for control groups. Nevertheless, funding should be provided for extensive controlled testing.

Be that as it may, consider the approval of drugs by the FDA. We are led to believe that thousands of patients are tested in controlled studies for months or years, when the truth is usually a few hundred people are tested for a few weeks. In his revealing book **Toxic Psychiatry**, Dr. Peter R. Breggen states that only weeks was the extent of the testing for the drugs Prozac and Xanax, as well as the "extremely brain-disabling and sometimes life-threatening drug Clozaril which was tested for only a matter of six weeks, yet will be administered for years. The drug Anafranil, for obsessive-compulsive disorder, was studied for only 10 weeks when it frequently will be administered for months or years." The FDA warns physicians that they should periodically reevaluate the long-term usefulness of drugs for individual patients, but this advice usually goes unheeded or ends up, over the long-run, being nothing more than an anecdotal experience of which physicians, ironically, are so much opposed. Without admitting it, doctors are now using this type of medicine as an art form, simply testing efficacy as they proceed over the long-haul. At least with magnetotherapy we are dealing with a treatment essentially risk free when some very simple guidelines are followed—not so with most drugs.

In past decades before requirements for FDA approval, general consensus from medical practitioners was all that was necessary in order to make use of a particular medicine, as long as no question of safety or lack of value was raised. An example of such consensus is bright light therapy that is simply a naturally occurring electromagnetic energy in a limited area of the frequency spectrum and which has FDA approval today. Magnetotherapy and its energy are in the same class. Some controlled studies exist for magnetotherapy, but greater affidavit documentation would help this medicine achieve its rightful role.

Affidavits would have legal value under our Constitution. Users of magnetotherapy are encouraged to provide documentation by recording details of treatment before, during and after. Paper and laboratory work should be outlined in a diary of progress, including type of magnets used, strength, duration and any other pertinent data. Physician comments before and after would be helpful. A witness to sign the document makes it more authentic. Magnet-X Corp. of Calgary, Canada, and other providers now ask for affidavits. Thousands of such affidavits would help to confirm the validity of this medicine.

Many of the cases described here commenced over a year and some several years ago with the latest possible results reported. Several depict safe and effective results from treatments administered ten or fifteen years ago. Because a case is self-help, it should not be automatically discredited. Most people don't lie about their recoveries. In addition, a number of controlled tests described here show efficacy from permanent magnetic treatment. Below is one such study from Japan involving magnetic beds. I start out in Exhibit 25 with a controlled, double-blind study, then proceed to describe cases reported by individuals and doctors in and out of clinics.

Exhibit 25 Magnetic Pad Efficacy Test Results
(Nippon Kenko Zokhin Kenkyukai Health Pad)

In this controlled study, 154 outpatients and a number of inpatients were divided into two groups, one provided with magnetic pads, the other with pads without magnetic devices. Assessments were performed one month after use. The patients with stiff shoulders were the primary goal; many had lower back pain as well. Radiographs were taken of the cervical vertebrae for presence of osteophyte formation, narrowing of intervertebral discs, and alignment asymmetry. Muscle tone change was measured with a Sakurai-type muscle tone instrument (JOURNAL OF ORTHOPEDIC SURGERY 26:163, 1975). Urinary glucose and proteins, and blood pressure were also measured.

Effect was noted in some cases within one week, most within three weeks, and others four weeks. Efficacy of the magnetic pad was found at the 1 percent significant level and no untoward effects observed. Conclusion was that pads with magnetic devices were significantly effective for those using them as opposed to the control, non-user group. In addition to an effect observed in patients with stiff shoulder caused by chronic rheumatoid arthritis, an effect was observed for those with traumatic cervical syndrome, osteochondrosis of the cervical vertebrae, and stenosis of the vertebral canal, an unexpected result.

Source: Conducted by Professor Akihero Myozaki Kagoshima University School of MedicineDepartment of
Orthopedic Surgery, in conjunction with the Kagoshima National Hospital, Japan, 1992.

Magnetotherapy Case Studies

Following is a variety of self-help and professionally administered cases to give the reader an idea of the possibilities of treatment. These are mostly personal experiences from the use of magnetic devices from various providers such as Nikken, Japan Life, Ameriflex, Magnet-X Corp., MagnetiCo Inc. and others. Various polarities and techniques were used by these subjects, their technical nature discussed in other chapters.

It is important to note that relief or cure was achieved with both bipolar and singled pole magnets of both polarities. Many of these successful cases were with Nikken bipolar and checkerboard devices and mattresses, mattress pads, and car seats. c

Case success does not necessarily mean that an another individual will realize the same results. As medical technicians state over and over again, the individual body is quite different from person to person and cures depend much on bodily condition and the immune system, as well as a desire to achieve success. Therapists believe that at least magnetotherapy gives a non-risk opportunity to realize meaningful results. One should always seek out expert advice from a physician, but if one therapy doesn't work, the patient should take enough control to search out a safe therapy that might.

Broken Neck, Crushed Discs, and Torn Rotator Cuff

Robert and Gloria H. were very skeptical when asked to try magnetotherapy, but they did and, after twenty years of suffering, it changed their lives. It doesn't mean it will happen to another even with a similar condition, but they say, if all else has failed, it is worth a try. The husband was in an automobile accident twenty years ago and had suffered a broken neck and a crushed disc in his lower back. After three surgeries on his neck, he continued to suffer severe headaches, loss of hearing, and nausea from pain. Medication for pain and twelve-plus Dramamine tablets daily for fifteen years were necessary. Two years after the automobile accident, he suffered a torn rotary cuff in the workplace. Waiting for Workmen's Compensation approval, he visited several physicians and physical therapists without results. In order to turn his head, he had to turn his whole body. It limited movement of his shoulder and resulted in lower back pain, anxiety chest pains and severe hot flashes, for which he took nitro tablets.

Robert was introduced to magnetic instruments—permanent magnets in a mattress bed. He was very skeptical and even sarcastic about the treatment potential because he had tried everything—pills, electric-shock, biofeedback, hypnosis, acupuncture, and whatever else was recommended. He laid on the pad for ten minutes and was able to get up and sit in the chair for the first time with ease. An excruciating headache was eliminated in twenty minutes by placing a bipolar, concentric magnet on the back of the neck for twenty minutes. The same permanent magnet on both shoulders allowed him to move his arms freely. Sleeping on the pad that evening, his wife noticed that he did not toss and turn as much and his snoring was greatly reduced. By morning, his lower back pain was gone.

Information Brief

Healing Power of Magnets

Magnetic fields work much more quickly and effectively than heat, infrared light, anti-inflammatory drugs, trigger-point injections or microwave diathermy. It's likely to be four or six months before an injured skier or other athlete is back in play again from the conventional treatment of ice, followed by heat to reduce swelling. Heat alone will not stimulate therapeutic repair of injured tissue or muscle. An ample supply of nutrient-rich blood is needed. Healing requires resumption of normal blood flow to the injured site, not simply pain relief. In magnetotherapy, knee braces can be removed more quickly; weightlifters can reduce lower back pain; sciatica (inflammation of sciatic nerve running down the hip and thigh) and carpal tunnel syndrome can be relieved. Osteopathic physician Sanford J. Paul, Mercerville NJ, is convinced of the effectiveness of magnetotherapy. "Though I use conventional medical methods I find that the application of biomagnets has helped in some difficult traumatic-injury cases. I feel that biomagnets should be part of the total armamentarium of future physicians," he says. However, "Unless used properly, their value is no greater than that of a regular magnet."

Orthopedic chiropractor Kurt Vreeland, White River Junction, Vermont, physician for the U.S. Olympic ski jumping team, uses magnets for ski and other injuries. "I have used magnets with good results on everything from rotator cuff injuries to what they used to call in football 'hip-pointer'." Nevertheless, Vreeland has limited success in convincing his medical colleagues of the efficacy of biomagnetics.

The problem with gaining general practitioner acceptance, says Dr. John O. Brian, M.D., Chief of Physical Medicine and Rehabilitation at the Hospital of Saint Raphael, New Haven, Conn., is "biomagnetics just hasn't had much exposure. I trained at one of the best rehab centers in the country, the Rusk Institute in New York, and biomagnetics never came up once."

Source: **Healing Power of Magnets**, *Fitness Magazine*, February 1992, Richard Dean Jenkins.

Robert left at 9 A.M. for his usual therapy session and was back at 10:30 A.M. overjoyed, speaking loudly to both his daughter and wife, saying "You're not going to believe this." The therapist could not understand what had happened. He found that Bob had full range of motion in his shoulder and no pain. He could turn his head and touch his chin to his chest, something he had been unable to do for twenty years. Robert can now hear the television at its normal volume and has taken no pain medication or Dramamine or nitro since magnetotherapy in late 1990. He has no headaches, sleeps all night well, doesn't snore, has more energy and his depression has lifted. The therapist was amazed and Robert's wife and daughter cried for a long while in happiness.

Back Injury

Nicole S., of Osprey, Florida, sustained a back injury from a fall down one full story of icy steps, damaging her tailbone. Later in life, she also fell off a ladder, badly twisting her hip girdle and spine, and unfortunately, still later, incurred an additional fall while horseback riding. The pain was particularly bad when she was tired or in a toxic state. With use of permanent magnets for four to five days, the pain completely left her. If she overworked or strained herself, the pain would come back again, but it was immediately relieved by applying magnets again for a few hours. Nicole says that she no longer needs afternoon naps because she sleeps longer and better at night, more in tune with the normal circadian rhythm. Her appearance has improved because a painful tenseness has been removed from her face and she has a more relaxed look. She wakes up more refreshed. She says she is in love, not with a person, but with a thing.

It is perhaps this kind of trial and error that makes the application of magnetotherapy uninviting for most doctors. They like precise solutions, almost always a drug; whereas, with magnetotherapy, the patient herself comes to know more about her condition and feelings than the doctor, and this takes time and personal experience. The patient learns when to apply or not to apply. The doctor cannot predict this. The magnetotherapist can only provide general guidelines. The patient begins to take control of her own life.

Chronic Fatigue Syndrome and Sleep Problems

In another case in Osprey, the patient, Karen H., was extremely negative about the fact of "wasting her time" lying on a magnetic pad to induce more energy in her system. She was programmed over the years against psychosomatic cures, prepared to resist and criticize. After ten minutes on the pad, she accused the therapist of not telling her that there was a heater in the pad. Of course, there was not, as the magnetotherapy made her feel warmer and more relaxed. In fact, she fell asleep for a good ten minutes and awoke feeling revitalized, now very much impressed with the results. Karen now enjoys her work more, even the double shifts, as the energy level has been raised from the sleep she has obtained on the magnetic pad each evening. This is another case of the person feeling out her own condition and handling it from her personal experience, something perhaps which the former family doctor might have done in the good old days.

Many fatigue and sleep problems go hand-in-hand. Joanne W. Elston, Calgary, Alberta, was introduced to a magnetic bed by her father because of poor sleep. Trying to sleep or staying asleep, was a losing battle for her. Every morning was the same old story of feeling tired, irritable, impatient, angry and the energy level at zero. Joanne says her first week on a magnetic sleep pad was nothing short of miraculous. "I was completely astonished at how fully rested, light and relaxed I felt and how much energy I regained. To the critics, I say this, "Don't knock it until you try it."

Back Injury and Sciatic Pain

The case of M.L.D. of Indialantic, Florida, who hurt her back in 1956 by backing into the bottom edge of a bathroom counter corner as she rose from bathing two of her grandsons, is another typical success of magnetotherapy and the use of permanent magnets in a magnetic bed. After visiting doctors and chiropractors and massage therapists for all the years since 1956, plus supplements of minerals and vitamins, nothing worked.

Her daughter introduced her to permanent magnets on December 17, 1990. The mother slept on the mattress pad and taped a mini-magnet to her sore spot on one side and a matching location on the opposite side of her body, midway between the breast and waist. Within two days, the pain was completely gone and she went off to enjoy a three-week vacation on the west coast of Florida pain free. Of course, when she came back, she again used the magnets in a maintenance program.

She also had irregular but frequent attacks of sciatic pain, but with the use of permanent magnets on each hip and using a magnetic seat as well, this pain was reduced and finally eliminated within two weeks. All of this occurred by living the same lifestyle, eating the same foods, and taking the same supplements. Nothing changed except the use of magnets—after 34 years of suffering. Now, what doctor would deny her the use of magnetotherapy? She says, "Don't fall into the same trap of judgment before giving it a real trial."

Arthritis

Fourteen year old Bob Glen, of Lundbreck, Alberta, with arthritis pain in most joints was relieved of almost all pain after two days of sleeping on a negative field magnetic pad. When he went on holidays without the pad, his pain returned and he could hardly walk. Now he doesn't go anywhere without it and says he feels 100 percent better after five months of use. No one appears ready to stand up and claim a cure for arthritis, which most physicians might agree would almost be a miracle, yet there is little question that pain was dramatically reduced.

In many cases, muscular and joint motion improve. Previously, I mentioned the case of Dean Bonlie who had arthritis since the age of 21 and experienced almost total relief of pain, after three decades of suffering, by sleeping on a negative oriented pad for three months. Anecdotes don't mean very much but even if efficacy occurred in only ten percent of cases, that would amount to millions of people. Dr. Philpott has recorded numerous arthritic successes in his Institute, citing reduced inflammation and increased fluid flow in muscles and tissues from magnetic fields. None of this means a cure, only that by using magnetic devices in an ongoing maintenance program, one might very well experience lasting relief.

Sports Injuries and Energy Lifts

Professional therapist and athlete, Don Caldwell from Bellevue, Washington, has used magnets successfully on Olympic team members and many other sports figures. Football players find the permanent magnet excellent for injured knees; and baseball players and bicyclists find magnets effective for swollen joints and painful muscles. Caldwell has used his therapeutic methods on people who have been in industrial or auto accidents with whiplash, hip problems and other forms of chronic pain. Relief comes about in 10 - 15 minutes of application in most cases. What he likes about magnetism is that it is portable—one can walk around while it is on any part of the body.

Magnets are not just for injuries. Remember that over 90 percent of the population is not in sports. Magnets can bring body recovery, not just "good rest." The first two hours of sleep, Caldwell says, are the most important. Putting in eight hours of sleep is not good enough if it's the wrong sleep. We need deep sleep. He has had chronic injuries and scars from an auto accident himself, whereby pain is eliminated and the body rejuvenated every time he uses the magnetic sleeping pads. Toxins are eliminated during the sleep period so one feels more comfortable in the morning. A tranquilizer user can reduce his intake, he reports. Caldwell says that the process facilitates the body's potential for recovery, helps to get more oxygen and nutrients to the cells, dilates arteries and brings more blood to the area. Particularly over age 50, capillaries begin to fold up, he explains. Electric blankets and heat pads won't do the trick because they don't penetrate deeply enough. Caldwell is convinced of this.

Caldwell says that the methodology is especially appropriate for desk people, CPA's, engineers, secretaries and computer operators with a desk posture and consequential misalignment of the spine. Nursing homes are great candidates for magnetotherapy because bedsores materialize for almost everyone; just putting salve on the patients won't do the trick. Rolling the patient over occasionally does little to alleviate the condition which can become quite serious, even dangerous. Magnetotherapy circulates the blood and heals sore areas.

Double Rupture of Back Discs

Lena H., from the State of Oregon, fell off a roof, slipping from a loose shingle at the age of ten while helping her family make repairs. She incurred a double rupture to her back disc that bothered her for the rest of her life. Later she developed arthritis, and in her sixties, osteoporosis. She was seeing a chiropractor several times a month, was in and out of hospitals, and had over $300 of drugs prescribed monthly. The drugs made her terribly ill; at one point they made her deaf for three days, reversing only when she was taken off the medication. She was introduced to permanent magnets at the age of sixty-six, using a small, silver dollar-size, 555 gauss, bipolar magnet in the small of her back for thirty minutes daily, and a single-pole magnetic mattress pad while sleeping at night. She also occasionally tapes the flat, thin magnet to her back while sitting in a chair. Surprisingly, the first thirty-minute application had her walking erect for the first time in many years. Apparently, the magnetic fields limbered the spine sufficiently to straighten somewhat, which also lengthened her right leg to within only one-half inch difference from the left, where there had previously been a two-inch difference that caused her to drag one leg. It not only lengthened the leg, but it also eliminated the pain. She turned 67 in June and has had relief since September, 1990. Of course, if she overdoes strenuous work by her own doing, she can feel pain again, but she reports a simple application of the magnets puts her right back into proper condition. She cannot seem to use a magnetic pillow, however, because the shape of the one she tried was too high and stiff. In any case, this is the first time in her life that she found anything that worked. She reports that if she feels any stress from overuse of the magnets, she simply stops using them for several days.

The magnets she is using are either bipolar or positive exposure. For short periods of time at low gauss, before possible habituation sets in, results have been highly satisfactory.

Diabetic and Lack of Circulation

Wally E., from Marysville, Washington, was ten years in pain and had five toes cut off his left foot. Now with the use of magnetic insoles, he has no pain in his feet and believes it probably could have saved the toes on his right foot if he had known about magnetotherapy before. As a diabetic, he has virtually no circulation in the feet, which turn white at times. With the magnetic insoles, his feet feel ticklish and now have feeling in them when he walks. Two of his friends, he recalls, fell off ladders and their pain was eliminated after brief treatments. His daughter, who works in a bank with cement floors, uses the magnetic insoles for comfort and better circulation.

Stiffness, Soreness, Lack of Circulation

Escha T., from Toledo, Washington, a nurse practicing alternative therapies, did not need to be convinced of the therapeutic effects of magnetism. She started on her own back pain to increase circulation with a magnetic pad. For the first time in years she awakened in the morning without a stiff back. One of her patients could not lift her arms because of a terrible problem with bursitis; but after only thirty-six hours use of magnets, she was able to lift both arms, changing her entire character and lifestyle. She and her chiropractor husband recommend a daily maintenance program for the use of magnets, besides sleeping on the pad. It eliminates toxins at night and that feeling of old age. It's good for you, she says, whether you have pain or not. It gives you energy.

Hip Injury

Bob S., from Boise, Idaho, spent 30,000 dollars on a hip injury he received thirty-five years ago. The permanent, bipolar magnet took the place of pills and eliminated the pain after only a few short, 15 minute treatments. He has been pain free since August, 1990. He uses a magnetic bed pad and pillow. Treatment usually takes one or two days until the swelling or pain is eliminated.

Shoulder and Body Pain

Some people get too much of a reaction at the beginning, from magnetic beds. One case, Elsie H., from Minnesota, had such a sufficiently adverse reaction that she had to get off the bed pad. Even the negative polarity can develop a stressful feeling as the body detoxifies. This may last several nights or even longer depending on the severity of the patient's condition. But one should not give up the therapy. She found greater success with permanent magnets placed at the site, including for shoulder pain even though her shoulder had to be largely replaced. She also used magnets on her jaws to relieve pain throughout the body.

Information Brief

Unfounded Arthritic Claims

The following is an example of unfounded claims by drug companies and how they attempt to convince a naive medical profession of efficacy by buying off consultants, expert panelists, and so-called respectable medical journals that physicians admire like little bibles.

The FDA is requiring Syntex Laboratories Inc., makers of Naprosyn and Anaprox (half of Syntex's $1.8 billion in sales last year) to carry out a multi-million dollar advertising campaign retracting unfounded claims about curing arthritis. There is no clear evidence that it results in anything more than relief of inflammation, which can cause pain. They attempted to plant in the minds of physicians that Naprosyn could prevent the joint degeneration that depicts arthritis. The research was preliminary, based on studies in test tubes and animals that are not adequate to support any conclusions about how a drug might work in humans.

Syntex assembled an advisory board staffed with scientists who were paid as promotional consultants and independent arthritis researchers who appeared on sales pitches on cable TV and video tape. Ads stating that studies showed the drug "significantly reduced degenerative enzyme activities by as much as 80 percent," were published in 18 medical journals. The company sponsored speakers at medical meetings and gave them slide shows. Physicians were taken to dinner or invited to join promotional panels. Syntex signed a consent decree to stop making false claims, but the drug is still being sold while many of the 37 million Americans who suffer from arthritis will still use it under a misperception. The FDA states that while some drugs can relieve pain and inflammation, there is no known treatment that prevents or stops progression of arthritis.

Source: *Washington Post*, October 11, 1991; author.

Chronic Neck and Back Pain

Minnesotans Chris and Jim N. had chronic neck and back pain from an auto accident. With magnetotherapy, each day their conditions improved. They say that there quality of life has improved 200 percent.

David C. Brodeur B.Sc., D.D.S., M.P.H, of Calgary, Alberta, injured his back over 25 years ago at his university, suffering a degenerative disk disease as well as osteoarthritis in the lumbar vertebrae. He began to feel pain relief after the first two weeks of sleeping on a negative polarity magnetic bed. Improvement in pain levels and mobility have continued. He let his parents sleep on the bed for several weeks, both in their 70's, and they have experienced considerable reduction in body aches and pains, while eliminating pain medication they had been taking.

Sgt. George Breen (retired, 58 years old), injured his back in the Canadian Armed Forces three times—in Korea 1953, Germany 1959, and in Canada 1965. A spinal fusion (lower lumbar) was done in 1966 but he was unable to cope with his duties and was honorably released on medical grounds at 48 percent disability. He suffered a lower back pain for over two decades as it took its toll both physically and mentally. Medication, heat treatments, physiotherapy, chiropractic sessions and long periods of bed rest offered only temporary relief. Finally, he tried magnetotherapy by applying a four inch by six inch negative pole magnet directly to the injured area and in twenty five minutes most of the pain was eliminated. It was exciting for him to stand up and not be subjected to the usual flash of burning pain under the muscle of the upper portion of the right leg. He now sleeps on a magnetic bed every night, feeling much more relaxed and at peace with himself. He is free of back pain for the first time in 25 years.

Multiple Sclerosis Victim Pain

Jackie S., who has multiple sclerosis with tubes sticking in her back used permanent magnets for one evening. The next day she awoke without any back pain. As mentioned earlier, Dr. Harry Park M.D. has found unusual success in treating MS cases, even to the extent where some patients have had the good fortune of being able to rid themselves of wheel chairs. In the case mentioned here, Jackie used a south pole Nikken pad. In Dr. Park's cases, patients were treated for about 10 minutes with the south polarity to stimulate muscular movement and then negative magnetic fields applied from then on to achieve polarity balance and to prevent any adverse effects.

Wrist Pain

Mary Lou H., of Minnesota, was in an auto accident and broke her wrist, which would hurt mostly when it rained. A small, 350-gauss bipolar, flat magnet took the aching away in her fingers and also her wrist pain by the next day. After several months, there was still no return of pain. Her daughter, who had palsy in her face and an unstable stomach, lost almost all pain in a few short months with magnetotherapy

259

application. Quite frequently, she also had an unstable stomach. The sleeping pad has eliminated problems in that respect.

Knee Pain

Rich E., from Sioux Falls, South Dakota, at age 85 has had a pain in the knee from a football injury during his college days. A small, bipolar 555-gauss, flat magnet placed on the knee has eliminated the pain. Whenever pain returns, usually a week later, a mini-magnetic pad eliminates the pain immediately.

Shoulder, Hand and Speech Ailments

A young woman, Barbara S., from Hillsboro, Oregon, with a shoulder injury, numbness in the right hand and nerve damage from a 1968 auto accident, had seen doctors and chiropractors who told her they had done all they could do. This meant she had to live with pain for over 20 years. A simple 550-gauss magnet in one hour took the numbness and pain away. The same treatment healed her cabinetmaker husband, who couldn't bend his fingers from tedious carpentry work. He can now double his fist without pain. He carries a small magnet with him at work for whenever he needs it. He hasn't had to see a chiropractor since, except to set bones in place after an accident.

A sister in his family, with lack of coordination in her speech, was able to return to the normal use of her voice within a three-hour period with the application of magnets. These small magnets were bipolar and only used for short periods of time at low gauss strength, so the habituation effect never had a chance to take hold.

Tumors and Hyperventilation

One woman, Diana I., with a tumor in her back, applied a bipolar magnet and within two days time noticed a reduction in the tumor. In one week the tumor was itching and in one month, there was a 70 percent reduction in the size of the tumor. She also hyperventilates upon waking in the morning, a condition she had for several years. The magnets eliminated the hyperventilation completely. Both the husband and son can't believe the reduction in tumor size and the increased energy of Diana. Also both the husband and son got rid of backaches by sleeping on magnetic pads. They have been pain free since September, 1990.

Severe Pain and Migraines

Elsie H., of St. Paul, Minnesota, eliminated the pain in her right arm following surgery from application of magnetic fields. Her close friend, who experienced three-day migraines, eliminated them entirely with magnetotherapy.

Stiff Joints

Automobile accidents are probably the main cause of paralyzation of individuals. About 50,000 Americans are killed every year in the deadly automobile and a quarter of a million seriously injured. Over the years, the seriously injured number into the millions. Most cannot seem to find the relief they desire.

Jacqueline W., of Sarasota, Florida, had a serious auto accident several years ago requiring weekly visits to a chiropractor and a neuro-muscular therapist just to minimize the pain. Every morning she had to do stretching exercises to limber her joints and lower back, in order to reduce pain. After using a magnetic mattress pad, her pain almost dissipated completely and those morning exercises were hardly necessary. Also, now she has considerably more energy throughout the day.

Glioblastoma

Dr. Philpott cites the case of a 20 year old student who was diagnosed by traditional techniques to have a glioblastoma which had infiltrated the brain tissue so extensively it could not be surgically removed. The patient was incapable of making any response to environmental stimuli. Philpott applied a 4"x6"x½", solid-state, ceramic magnet on the back of the head where the tumor had initially started. Negative fields were continued 24 hours a day. In three days, the patient was able to wiggle his fingers in response to questions. In three weeks, he walked out of the hospital with the assistance of only a walker. Six months later, he was reported doing well, other than a residual imbalance problem. Magnetotherapy was not the only treatment utilized in this case, but was the primary treatment. The patient continued negative magnetic exposure of the brain five hours per day for a set period.

Melanoma

Another Philpott case involved a young man thirty years of age with melanoma, which had been surgically removed, plus a metastasis which also had been removed. He treated himself by the general body method with negative magnetic energy daily for a minimum of three hours. Chances of metastasis with melanoma are high, however, after three years no evidence of further metastasis is present in this patient.

Sore Shoulder

A close friend, Karen S., of Alexandria, Virginia, was able to stop seeing the chiropractor altogether, after applying a bipolar, permanent magnet to her severely painful shoulder derived from her office/home cleaning business, where she constantly uses her arms and shoulders. She eliminated a continual monthly bill of $150 with a $20 permanent magnet that will last almost forever. Whenever there is a pain, the doctor is there in her purse to be attached to her shoulder for ten to fifteen minutes. She now knows her problem and how to treat it. She has taken control of her life, saved her modest but life-supporting business, and is happier as a result. Her confidence is also way up.

General Use of Magnetotherapy

Many therapists and M.D.s use magnetotherapy. Chiropractors and neuro-muscular specialists in almost every metropolitan area of the country utilize this therapy. Many are quietly using magnets as part of their regular protocol without fanfare.

Many therapists, and especially M.D.s, fear ruining their reputations or dread being called quacks if they choose to use magnetic fields, yet over 100,000 operations are performed every year with magnetotherapy by orthopedic surgeons who draw salaries of as much as $400,000 or more. For some reason, if a doctor cuts open a leg and manipulates a fracture, then heals by electromagnetism, this is more acceptable than simply placing a permanent magnet on the patient's body to assist bone fusion or to reduce inflammation and pain or to stimulate acupuncture points. Yet the same level of cure or relief can occur in most cases with either electromagnetism or permanent magnets. It appears that drawing blood or using some weird, technological-looking instrument is required to gain credibility and a big fee.

Dr. Harry Park, Vancouver, Washington, uses permanent magnets in almost every case in preference to acupuncture needles. In many cases he uses a combination of the two. He utilizes a powerful 12,300 gauss neodymium magnet on breast cancer patients resulting in reduction of tumors. For certain other critical problems, Dr. Park uses a specially designed 12 inch thick solid magnetic bed of 20,000 gauss—weighing over 2,000 pounds—for about one hour of treatment with magnetic north (negative) facing the body. He supports use of the negative polarity, citing over two dozen studies that show blood sugar levels rising rapidly under positive field use and coming down from the negative magnetic fields. He reports that symptoms are reproducible for many ailments, citing epilepsy as one disease whose symptoms appear when positive fields are used and go away under application of negative fields. This is certainly strong evidence of the differences between these two fields.

On the other hand, some have expressed concern that over application of negative fields might slow down ilieus and dry up fluids. However, Dr. Dean Bonlie does not believe this to be true. As reported earlier for a number of people, withdrawal symptoms of stress or other reactions can occur from application of the negative polarity as well as the positive until toxins are released from the body. A gradual increase in the amount of time one sleeps on a magnetic bed, for example, is recommended—from one or two hours, to three or four, and finally a full night. Dr. Park supplements his treatments with natural herbal drinks that reduce withdrawal effects considerably and remove toxins 10 times more quickly, according to his results. This sounds like excellent advice to be used by all magnetotherapists. Too great a stress at first could discourage one from sleeping on a magnetic pad.

One Physician's Approach

Many of the cases cited in this chapter represent individuals treating themselves without much medical assistance. It is recommended that anyone with a serious ailment first get medical advice, then proceed on to alternatives, preferably under observation.

Treatment protocols of several physicians have already been enumerated. Here is discussed in greater detail the treatment regimen of one doctor in order to give an idea of a comprehensive approach. Although this relates to how Dr. Philpott would approach cancer treatment, the procedures are very similar for most diseases and therefore is a good, typical example.

In this protocol, Dr. Philpott first exposes a cancerous lesion, as the case in point (or other illness), to a negative magnetic field for as many hours per day as possible. This is combined with the pacing of the basic circadian biorhythm with a bright light in the morning and a negative magnetic energy directed towards the crown of the head during sleep. These two elements combine to help create valuable defenses for a non-toxic, non-addicting, non-allergic, non-infecting, and a well-nourished and mentally optimistic state. Since approximately 70 percent of the body's energy is derived from nutrients, a proper diet is essential, including important levels of vitamins C, D, E, A, B_6 and B_2, as well as niacin and various minerals. Good nutrition tends to keep the body's pH level up and allows magnetic fields to function more effectively.

Simultaneously to the above, the patient should engage in imagery for 15 - 30 minutes daily or for 10 minute periods several times daily to visualize the receding of the cancer (or other illness), along with relaxation techniques. Dr. Bernie Siegel, mentioned earlier, whom millions have followed to acquire a positive mental attitude, underscores the value of good mental imaging and a happy outlook on life to effect cure and to make it long lasting.

Dr. Philpott states that we know that cancer is electrically positive, verified by the body's concentration of negative energy to try to heal this disease. He stipulates that negative electric energy and negative magnetic energy have similar, beneficial biological effects. The application of negative magnetic energy to the body generally, and more particularly to cancerous locales, can materially aid the body, since cancer cells (or tumors) have lost the magnetic characteristics of normal cells.

As researchers have pointed out, positive magnetic energy (in contrast to negative energy) has no capacity to heal on its own, but rather attracts negative ions to the site for healing in performance of the counter-irritant function. Certain doctors (Dr. Gusta Wollin and Dr. Eric Endy as reported in the journal, *Magnets in Your Future*) advocate using positive energy directly over the sternum to stimulate the thymus gland. Philpott believes that it is theoretically possible that this could stimulate the production of T-cells and so aid the immune defensive system. Yet if positive fields are used, Philpott would limit them to three minutes of application several times daily and would ensure that the negative fields were applied as many hours of a 24-hour day as possible.

In regard to cancer, Philpott makes no claims statistically that there is scientific proof that negative energy application cures cancer. He says that "there is probably no quicker way to lose professional reputation than to claim a cure for cancer." On the other hand, he can cite numerous successful case histories. His wife of age 71 incurred basal cell carcinoma (diagnosed by a pathologist) on the forehead from sunburn which periodically needed to be removed surgically. In time, he began treating the lesion nightly during her sleep with a small neodymium magnet; in six weeks, the pathological area had dried up and peeled off without a scar. Other cases involve glioblastoma of the brain and melanoma.

These patients could not wait for controlled tests, especially after all else had failed. Philpott has meticulously documented numerous cases in his clinical practice from a point prior to treatment to a satisfactory period after therapy. In our modern-day science and scrambling for cures, one would think that the appropriate studies to verify these findings would already exist, but they don't. Checking with the National Cancer Institute, they report that no studies are being conducted on the possibilities of magnetotherapy as a cure for cancer and no studies are planned. Surely some tax dollars could be put to this use.

Exciting Discoveries for
Drug and Alcohol Addiction

Turning from individual cases and a typical protocol for treatment, let us look at an important clinical study that tends to verify the kinds of claims self-help people make. When an individual tells his health healing story, it is anecdotal. But when doctors cure thousands of patients with magnetotherapy with a success rate as high as 70 percent, it's more than anecdotal. Clinical trials under skillful investigators and proper record-keeping make good evidence. One such trial is discussed here involving drug addiction.

More appears to be taking place in England, Canada, China and a number of other countries than in the United States in the use of electric or magnetic therapy in the treatment of a variety of diseases, including drug addition, alcoholism, tobacco addiction, and certain other chronic diseases.

The first description for the treatment of drug addiction by electric-acupuncture was done by Dr. Wen in Hong Kong in 1973, following a visit to China to study the techniques used there. As we have already described, electro or permanent magnets can stimulate acupuncture points, and magnetic fields pass through skin and tissue without damage or pain and in a wider area for even greater effect. Philpott and others say that the permanent magnet does essentially the same thing as electro-intrusion. In this treatment, Dr. Robert O. Becker suggested to Dr. Wen's assistant at the time, Dr. Margaret A. Patterson, that the use of a flat, non-intrusive electric (or magnetic) base would work just as well as sticking one with a projectile. And he was right. It worked.

Acupuncture, for example, can take place through a set of headphones consisting of blunt electrodes (in place of needles) or magnets to stimulate points in and around the ear. With this method, there is no danger of infection or hepatitis, and the use of repeated needles is avoided. Dr. Patterson calls such surface electrodes, neuroelectric therapy (NET). Since all currents produce magnetic fields, we are talking about both electric and magnetic stimulation.

Information Brief

Alcohol Addiction and Rehabilitation

Jon H. S. , Portland Oregon, took a New Year's resolution January 1st 1992 to stop using alcohol which he had abused for 15 years (10 - 12 drinks per day). Upon using a negative oriented magnetic bed, Jon was surprised not to experience any withdrawal symptoms—no shakes, headaches, chills, or discomfort of any kind. The only side effect was increased sweating the first night.

In his previous attempts to quit drinking, he experienced the above type of symptoms on every occasion. This time he did not need aspirin or any other pain relievers. Instead he had the benefit of "A very sound sleep and increased energy." He is now on a very vigorous exercise program and has been surprised that even after strenuous exercise, he does not experience sore muscles because of the magnetic bed.

Source: MagnetiCo Inc., Calgary, Alberta, Canada, February 1992.

The clinical trial, described in Exhibit 27, uses electro-acupuncture to the ear, demonstrating success in detoxifying drug addicts without the usual side effects. The success of electroacupuncture has been documented in well over 100 journal articles since 1970. The U. S. needs to do more in this alternative system in order to make it available in all drug treatment centers across the nation. It's the first step in getting an addict on the road to recovery and setting him up for effective counseling and follow-up, which could never happen if he were not drug-free. (More is discussed on

Exhibit 26   Sampling Dr. Philpott's Case Histories

Five hospitalized patients with intractable headaches, not responding to traditional pain medication, were all relieved with the application of a negative magnetic field from a solid state magnet placed over the painful area. The longest time to obtain relief was 15 minutes.

A man with a toothache and perodontal abscess, exuding puss, obtained relief from pain within ten minutes of exposure from the negative field of a solid state magnet. The magnet was left on the infected area for four days, at which time he was examined by a dentist and no infection was found.

A deteriorated diabetic with diabetic neuropathy, producing a severe burning pain in the soles of his feet, was promptly relieved of his pain by placing his feet on the negative magnetic pole of solid state magnets. Three treatments a day of 10 minutes duration kept the pain relieved. After three weeks of treatment, the pain no longer returned.

A dog with cataracts had a resolution of the cataracts within 72 hours of exposure to the negative magnetic field of a magnet. Several humans have also been observed to have cataracts resolved with negative magnetic energy exposure to the eyes. (Albert Roy Davis also reported cataract resolution in

A man in his 70's with arteriosclerosis of his heart and brain obtained relief of pain in his heart within ten minutes of placing a magnet over his heart with the negative magnetic pole facing the heart. Sleeping with a negative magnetic field at the crown of his head relieved anxiety, depression, thick speech, unsteadiness on his feet with stumbling, as well as getting lost in familiar surroundings.   *(Cont'd)*

An Alzheimer's victim obtained relief from mental confusion when her head was exposed to a negative magnetic field. The mental confusion returned several hours after removal of the magnetic field.

Many subjects have reported remarkable relief of insomnia as well as increased energy when sleeping with the negative magnetic pole of magnets facing the top of the head.

A woman with candidiasis of the vagina obtained relief of symptoms and evidence of the fungal infection dying out with daily sitting on the negative pole of a magnet.

A man in his 70's with sleep apnea had a correction of the apnea when sleeping with a negative magnetic field at the crown of his head. He slept deeper and his fingernails, toenails and hair grew faster.   *(Cont'd)*

the number of centers that have undertaken this treatment in the U.S. in the next chapter.)

Exhibit 26   **Sampling Dr. Philpott's Case Histories** *(Cont'd)*

A woman in her 70's, while sleeping with a negative magnetic field at the top of her head and on a negative magnetic bed pad increased depth of sleep and increased energy. Brittle head hair developed normal texture, body hair that had lessened after menopause regrew, and a fibrous marble sized nodule in the left groin area which was residual to a post-birth blood clot 33 years before was resolved.

A woman in her 70's with basal cell carcinoma of the forehead, residual to a sunburn of the forehead some years before, treated the cancerous area every night while asleep with a negative magnetic pole of a magnet and in six weeks the cancer dried up and peeled off.

A young man with post-brain injury grand mal seizures occurring every two hours, day and night, without control by any medication, was seizure free with bitemporally placed magnets.

A teenager with temporal lobe confusion type seizures, evoked during a deliberate food test meal of eggs, had no seizures on a subsequent test meal of eggs when the negative pole of a magnet was placed on the temporal areas.

A man in his 60's, in a state of depression, had not eaten food or drunk water for six weeks and was being sustained by intravenous feedings. Tranquilizers and antidepressants were of no value. Electric shock was being considered as a necessity. He had reversal of his depression with one hour of exposure of a negative magnetic field applied to the back of his head.

Source: William H. Philpott, M.D., Choctow, OK, Feb, 1992.
(These cases were observed or administered by Philpott and clinically recorded over a period of time to verify results.)

The major significance of the treatment in the Hong Kong study is that 100 patients were treated for drug addiction—with no counseling or social support and no psychotherapy—and there was complete success in taking them off drugs without any medication. Withdrawal symptoms ceased within 15 - 20 minutes of starting the treatment. Treatments were for forty minutes over a 10-day period, after which the addicts reported no desire to take their drug of addiction any longer. Other successful cases were reported in the *Medical Journal of Australia* by Dr. Sainsbury, with results witnessed by independent psychiatrists. Dr. Patterson has repeated the same 100 percent rate of success in England with 60 patients.

SCIENTIFIC DIGEST

Drug Addiction and the Brain

Paul Tyler brings us up-to-date on findings related to electromagnetism. He reports that the National Institute of Mental Health studied rats addicted to morphine and found that current stimulation to the lower part of the concha (posterior to the external auditory meatus) precipitated signs of morphine abstinence. Researchers (Sjolund, Clement-Jones, Salar and others) have reported an increase in B-endorphins in cerebrospinal fluid following electro-acupuncture and other forms of electrotherapy. Increased rat brain levels of serotonin, tryptophan and hydroxyindole acetic acid have been reported. Numerous studies show changes of calcium ion levels in the brain following the use of magnetic fields.

It is believed that the body's own production of B-endorphins is turned off by drug addiction and that electro or magnetic stimulation enhances the natural production and release of encephalins and B-endorphins by the body, preventing the onset of withdrawal symptoms. Tyler speculates that calcium is the critical factor and not the endorphin system. He further states that modern medicine has studied and treated the chemical side of the equation but has almost completely ignored the electrical/magnetic side. The body's natural chemicals are released by an electrical signal so it seems plausible that an external signal can do the same at a specific site without drugging the rest of the body.

Source: **EMR and The Brain; A Brief Literature Review**, Paul Tyler,1990, prepared for an FDA conference.

Exhibit 27   Effects of Neuro-Electric Therapy and Drug Addiction

Case	Age	Sex	Main Drugs	Maximum daily dosage	Duration of drug use (in years)	Neuro treatment (in days)	Hours of daily treatment	Follow-up period (in months)
1	28	M	Heroin (snorted)	2g	12	35	2 - 6	21
2	22	F	Heroin (snorted and I.V.)	2g	6	28	1 - 3	20
3	31	M	Heroin I.V. Cocaine I.V.	2g 2g	3 10	10	2 - 6	19
4	22	F	Heroin I.V. Methadone oral (prev. heroine I.V. & cocaine I.V.)	600mg 1g 60mg 1g 3g	11 3 3 3	10 Relapse	6 - 7	--
5	43	M	Methadone oral (prev. heroin I.V. & cocaine I.V.)	500mg 1¾g 2g	3 23 23	28	1 - 3	5½
6	26	M	Heroin (snort) cocaine (snort)	1g 1g	3 10	10	1 - 10	1½

Note: Subjects were given some sedatives during initial treatment. Only two or three relapses occurred over one month, while over 90 percent of subjects were drug free two years later with fair to marked improvement in character. Range of treatment frequency varied from five to 2,000 cycles per second with the optimum under 100 c.p.s. with no clear indication that frequency or waveform had any real effect.

Source: Summarized from *Bulletin on Narcotics*, Vol XXVIII, no.4, October-December 1976. Study conducted by Dr. Margaret A. Patterson involving 60 patients, England, Britain. This exhibit shows a sample of just six of the 60 subjects.

The method used in these demonstrations consists of electrode contact in the concha of each ear and a current of 1 to 2 milliamps range and frequency of 5 to 2000 cps. Success may be due to the actual reconditioning of certain brain circuits. To prevent recidivism, intense counseling and rebuilding of lives are also essential. With this treatment, the patient is significantly more receptive to rehabilitation. Sleep patterns return to normal far more rapidly, eliminating one of the major problems of other forms of withdrawal. Most importantly, consistent increase in optimism is generated rather than the usual depression. In any case, some evaluators would like to have more specifics, such as frequency, type of pulses, repetition rate, etc. By using a steady-state magnet this is all irrelevant in any case, since only the gauss strength and polarity are significant. However, use of correct frequency would likely make results more efficient and effective.

It is hypothesized that drug addiction turns off the body's own production of B-endorphins and, upon acute withdrawal, distress is caused by the failure of the body to produce endorphin and encephalin. Electrotherapy enhances natural production and release of endorphins, thus preventing withdrawal symptoms. Dr. Patterson claims that electro-stimulation is effective for most drugs, including heroin, cocaine, barbiturates, alcohol and nicotine. *

With the serious drug problem prevalent in the United States and the world, more study and application of electro and/or magnetotherapy needs to be undertaken as soon as possible. The U S has concentrated too much on supply and interdiction and too little on the physical cause of increased drug addiction. Federal agencies have not seemed interested. Perhaps this is because they feel people should not try drugs to begin with and, perhaps, fear that electromagnetic treatment may tend to increase the endorphins in the brain, mimicking the effects of illicit drugs, a process called "wire-heading." Some may use the science foolishly and dangerously; yet, under professionally supervised clinical treatments and after only six weeks of care, patients have turned drug free. Most remain so with proper follow-up and counseling, job programs and other support. Certainly these findings are worth further exploration.

---

* The italicized text refers to more complex information.

Chapter 9

Magnetotherapy Helping the Health System

Here we have a new understanding of a historic treatment—magnetic energy used by millions, with the intake of chemicals and drugs within the body an anathema to our lives. In magnetotherapy, no medicine is orally fed or injected into the body. It is essentially a natural cure, even free from the intricate procedures of such therapies as acupressure, acupuncture, homeopathy, hypnosis, elaborate diets, or mind control. It is the simplest, least expensive, and most painless and safest therapy known. A magnet is the only instrument used. It is not magic. It doesn't heal anything, rather it stimulates the body to heal itself. It allows body cells to function at their peak levels as a wholly natural event.

One of the questions posed is how many conventional doctors would ever recommend natural therapies? Too many strive for the highest paying positions—radiologists, oncologists and pathologists. In Canada, over half of the doctors are family physicians; in the U.S. only 12 percent. If we all had a good family doctor, most of the unnecessary testing and padding would flatten out and our national health bill would drop. Several states now have plans, such as the Maryland Access to Care, that require all low income residents on Medicaid (300,000 in Maryland) to have a personal physician in order to guide patients to preventive care, immunizations, mammograms, checkups, and the elimination of unnecessary, expensive treatments. These doctors get higher pay for being available after office hours and for treating patients with a sense of special care and warmth, and providing preventive education. They also look for safe, natural treatments. The problem is that there aren't enough of these doctors. Certainly it is a failure of the medical schools and medical associations.

The federal government started a new program in 1992 that will fundamentally change the way we think about medical services. Medicare will pay doctors more for spending time with patients and for listening and talking and evaluating conditions together, and less for operating and employing instruments and other costly procedures. Private insurers may begin to adopt similar standards. This will benefit the family doctor where one in four netted less than $65,000 last year. The medium income for family physicians was $93,000, internists $120,000 and surgeons $200,000. But 25 percent of surgeons earned $300,000 to $400,000 and above. Under the new plan, family physician fees will rise 28 percent by 1996, while fees for neurologists, radiologists and pathologists will drop by 20 percent. The forward looking Joseph Boyle, executive vice president of the American Society of Internal Medicine, pushed for this change long ago. Now, finally, we are headed in the right direction.

Ethically, it is the responsibility of the doctor to become knowledgeable about all cures. Unfortunately, magnetotherapy is not taught in our medical schools and only a relatively small number of M.D.s are familiar enough with it to use it. A patient should not have to wonder if his skilled doctor is fully cognizant of all medicines, is well read and trained, or is making the correct judgment in each case, regardless of time or financial return. No longer should General Practitioners (GPs) be considered mentally deficient "bumpkins" because they haven't chosen to enter the more lucrative specialties of surgery or radiology. It is time to touch the patient, express love and understanding, and tell him or her the details. Some believe we need a specialty of "generalization," where medical sensitivity and a total approach to healing predominate.

The family doctor's caring characteristics are exemplified by Dr. Bernie Siegel who advises the dissatisfied patient to give the doctor a hug to make him more willing to respond to what then becomes a warm human being rather than a disease. But if it doesn't work, he says, it's time to get another doctor in place of a mechanic who deals only in cases, charts, remedies, prognoses—but not real people. Recall that Hippocrates said that "he would rather know what sort of person has a disease than what sort of disease a person has." Siegel throws out an idea for training doctors that suggests physicians initially should not be allowed to prescribe medication or consider an operation, rather first simply engage in helping, caring and sharing on an emotional level—then proceed to the more conventional steps. Furthermore, full participation by the patient should be paramount. (See Exhibit 28, **Yale Physician's Oath 1991).**

Exhibit 28 Yale's Physician's Oath, 1991

> Now being admitted to the high calling of the physician, I solemnly pledge to consecrate my life to the care of the sick, the promotion of health and the service of humanity.
> I will practice medicine with conscience and in truth. The health and dignity of my patients will be my first concern. I will hold in confidence all that my patients relate to me. I will not permit considerations of race, religion, nationality, or social standing to influence my duty to care for those in need of my service.
> I will respect the moral right of patients to participate fully in the medical decisions that affect them. I will assist my patients to make choices that coincide with their own values and beliefs.
> I will try to increase my competence constantly and respect those who teach and those who broaden our knowledge by research. I will try to prevent, as well as cure, disease.

The first hand experience of Siegel, formulated from his dealing with thousands of patients, has revealed that about 15 to 20 percent of clients with serious illnesses, unconsciously or consciously wish to die in order to escape their problems. In the middle of the spectrum, about 60 to 70 percent perform like actors to satisfy the doctor and do whatever they are told, unless, of course, it requires a radical change in lifestyle. This middle group would rather be operated on than actively work to get well. Yet there is a final group of 15 to 20 percent who are exceptional and refuse to play victim. They educate themselves and become specialists in their own care, without the regimentation of years of medical school. They understand that there are choices.

My father-in-law is in the last category, refusing to play victim. When he was hardly able to walk, shuffling across the floor and diagnosed as seriously diseased and old-aged at 75, he educated himself about every technique of healing, reading a dozen medical books and consulting with experts and searching alternative therapies. He found the answers he needed largely on his own and lived well into his eighties in a vigorous lifestyle. He remained spry as ever through his eighties, taking his sailboat out with his wife on weekends. He's a prime example of a positive attitude of wanting to live, to see his grandchildren, to sail, and to enjoy life to it's longest end.

Hope may be alive for the specialty of "generalist," as the trend for more personal care turns to the patient's favor in psychiatry. Women constitute 24 percent of practicing psychiatrists but are more than 40 percent of psychiatric residents in hospitals. In the not too distant future, the majority of psychiatrists may be female. "Women in our society are enculturated to be empathic, and psychiatry depends in part in its practice for that," says Paul McHugh of Johns Hopkins Medical School. Psychiatry is interesting, particularly for women, and allows for a more flexible schedule for dual careers that suit women more as homemakers than professionals. Women "are so devoted to their patients, I often have to bail them out; they've taken on so much," he says. This sounds like the kind of doctors we need, sensitive and caring, professionally honest and more willing to resist pressure groups lobbying for special interests.

Nevertheless, leadership roles are still male dominated, and training programs have not changed. Fortunately, the stigma of mental illness and diagnoses and treatments are better understood. And women are more likely to engage in healing by means of listening and touching and showing compassion. The whole philosophy of dealing with the mind and body equally for healing applies—physical and mental problems resolved as a unitary element. Bill Moyer's book **Mind and Body** and a recent PBS television series on this subject has helped to dispel some of the mysteries, daring to show the efficacy of alternative therapy.

Passive emotions, such as grief, feelings of failure, and suppression of anger produce over-secretion of hormones by the adrenal glands, suppressing the immune system, says Siegel. One of the most widely accepted explanations of cancer is the "surveillance" theory that postulates cancer cells are developing in our bodies all the time but are naturally destroyed by white blood cells before they can develop into dangerous tumors. Anything that adversely affects the brain's control of the immune system, Siegel believes, will foster malignancy. And as already stated, it has been shown how magnetic fields can improve the functioning of the immune system and also help in dealing with Chronic Stress Syndrome and other depressive diseases.

Mental and physical attributes go hand-in-hand. Dr. Robert O. Becker found that hypnotised patients can produce voltage changes on command in specific areas of the body to affect both chemical and cellular processes of healing, which may help to explain the placebo effect associated with a variety of treatments. Today, bioelectricity and biomagnetism have enabled us to reach our body's controllers directly in order to treat tumors and other ailments. Since many people have difficulty accepting loving and hugging or mind therapies, magnetotherapy and other alternatives are also necessary ingredients. Most people are simply unwilling or unable to heal by mental attitude alone. We need to use all options. We must ask, if drugs don't work, should we pass up hypnosis or acupuncture or magnetotherapy!

Physicians have an ethical responsibility to explore all reasonable alternatives. For example, about 10 million Americans suffer from depression every year at a cost of 27 billion dollars in productivity. A survey conducted in 1991 for the National Mental Health Association found 43 percent of people believe depression is a personal weakness, yet health experts know it is essentially caused by biological, chemical and environmental factors. Government studies show that a combination of psychotherapy and drugs can successfully treat 80 percent of depressions that have symptoms of hopelessness and sadness, sleep or eating problems, loss of interest in normal activities, aches and pains, chronic headache, loss of sex drive, feelings of worthlessness or thoughts of suicide.

In clinical depression, patients will start slipping further and further very early, blaming themselves, and getting caught up in guilt and self-deprecating beliefs. Yet various treatments can help. Clear evidence exists that magnetotherapy improves sleep, relieves aches and pains and headaches, increases energy and consequently sex drive, and generally makes one emotionally stronger.

The System is Failing Us

The recent chief executive of the AMA, James S. Todd, recognized that the private health system has not worked. The profession is splintering. Surgeons and radiologists have ignored AMA calls for health expenditure boards to set fees or to negotiate budgets among physicians and hospitals and other providers. He says, "If it becomes every man, woman, and child for themselves, then let's stop fooling around, let's get National Health Insurance, go to work for the government and be done with it because that is exactly what will happen. They will chew us up, piece by piece by piece—until we don't have any resemblance of the profession left."

276

From another point of view, John R. Ball, executive vice president of the American College of Physicians, representing 72,000 internal medicine specialists, says, "Politically the AMA has for too long fought change, rather than accept that physicians are only part of the system." Nurses, psychiatrists, chiropractors, physical therapists, home care providers and alternative therapists are all pushing for better ways to care for America and their numbers are growing. Chiropractors, for example, grew from 13,729 in 1970 to over 20,000 today, treating 8 1/2 million new patients. With the advent of new knowledge from a variety of alternative therapies, we may see a doubling of these figures in another decade.

A recent Gallup poll shows 69 percent of Americans have lost faith in doctors. People are worried about unnecessary surgery, over-prescribing of drugs, and investment by doctors in the same laboratories to which they refer patients, observes Dr. Sydney Wolfe of Public Citizen Health Research Group. Now the AMA has announced an image campaign: "If you, like many Americans, think doctors are a bunch of inattentive money-grubbers, then the American Medical Association has a message for you." AMA plans to spend millions of dollars in ads over the next couple of years to "highlight the caring, sharing, sensitive side of members." They say that the public does not fully understand or appreciate the work they do.

However, humans need a deep, personal touch. The Pathways health chronicle reports that people become emotionally sick when preoccupied with their own special problems brought on by illness. Therefore, they often feel guilty or angry at a higher level than usual—confused, depressed or nauseated. They complain of physicians' lack of compassion that makes them feel humiliated and the use of doctor jargon that leaves them confused. "The doctor never looked at me during the entire encounter," is a common complaint. "They continually interrupt, disrupting the patient's attempt to complete a thought."

Most diseases involve, at least in part, stress, psychological and social factors—considerations lost by most doctors for improving health. Risks from chronic hostility or depression may be greater than we expect. The NIH recently issued a list of cardiovascular risk factors—family history, previous circulatory disease, smoking, diabetes, obesity, high blood pressure—but incredibly, says Dr. Howard S. Friedman, author of "The Self Healing Personality," there was no mention of stress or hostility or any psychosocial variable! Of the $3.5 billion spent on this type of research each year by NIH, we wonder why there is a lack of concern for life's social factors and alternative therapies that have proved successful.

Authors Jim and Andrea Fordham, in Pathways, recite a story where a merciful doctor offered to make house calls occasionally to the home of an 80 year old man who could not drive very well any more. "Some weeks later I drove to that small town, followed his directions to the outskirts, found the house trailer and concrete block that Mr. and Mrs. Henry called home," the doctor recalled. "I was greeted with a smile and a special handshake. As I left, I felt absolutely wonderful." This care for the person rather than trying to stamp out a disease cannot be legislated in any national health plan. Doctors must find it within themselves.

Why can't more physicians accept the fact that alternative treatments are real and at times more effective than conventional methods? Why can't doctors say that it is okay to omit treatment on occasion or say that it is all right to let people die gracefully on occasion? Why can't doctors talk about prevention more often? Why are millions of Americans engaged in their own nutrition and exercise programs, acupuncture, homeopathy, and magnetotherapy? Prevention education is almost unknown to physicians or unimportant to their income or patient care. Prevention has failed our system while the average individual must take health into his or her own hands. It is paramount for physicians and the health insurance industry to begin to promote prevention and alternative therapies.

Private health insurance can no longer provide us with security and peace of mind. Over 81 million Americans under age 65 have medical conditions that health insurers can use as an excuse to raise premiums or to deny coverage. These include arthritis, heart murmur, ulcers, arrhythmia, multiple attacks of bronchitis, diabetes, cancer, and a wide variety of other conditions. Does this mean more and more Americans must turn to alternative therapies? It may very well be the case, as we see the system is failing us for major illnesses and even ignoring the most serious. Most insurance won't pay for sleep disorders or simple stress. These are all reasons that we may have to turn to National Health Insurance unless some more responsive answers crop up from the medical profession soon.

The bulk of the medical profession seems to have forgotten about prevention altogether. The, August 1991, Harvard Health Letter called prevention philosophy AWOL, saying if you need a pap smear, mammography, update on shots, cholesterol profile, or counseling on such things as diet, drinking habits, emotions, or exercise, you must get out your checkbook. But if you need a heart bypass at $30,000 from a bad diet or lack of exercise, or you need a liver transplant at $250,000 from drinking too much, it's "on the house."

Fortunately, some companies are coming around. Mark Bricklin, editor of the Harvard Health Letter, reports that Blue Shield's Health Trac Program encourages better health behavior at a cost of $20 per person and shows a saving on the average of $166. Also Kennecott Copper's Wellness Program shows a drop of 55 percent in medical costs. The Prudential Life Insurance Fitness Program reduced disability days from 8.6 to 3.5 days, and one of its high blood pressure programs reduced claims 78 percent. In a program of lifestyle advice and blood sugar monitoring for women with diabetes before pregnancy, the birth defect rate was reduced 90 percent. Good signs, but every physician needs to incorporate prevention techniques into her practice.

If we wish to cut the nation's health bill way down, we may need mandatory or at least incentive-type wellness programs sponsored by companies and other employers. People quit smoking and begin exercise and good nutrition habits when they are observed and encouraged. Not many will do it on their own. More than half of all deaths in the U.S. are directly related to lifestyle, according to the Center for Disease Control.

A wellness program created in 1978 by the Associated Group, an Indianapolis based insurance and financial services company, provides a brief exam of blood pressure and cholesterol screening and behavior modification programs of weight control, smoking cessation, and nutrition. About 80 percent of the group's 2,400 employees enrolled and more than a third attended classes. Findings show reduced health risk factors, absenteeism and subsequent health care costs.

A two-year study at Reynolds Electrical and Engineering Co., Las Vegas, showed that the wellness program can be transferred to other companies. Anthem Health Systems expects to market its Stay Alive and Well Health program, with the claim that $2.51 is saved for every $1.00 of expense over five years. Johnson and Johnson, the world's largest maker of health care products began a wellness program in the late 1970's and now markets it to companies, including International Business Machines Corp. and General Motors Corp., showing it has saved them $154 in health care costs for each employee.

Promise of a Unified Approach

At one point, psychiatry held the promise of the discipline that might integrate the entire body into a unified protocol of treatment. That has not happened even though efforts continue. Some psychiatric M.D.s have come close to that ideal. They treat pain and disease while assimilating the implications of the mind. It seems a travesty that any physician would treat a cancer or heart condition in a localized physical sense and not even consider one's state of mind and the entire body. Psychotherapy and various alternatives allow a physician to treat the patient in an integrated fashion. Magnetotherapy makes the total body approach relatively easy because of little fear of any adverse side effects.

A more unified treatment is slowly beginning to take shape. Doctors at Sloan Kettering in New York and M. D. Anderson in Houston routinely urge patients into group psychotherapy meditation and visualization classes. Heart, angina and high blood pressure sufferers are sent to biofeedback and stress-reduction programs as a supplement to drug treatments. An interesting analysis by U. S. News and World Report (September 1991) shows improvements in the integration of therapies, such as in acupuncture, hypnosis, biofeedback, naturopathy, reflexology, massage and other treatments designed to keep physical and mental life forces in balance. In fact, all of the relaxation methods, including warm baths, yoga, meditation and so on help to dilate the blood vessels and capillaries to increase blood flow. This is what magnetotherapy does in addition to building stronger cells.

A ten year study by psychiatric professor David Stiegel, Stanford University, found that breast cancer patients who took part in support groups and self-hypnosis to ease the discomfort and trauma of surgery and chemotherapy, survived twice as long on average as those who did not. "I am convinced that the psychological measures used to treat or prevent heart disease are just as important as anything else we do," says Dr. Dean Ornish, preventive medicine specialist.

Dr. Bernie Siegel talks about nerve fibers that enter the hypothalamus to affect our intellectual and emotional processes, stimulating or shutting off the pituitary gland's production of growth hormones. "Psychosocial dwarfism had been found in children caught in a crossfire of hostility, low self-esteem, and other emotional factors that act upon the brain's limbic system," he says. Of course, as shown in these pages, we now more fully realize that magnetic field therapy can reduce stress, create better sleep and rest, and increase growth in humans. A combination of mental and physical therapies works hand-in-hand. Some of the more potent therapies need to be examined along side the more benign. For instance, can it be possible that magnetotherapy is more predictable in treating emotional and mental illnesses, seizures, and other disorders than medication or is as effective but safer than electric shock? Some more answers are needed for an illness that costs the U.S. $250 billion annually and affects one in six Americans.

Information Brief

Drugs, Electric Shock, and Permanent Magnets

"A brain is a terrible thing to waste," shouted over 100 people representing various organizations from the U.S. and around the world at the gathering of the 1992 convention of the American Psychiatric Association in Washington, D.C. Protests were over treatment with drugs and electroshock. "What I expected to find in psychiatry was a good listener, instead, I got drugged. The main purpose of the treatment was to get me into a state of mind that would make other people—not me—comfortable," one speaker told the crowd. Another said he was mentally abused, having been prescribed 17 different psychiatric drugs. What finally worked for him was living with a group of people in a self-help community house. For psychotic illnesses, psychiatry seems to believe drugs or electric shock is best. Yet little attention has been given the more benign magnetotherapy.

Source: *Washington Post*, May 4th, 1992, David Brown; author.

Electroconvulsive Therapy

Consider the relationship between electric shock treatment and magnetotherapy. Shock treatment or electroconvulsive therapy (ECT) is a favorite with the American Psychiatric Association (APA). Most specialists believe that patients are damaged by this jolting of the head, with the exception of the psychiatrist who administers these shocks and never sees a bad outcome. Yet psychiatrists admit that there are some patients who are "just too nice for us to put under shock therapy." Dr. Breggen calls it, "electrically-induced closed-head injury or electrical lobotomy." It is celebrated at the annual conventions of the APA, Society of Biological Psychiatry, Royal College of Psychiatrists, and International Psychiatrist Congress.

Psychiatrists typically charge $200 per treatment several times per week for ECT for as many as five to ten patients weekly. For the short hours involved, this can add up to a quarter of a million dollars annually for this therapy alone. One California psychiatrist says he shocks about 10 to 15 percent of his patients, relates Breggen, who estimates that over 100,000 persons in the U.S. are subjected to it annually.

Many doctors believe that it can cause brain damage and memory loss. Certain studies conclude that there is no meaningful evidence of any beneficial effect, while other studies show positive results in serious cases where nothing else has worked. Many doctors, says Breggen, act on the axiom that the brain damage does the trick. Furthermore, modified ECT that involves sedation and muscle paralysis and artificial respiration, is no safer, in his opinion. In fact, it may be more dangerous because the current needs to be stronger to overcome the anticonvulsant effect of this sedative, Breggen concludes.

Dr. William Philpott, psychiatrist M.D., gave up electric shock treatment some years ago. He believes that in some very serious cases there still may be reason to use pure electric shock treatment, but he would encourage psychiatrists to turn to the more benign therapy of permanent magnets in almost all instances. He recommends using negative, steady state magnetic fields that are considerably safer and that have proved effective on thousands of his own patients after years of observation. Natural, solid-state magnets do not create shock, rather balance the brains energy field without electric current and at low field intensity more receptive by the human system. In most cases, gauss strength can be increased according to the need to produce results without adverse effect, according to Philpott. Many conditions are immediately relieved—depression, refusal to eat or work, deep seated anxiety, hysterical beliefs, psychosis and other conditions. He states that there is no change in respiration or heart frequency, and no stress created by using permanent magnets. He is working on a static magnetic device of sufficiently high gauss strength to be able to replace most everything that electric shock therapy now does. Gauss strength of 30,000 or more may be needed to treat some problems, a power close to that achieved (45,000 gauss) by MRI used for diagnostic purposes that utilizes both polarities. It seems reasonable that the same strength can be transformed to serve therapeutically and in the safe, calming negative polarity.

In 1979, the FDA put shock machines into Class III safety category, reports Breggen, which means "an unreasonable risk of illness or injury," the most restrictive category. But APA lobbyists succeeded in convincing FDA to reclassify the procedure into Class II, at least in the area of depression—in effect approving them safe and efficacious. This has satisfied no one.

Psychiatry will fight to the bitter end against any kind of reform, says Dr. Breggen, "To this day it resists even the slightest control over its most obviously abusive practices, such as state or mental hospitals, involuntary drugging, electroshock, and lobotomy, and it fights against every attempt to increase patient's rights." He is sadly pessimistic that they will ever change their attitudes.

The work of Dr. Philpott in this respect might change some minds, especially in more moderate cases that require a simple shifting of positive field electric forces in the brain to the negative field. This balance sometimes takes only a few minutes, as demonstrated in Philpott's offices over the years on many patients. We cited the case earlier where a professor from the University of Michigan, who would not eat or drink (fed intravenously), was turned around in several minutes with application of permanent magnets to the head. To stimulate a national modification in this controversial treatment would be worth all the effort that one person has ever put into his work.

It is important to recognize that the therapy prescribed is related to the mental condition. Schizophrenia, manic depression, epilepsy and certain other mental conditions are organic and viral, according to most mental health experts and also accepted as such by the NIH. For these, it matters not what you did in your childhood or how your father and mother treated you, says Philpott. A research project for every case or a formula for trying to make some sense out of one's background is foolishness, he emphasizes, which may appear somewhat in conflict with Dr. Breggen's view. Certain diseases are toxic in nature. In some cases, the brain did not develop to its proper potential and may experience electrical imbalance. Certainly patients respond when delving into their backgrounds and

Exhibit 29   Case Study of the Value of Magnets in Psychosis

In 1972, John had the delusion he was Jesus Christ. His psychosis developed in response to exposure to pesticides that he had sprayed on his apple orchard and the fumes from a propane fueled fork truck used in his warehouse. He was also reactive to several foods. He would become sane when detoxified with intravenous Vitamin C and the avoidance of auto exhaust and specific pesticides used on his orchard. Deliberate test exposure to these elements provoked delusions. Treatment involved eight weeks of hospitalization.

From this period, John remained mentally well for several years until his next door neighbor repaired his roof with a hot smelly tar, which contained petrochemicals maladaptively reactive to him. He became delusional, believing someone was going to hurt him. He was intent on finding the person whom he believed intended to harm him, "Seeking to find his enemy and doing him in first." His protective wife hired two attendants to keep him from leaving the house, but after several days had to arrange for hospitalization again. But before taking him to the hospital, she called Dr. Philpott for advice. She had been Dr. Philpott's nurse for five years and remembered how they had used magnets on the temporal areas in similar cases. With this in mind, she placed a small (.866"x.394") round neodymium magnet (gauss strength 12,300) on both temporal areas. Within ten minutes her husband was no longer delusional and there was no need for hospitalization.

The magnets did not alter the patient's level of consciousness. For one week, the magnets remained bilaterally on the temporal area day and night. The second week, a magnet was stationed on the left temporal area only. This magnet was then removed and the patient remained sane. He now sleeps with magnets at the crown of his head, composed of four (4"x6"x½") ceramic magnets held upright one inch apart in a carrier. The magnetic field is nineteen inches across and six inches high, applied at the crown (top) of the head. The top of the head is no farther than three inches from the magnets.

As a point of interest, hospitalization for this case in the early 70's, would have cost several thousand dollars; seventeen years later, the cost is $100 worth of magnets, no hospitalization, and sanity in ten minutes. Also at this later date, it was not necessary to be removed from the chemicals that evoked his delusions. Nevertheless, by the end of the two week period, the odor of the chemicals no longer was present. Toxins had also been processed out of the body. Negative magnetic energy, as in this case, oxygenates human cells which materially aid in the detoxification process.

Dr. Philpott states that, "I have documented numerous patients, who, with proper placement and appropriate magnetic gauss strength, have had serious ailments controlled, such as delusions, hallucinations, depressions, obsessions, compulsions, panic behaviors, phobias, anxieties, psychotic depressions, grand mal seizures and temporal lobe seizures, all without the use of any medication. Magnetic energy can succeed even when tranquilizers, antidepressants, and anti-seizure medications fail. The explanation for this is the control of an abnormal degree of electrical activity of the brain. It has been documented that an external

Source: Dr. William H. Philpott, Chactow, Oklahoma, 1992.

284

administrating counseling that is gratifying and repairing. But the best treatment considers the organic nature of mental disease as well.

Epilepsy, for example, is caused by abnormal electrical activity of the brain and can be treated by negative magnetic energy, according to Philpott. He originally treated epileptics with various medications but eventually turned to magnetic fields when he found he could control all types of seizures more effectively, even those where medication had no influence. Of course, the initiating causes of epilepsy—trauma, infection, nutritional or maladaptive reactions to food, chemicals or inhalants—must be addressed for long-term healing in contrast to simply controlling seizures. Assessment also needs to be made for appropriate intake of vitamin B6, magnesium, calcium, taurine, and other nutrients. Philpott says that over 50 percent of seizures can be controlled by avoiding allergic, environmental substances that affect the central nervous system. Some doctors still prescribe carbamazepine to control electrical activity in the brain whereas he believes that the safer permanent magnet could be used.

Philpott tells us why general anesthesia can replace electric shock. No matter how the anesthesia is produced, its effect is to switch the occipital lobe of the brain's polarity from the positive to the negative. Anesthesia is more health strengthening than sleep and therefore more capable of countering allergies, addictions, inflammatory secretions, toxic states, epilepsy and a variety of mental disorders. He says that it is the electric shock therapy that produces the undesirable effect and that there is no need to use electric current. The success rate of natural, permanent magnetic therapy will be double that of electric shock or drug treatments, and the expense several times less, with any hospitalization requirements minimal, Philpott predicts. He believes this from his own experiences involving thousands of cases where he has found a success rate of over 70 percent. In epileptic cases, he has never had a failure.

A negative magnetic field is not an analgesic, rather a normalizer of disordered metabolic functions. Anesthetic states produce a switch in the brain's magnetic field from positive to negative, thus general anesthesia occurs when the brain is in a negative magneto-electric field. Animal models using solid state magnets can produce general anesthesia. Eventually this may be possible to do with humans which would minimize or eliminate disorders of the heart and respiration functions prevalent with other types of anesthesia.

Information Brief

Treatment of Central Nervous System
With Permanent Magnets

Dr. Donald L. Dudley's practice consists of severely ill patients with central nervous system problems, many who have not responded to drug or surgical treatment. We are hopeless and helpless given our current level of knowledge to treat some of these patients.

We have made the magnet treatment protocol (essentially Philpott Medical Services protocol) available to several patients with brain injuries, central pain and/or seizures. No known medication had provided these patients relief from their symptoms. Patients are reporting improvements in their conditions after utilizing the magnets and we have been able to objectively measure the effects of this new treatment option on the individual EEG's and mapped Evoked Potentials.

I am astonished that a treatment which is nearly as old as mankind can remain unknown to the general public. We have demonstrated a viable treatment option for certain patients with medical conditions of the central nervous system. Magnets are a valid medical treatment and as such should be covered by insurance and made available for self-help and by prescription from trained physicians.

Source: Dudley, Donald L. M.D., Neuropsychiatrist, Washington Institute of Neuroscience, Inc., Seattle, Wash., August 1992; Neurodiagnostic Services, Biological Psychiatry, Internal Medicine, Cardiology, Clinical Research, Mental Health Care.

Negative fields can control electrical activity, calm the brain and stop symptoms associated with hallucinations, delusions, seizures, panic, etc., without disordering mental alertness and orientation. Philpott believes that in the near future we will be able to implant a small, thin magnet under the skin for control of seizures, tremors, depression, panic, delusions, etc., much like the solid state magnets implanted under the skin over the mastoid to enhance hearing.

For schizophrenia, Philpott enumerates primary and secondary causes in his treatment methodology:

Schizophrenia (Causes and Treatment)

Primary causes

1. Viral infection causing mild encephalitis early in life while the brain is developing, and can occur during gestation or shortly thereafter. Possibly B6 deficiency can be a cause.

2. Viral infected immune system, especially B-lymphocytes that make antibodies.

3. Viruses, such as the herpes family, Epstein-Barr, cytomegalovirus, human herpes virus #6, herpes zoster (chicken pox), herpes simplex I or II, or Rubella and mumps.

Secondary causes

1. Nutrition becomes disordered or maladaptive reactions to foods, chemicals or inhalants.

2. Genetic errors, such as celiac disease, homocystinuna, carcenuria, etc.

3. Learning disabilities, such as dyslexia, hyperkinesis, Tourettes syndrome are a continuum to schizophrenia.

4. Type 2 diabetics, amyotrophic lateral sclerosis and alzheimer all have laboratory measurable evidence combined carbohydrate disorder and hyperamminemia leading to serious neurotoxin symptoms.

Treatment

1. Sort out maladaptive reactions and use avoidance and spacing to control symptoms.

2. Review nutritional state of vitamins, minerals, amino acids and essential fats.

3. Evaluate degree of activity of viruses and fungi.

4. Apply magnetotherapy specially to crown of head to gain deep sleep, and bright light therapy upon awakening, gaining control of abnormal electrical activity of the brain to the level of anesthesia as necessary.

5. Engage in such techniques as relaxation training, desensitization of anxieties and phobias, behavioral training, imagery, psychotic preoccupation and acting out.

SCIENTIFIC DIGEST

Schizophrenia Demystified

Every year, 100,000 are newly diagnosed as schizophrenic while 600,000 Americans are in active treatment and several millions suffer from it—as many people as are in Oregon, Mississippi and Kansas combined. Three-quarters develop this disease between 16 and 25 years of age. Occurrence over age 30 is uncommon. It is definitely a brain disease, a biological entity clearly as diabetes, multiple sclerosis and cancer, exhibited by impairment in thinking, delusions, hallucinations, and changes in emotions and behavior. One may think he or she is being watched, followed, controlled or persecuted. The physical result is apathy, slowness, lack of drive or behavior that becomes ritualistic, with posturing, gesturing, parroting, repetitive movements. It is not a split personality or idiosyncratic way of thinking, correctable through psychoanalysis or family interaction theories. It is no one's fault. And there are several different kinds of schizophrenia of the brain.

Schizophrenia has its roots in disordered brain function that produces erroneous sensory data and disordered thinking. The proper response from others is patience and understanding. It is not bipolar illness (formerly called manic-depression), a periodic, recurrent mood disorder with intervening periods of complete normalcy. It is not schizoaffective disorder, an intermediate disease category between bipolar disorder and schizophrenia, nor is it brief reactive psychosis, usually precipitated by severe stress that lasts less than two weeks. Some symptoms may mimic schizophrenia, due to other diseases such as brain tumors, temporal lobe epilepsy, and viral infections of the brain.

About one-third recover, one-third are improved, and one-third unimproved. Early age of onset, family history, marked thinking disorder, withdrawal and apathy point to a poor outcome. Drugs certainly influence outcome but no one can say how much. Drugs have decreased relapses and rehospitalizations but whether any brain damage is prevented is unknown. One-third would have probably recovered without drugs in any case. Others may be stabilized or chances of rehospitalization cut as much as 60 percent. Supportive relationships, friendships, advice are useful adjuncts. Family members should not blame each other for the problem nor misconstrue symptoms or minor incidents that might grow out of proportion.

Source: Excerpts from Surviving Schizophrenia: A Family Manual, 1983, E. Faller Torrey, M.D.

Addiction Therapy

I have already discussed the fascinating results of electro-magnetic therapy in clinical studies in both China and England where drug and alcohol addicts were detoxified from their addictions without any withdrawal symptoms and who remained free of addiction. The long-term success of being drug-free still depends on such things as group therapy and a variety of other counseling and treatment programs. Psychotherapy is much easier and successful when patients are drug-free. One method of detoxification is from electric or magnetic stimulation of the concha behind the ear. Such experiments are needed in the United States to help tackle perhaps the nation's most serious domestic problem—drug and alcohol addiction.

To reinforce the success of alternative treatments, many now understand that the body is a bioelectric system with defined pathways of energy and magnetic forces in every cell. More and more doctors are beginning to realize this. A study published by JAMA of research done at the City of Hope Medical Center in Duarte, California, confirms that severe alcoholics carry a DNA marker or possibly a number of minor genes that create a cumulative effect on this disease. Further study might show how extended therapeutic procedures could effect the DNA and surrounding cells.

In addition to magnetotherapy, acupuncture is now being used to ease withdrawal pain for both alcoholics and drug addicts. Once the energy flow is rebalanced, the brain's chemical endorphins are released to block or override any pain, inflammation, or other signals. Studies this year at Lincoln Hospital in the Bronx by Dr. Michael Smith, Director of Substance Abuse, show a 60 percent success rate of keeping hard core addicts straight for three months. The city of New York has allocated two million dollars to fund 25 other acupuncture treatment programs. Nationwide over 200 drug treatment programs are using acupuncture.

I have described how magnetotherapy can be used by therapists more effectively than acupuncture because the magnetic fields reach more body points and penetrate to greater depths. It would be a blessing for this nation and other nations of the world if thousands of therapists were to combine these treatments, especially since magnetotherapy does more than simply relieve pain or withdrawal symptoms for many. For a small cost and modest training, almost overnight we could have magnetic beds and devices in drug and alcohol treatment centers all over the nation. Of America's 550,000 doctors, 3,000 now use acupuncture, while ten years ago only 500 used it. There are also 7,000 non-M.D. acupuncturists and 5,000 certified C.A.s in the U.S. whose profession requires extensive training and three to six years of apprenticeship. Yet we find in 24 states, acupuncture must be performed by a physician. On the other hand, there are no regulations for the use of permanent magnets or any certification required, except in California where one must confine himself to treating pain or sleep disorders. Remember that instruction in magnetotherapy is much simpler and the methodology safer than most therapies.

Since addicts experience little or no withdrawal pains and feel relatively comfortable in an energy balanced condition from receiving certain alternative treatments, they could apply non-invasive devices in a self-help fashion as needed in the confines of their own habitats. This could enable some drug users to kick the habit on their own. Few addicts would apply piercing acupuncture needles, but, on the other hand, anyone can place a magnet near energy points and accomplish similar results without pain or a great deal of instruction. Remember the case histories we cited where a carpenter and a house cleaner take their little half dollar size magnets with them to work to arrest pain whenever they feel the need.

It is not unrealistic to imagine a drug addict carrying a magnet for application with him wherever he goes, if he feels the need for drug use or begins to feel the pangs of withdrawal which may force him on drugs again. We spend about three quarters of our 11 billion dollars of national drug allocations for interdiction. Surely it would make more sense to turn a larger piece of these funds over to reducing the desire for consumption by means of realistic treatment programs. Are we able to rise to the occasion? Hillary Rodham Clinton might be encouraged to put this into her national health plan. What better way to help children than to get parents and adults off drugs and alcohol!

Integration of Therapies

The unified approach of healing must involve non-conventional methods. One-third or more of the U.S. population uses some form of unconventional therapy, most of this growth coming about in the last few years. It is a 27 billion dollar industry, as reported by Time Magazine last year, while the baby boomers, disenchanted with regular medicine, cry for more. People are tired of waiting in clinics and doctor's offices, tired of blood tests, X-rays, insurance forms, and pills. They have begun to realize that if it is not a sudden crisis, most physicians really don't seem to help. Arthritis, osteoporosis, lower back pain, chronic fatigue syndrome, high blood pressure, coronary-artery disease, ulcers, and many forms of cancer are just a few ailments where doctors appear stymied. Too many medical problems turn to surgery. Quoting medical writer Abraham Muslow, "If all you're trained to use is a hammer, the whole world looks like a nail."

A whole series of therapies were identified by *Time Magazine*, including the following: great interest for crystals that are supposed to release tension in the body in tuned vibrations; the 1000 year old shiatsu that uses finger pressure; ayurveda that relies on a twenty minute warm dip of herbal oil; Alexander technique to improve posture, much like Rolfing's deep (and at times painful) massage to realign the body; iridology that diagnoses disease by looking for patterns in the eyes; macro-biotics that uses the discipline of good diet and balancing of yin (passive energy) and yang (active energy); and reflexology that works on the hands and feet for headaches and belly aches and gall bladder problems, etc.. Famous stars like John MacEnroe and Lisa Bonet partake of alternative therapies, as do millions of others. When the famous do it others seem to catch on.

Over 5,000 doctors now combine hypnotherapy with conventional treatment to ease such ailments as migraines and arthritis or to heal burns faster. The AMA's Council on Scientific Affairs labeled hypnosis as a legitimate therapy over 35 years ago, recognizing that "drugs alone cannot quench the fiery nerve pain" of surgery.

Over 1,800 credentialed psychiatrists, doctors, nurses, dentists, social workers, and physical therapists practice biofeedback. It is also used at the Mayo Clinic and the Cleveland Clinic. Insurance companies of Aetna and John Hancock pay for certain biofeedback treatments, while Blue Cross/Blue Shield recommends against payment, according to a study reviewed in U.S. News and World Report. Prudential Insurance Company reimburses for biofeedback treatment for migraines, muscle tension, hypertension, chronic pain and anxiety, and also pays for home treatment. As a patient watches a display monitor and his temperature in biofeedback, the subject sends messages to the hypothalamus in the brain, then to the blood vessels in the hands and arms to create more rapid blood flow. Induced energy and increased oxygen supply, very often through the biofeedback effect, are what magnetotherapy does so well and with a high rate of success. Perhaps in the near future insurance companies will also recognize the validity of magnetic field treatment, its preventive nature and it's ability to slash medical bills over the long-term.

Insurance companies have recognized bioelectromagnetic treatment for most ailments for over a decade, yet doctors fail to recommend it for many diverse ills as they prescribe for biofeedback, hypnosis, massage and other relevant therapies. The use of TENS (Transcutaneous Electrical Nerve Stimulation) micro-current discussed in an earlier chapter, is reimbursable by insurance companies and is listed in the physician's "current procedural terminology" (CPT) for reimbursement. It has been demonstrated that both electromagnets and permanent magnets are highly effective for treating many ailments and pains, restoring body energy balance, and improving immune function. They could be a prime new preventive maintenance therapy and a great insurance cost cutter. The nation awaits insurance endorsement.

A number of controlled trials have taken place for alternative treatments which should help gain acceptance of these therapies by the medical community. Over 105 controlled studies for homeopathy (reported in the February 1991 British Medical Journal) for example, found positive results in 81 trials. In the May 1991 Journal of the American Medical Association, a three page letter described positive findings for herbal and meditation treatment. One U. S. study found herbal compounds reduced the incidence of breast cancer in up to 88 percent of experimental animals. Numerous organizations and companies promote herbal compounds and can cite thousands of successful treatments for just about every disease. In the case of the science of homeopathy, we pointed out earlier that Dr. Philpott discontinued its use for the much easier and, what he states, the more effective magnetotherapy because he found they do essentially the same thing. Magnetic fields have the ability to override many other treatments.

However, as I have already suggested, if one is having success with a particular treatment, he should continue it, perhaps supplementing it with other methodologies. An advantageous turn for the nation's health would be for the thousands of homeopathic and herbal practitioners and their millions of patients to include magnetotherapy in their regimen, recognizing their similarities and combined potential. Together, these therapies could result in more creative and even greater healing. Physicians should become familiar with all therapies and be ready to recommend to their patients any one of them or at least advise them of findings and reported results. This is the only fair thing to do, since the average individual is caught in a messy, costly and uninformative system no fault of his own.

Nurses and physical therapists seem closer to an understanding of the problem. There are 1.1 million nurses in America today; yet there is a shortage of 200,000. Some hospitals are obliged to use friends and relatives to help with routine nursing chores to relieve staff for more important duties. This friendly help is an excellent progression of loving care as well as a big cost saver. But remember that not all hospitals and doctors are equally good. The medical community knows who the good and bad are but generally chooses not to share this information with us. The patient has to go off to such organizations as Public Citizen Health Research Group to determine who is effective.

Can more sensitive nurses and doctors pull us out of the morass?. They can help. Most nurses believe in personal care, love for patients, alternative therapies (including laying-on-of-hands), and a strong desire to control their work by staying with a patient from time in until time out. One analysis shows that the most important determinant of the hospital death rate is how effectively nurses and doctors communicate and, of course, the degree of cooperation that results from communication passed on to patients who want so very much to be part of the process but are usually left out. These elements were shown to be more important than technical capability or life saving treatments. It very much revolves back to the psychosomatic nature of the human element—desire for love and care, the need to know what is going on, and a chance to participate in decisions. Support groups, physical therapy, increasing the body's energy, laying-on-of-hands, and love and care are all legitimate parts of the healing process. Can anyone imagine what such a change in the nature of treatment could do to health costs?

"Physicians have overeducated and overpriced themselves for the kinds of services we are talking about," says the American Nurses Association (ANA). Patients seeking medical help for headaches spend up to $75 for a first visit to a nurse practitioner, $125 for a primary care physician and $235 for a neurologist. Five times more money is spent training a physician than a nurse. The ANA argues that the 300,000 nurses now providing some primary health care in the school, community and occupational settings should be given larger responsibilities to reach the millions of people who go medically unattended today.

SCIENTIFIC DIGEST

The Silence of the Hospitals

The American Hospital Association (AHA), which represents the nations 6,000 plus hospitals, recognizes a serious health problem: 1,700 hospitals fail to meet minimum standards, 51 percent did not adequately monitor for unnecessary surgeries or whether surgery was done safely, over 51 percent did not adequately monitor care of patients in intensive or coronary care or evaluate the quality of care by the medical staff. These among other faults are revealed in Walt Bogdanich's book **Great White Lie: How America's Hospitals Betray Our Trust and Endanger Our Lives**. Dr. Sidney M. Wolfe, Public Citizen Health Research Group, favorably comments on this book, citing Jefferson's articulation that "information is power," but that the American public is kept in the dark.

Bogdanich cites a Harvard study which projected nationally that 80,000 patients died in hospitals in a single year in the United States. He says that there is a shortage of hospital pharmacists and that their hours of work are dangerously long leading to patient deaths and medication mistakes; hospitals "dump" or scare off sick patients; fully trained nurses compromise care; billing error rates are as high as 90 percent; and that the Hospital Corporation of America gives payoffs to doctors for referrals. Investigators from the University of California, San Francisco, reported that 114 internal medicine residents at three major medical centers made 114 errors, 90 percent of the patients got sicker and 35 percent died. Nationally, as many as 200,000 patients die from medical errors.

Source: Bogdanich, Walter, **Great White Lie: How America's Hospitals Betray Our Trust and Endanger our Lives, 1992.**

The American Medical Association (AMA) believes the best relationship is a partnership between nurses and doctors, allowing the doctor to make the clinical judgment, but once made in more complex cases, patients should be allowed to visit a nurse directly. For simple headaches, colds and minor pain, a nurse or alternative therapist may be the best first choice for quality, caring care and lowest cost. It may be the only reasonable way the U.S. can reach the 50 plus million people under represented in health care.

Information Brief

Curing Bed Sores

Bed sores are a significant national problem. Pressure ulcers form where bone causes the greatest force on the skin and tissue, squeezing them against an outside surface, such as a mattress or chair. Federal guidelines call for frequent inspection, the use of creams and oils or antibiotics, minimizing moisture accumulation, changing position often, avoidance of knees and ankles touching each other, and never dragging a patient across bed linens. Never use doughnut pillows to sit on because they reduce blood flow and cause swelling. Also avoid massage over bony parts. Conventional wisdom has been that massage was a way to stimulate blood flow, but recent studies suggest that massage does more harm than good, says Nancy Bergstom, Professor of Nutrition and Nursing, University of Nebraska, College of Nursing.

A 1991 cost study showed treatment for bed sores, including hospitals stays, amounted to $6 billion a year. Individual costs range from $1,000 to $30,000 and one out of every ten hospital patients and about one-third of all nursing home patients develop such sores. Many cases are not even reported.

But users and providers of magnetic beds and seats report a high rate of success in minimizing bed sores. Instead of antibiotics or the now recognized obsolete massage after the fact, it has been discovered by many that magnetic fields increase oxygen supply to tissues without harm to bony parts or tissues. It may be time for both hospitals and nursing homes to consider use of magnetic beds and chairs. Certainly controlled research on 30 or 60 patients is in order. If magnetotherapy substantially reduces this single costly problem, its further exploration would be well worth it. Only these kinds of solutions to our health crisis will substantially cut costs and provide better, wiser care for patients.

Source: *Health Journal, Washington Post*, May 19th 1992, Sandy Rovner; author.

Home care is another option. It represents a trend in the direction of greater personal attention. It may be one way to cut costs and also substantially allow therapists sufficient time to provide less expensive, long-term therapy that so many patients need, including the alternatives of acupuncture, massage and magnetotherapy. Some believe we are in a basic redefinition of our health care institutions, as the hospital becomes more and more an outmoded vehicle.

The home care company of Caremark, for example, did $700,000,000 of business in 1990. Other public companies that do a large volume of home care are Critical Care America, T2 Medical, Inc., and

Home Nutritional Services, Inc. This industry creates a great opportunity to carry self-help treatment directly into the home.

Information Brief

Rise of Active Patients

Consumers are learning that they cannot put full faith and credit in every doctor, lawyer, or savings and loan accountant. Dr. Tom Ferguson M.D., in the *Futurist*, **Patient, Heal thy Self** (Jan - Feb 1992) describes surveys which show that in 1975 over 90 percent of patients were passive and only one or two percent active and responsible; while in 1988, the passive figure dropped to 55 percent and the active percent to 8; and the trend indicates that by the year 2,000, only 30 percent will be passive, 25 percent active, and 40 percent in the middle listed as concerned. The whole idea of the hospital as the medical factory and the patient as raw material is passé, he says. One needs to negotiate with the doctor, take turns talking, and agree as to what has to be done. Turn down the physician who says, "You needn't be concerned with that," or "let me worry about that."

The secret is that most health professionals were never comfortable playing God, Dr. Ferguson emphasizes. Active participation makes it possible for the doctor to come out of the closet, climb down off his pedestal, and allow the patient to get off her knees.

A lot of procedures done in hospitals, such as intravenous antibiotics and parenteral nutrition, for example, can be done as well in the home. Personal touch from a loving nurse or therapist can also come about much like true family doctors. The cry is, "I want to be a partner with my doctor." In home care, patients are monitored on a regular basis by a licensed physician, since some face-to-face contact with a doctor is necessary. Like any business, the system must be regulated to watch for illegalities such as provider kickbacks or unethical referrals or overcharging for drugs and equipment. For example, some providers have been known to charge $180 for a vial of antibiotic cytovene when you can get it at the local pharmacy for $40, or as much as $9000 for a monthly supply of liquid protein and nutrition that only costs $1300 wholesale. We would want, for instance, to prevent providers from charging ten times the cost of a $10 or $20 magnet, or $2000 for a $500 magnetic bed pad.

A case involving a neighbor of mine demonstrates an example of intimidation. The overweight mother experienced a serious backache for

Information Brief

The New Hospital

Self-help groups are now helping the passive and concerned patient. The Self-Help Clearing House, Denville, N.J., has helped set up over 550 such groups all over the country. One group, Commonweal Cancer Help Program, Bolinas, Calif., has surveyed 30 of the best known alternative treatment centers under a MacArthur Foundation "genius" grant and has found that the best, most common success characteristic is health active patients seeking to integrate the best of conventional and alternative medicine. When patients understand their conditions and the possibilities, it is less frightening. At the same time, greater healing takes place.

Some hospitals are changing. The Planetree Health Resource Center, San Francisco, plays classical music, patients wear their own robes and pajamas, sleep on colorful flower sheets, and sleep in as late as they want. There are no nurse's stations, rather a patient area where they can read and write and check their own health charts. Family members are welcome at all times, no set visiting hours, and families can cook for their loved ones and serve as active partners, as well as change dressings and flush out IV lines or whatever is help to the staff and patient. It's about time! We have been stuck with a century of bad practice.

many months without any relief from her doctor except temporarily when he jabbed her with a pain killing drug. It may mean that the patient must be on this drug forever. When the mother asked her doctor if it would be all right to try a magnetic bed, he advised her not to try; and, of course, this passive patient, at least so far, is taking the doctor's advice. There is little two-way communication. Yet the mother is using a plastic 3" x 5" negative oriented magnet which relieves pain wherever she places it on her body. If the doctor doesn't come through soon, she may take things into her own hands and begin to sleep on a non-invasive, magnetic bed. Certainly the success of that little magnet ought to demonstrate some validity of the procedure.

By the way, how many doctors have you ever seen in a hospital as patients? The movie **The Doctor** showed how one doctor couldn't stand the care he received while being a hospital patient and so rebelled against the system to increase the sensitivity of other doctors. Most hospital care could be handled at home if doctors and care takers would visit homes. Many doctors treat each other in parking lots, getting advice and then

Society should try to determine the right price for medical tasks, weighing inherent difficulty, performance time, training required and other semi-subjective variables, says Stanley J. Reiser, **Medicine and the Reign of Technology**. Why should a radiologist charge $24 for an X-Ray, $180 for a CAT scan, and $250 for an MRI reading when they each average only 5 to 10 minutes of the doctor's time? Some radiologists are making $300,000 annually plus bonuses, with relatively easy hours and liberal vacations. The total cost of the MRI study is $1,050, mostly because of the cost of equipment. It seems fair to cut the radiologist's fee and other fees to help pay for the technology quicker so the customer doesn't have to bear outrageous fees forever, or else purchase expensive equipment on a shared, regional and joint private-government basis. Even the radiologists can't understand why they make as much as they do for the time expended; but if the system allows them, they'll take it. And what about the poor family doctor working tedious, long hours?

going home to administer their own cures. If we had a larger dedicated core of family doctors, our health bill would drop drastically and our health sky rocket, a reverse correlation. Our National Health Service is struggling to meet demand and to encourage doctors to serve in the neediest areas. Surely we can pay the way for more people to enter the National Health Service where they are vitally needed, especially since we are running out of other jobs.

And we need to share technology. Expensive MRI and other testing could, as conveniently and at a fraction of the cost, be accomplished at a regional diagnostic center whose cost could be both publicly and privately shared. If profit were not the prime motive, a $1 million MRI machine could be shared by dozens of doctors and the cost for a test dropped to one-tenth the usual. Perhaps the federal health service could share in the original purchase of capital equipment or offer tax incentives that would eventually result in lower charges and greater sharing.

Hope is ahead. Doctors are improving in their approach to patients and are beginning to recognize preventive health to a greater extent, even for themselves. Most now believe in the risk of smoking, for instance, as only three percent smoke today, compared to eight percent a decade ago. Vitamins are not as important to them as a well balanced diet, as only 23 percent take vitamin supplements; but they do recognize the greater significance and need for minerals, especially calcium whereby 35 percent of doctors take a minimum of 800 milligrams daily, as reported in the Futurist. But new federal guidelines recommend 1200 - 2000 milligrams of calcium daily. Anyway, some have seen the light.

The Best Health Advice

As a normal human being, you might ask what is the best way to keep in good health. Not surprisingly, it is the same old way your mother taught you. McCall's Magazine reported an interesting survey done a couple of years ago of 7000 residents of Almeda County, Calif., concerning seven life-style practices that were shown to help people live ten years longer than those who did not follow these practices. So effective were these measures that 70 year old people who practiced them were as healthy as 35 to 40 year olds who did not. Yet there is nothing unusual about them:

- Eat regular meals, including breakfast.
- Don't snack between meals.
- Drink in moderation or not at all.
- Exercise about three times a week.
- Keep your weight within 20 percent of average.
- Don't smoke.
- Sleep 7 or 8 hours a night and be happy.

To sleep well is an important part of any health regimen. Poor sleepers are more likely to have trouble concentrating or remembering things, accomplishing tasks, driving a car or handling stress. This is why many providers feel magnetic beds can be so important in one's life, particularly for poor sleepers who toss or turn endlessly or feel tired when they get up even after eight or more hours in the sack. Even for sound sleepers, magnets will give them more energy than normal.

And, of course, we must stay happy because stress levels will be lower and we will heal easier. One might even have to improve his personality and attitudes. One study, conducted over five decades,

showed that the happiest people were 12 times more likely not to become chronically ill or die early, even taking into account alcohol, tobacco, obesity, and family history. According to a study of 118 male lawyers, these men were four times more likely to die by age 50 if they had a high hostility score. So smile, be happy, commit yourself to something, look forward to challenges as exciting rather than threatening. Take control of your life. Do not exist on the mercy of someone else.

All of this is good advice, but what if you have aches and pains and other ailments now? The answer is to do all of the above plus consider an alternative therapy suited to you. A magnetic field maintenance program is certainly one choice. Of all the habits, magnetotherapy probably is the easiest and perhaps the most pleasurable thing to do. If you have serious problems, surely see a doctor and get medical advice, but get someone who is familiar with all the alternatives who will discuss them thoroughly with you. You are not a pussycat.

Exhibit 30 Benefits of Exercise

Moderate exercise has been shown to be an effective cancer fighter, while very intensive exercise may actually be detrimental if it suppresses the immune system. So don't overdo it. One study shows prostate cancer more common among male athletes, reports the American Health Foundation. (Other studies have shown a higher prostate cancer rate among higher volume sex participants.) The equivalent of walking ten miles or more per week cut the risk of developing colon cancer in half in men compared to the less active. "The theory is that exercise increases the rate of transit of food through the gut," says I-Min Lee, a epidemiologist at Harvard University, as reported in the Journal of the National Cancer Institute. If cancer is caused by carcinogens in the fecal stream, there is less chance of contact with colonic mucosa where most colon cancer starts.

A long-term study of 5,400 female college alumnae, half of whom were former college athletes, shows that the active women had significantly less cancer of the breast and reproductive system and a lower incidence of benign breast disease. Non-athletes had 2.5 times the amount of reproductive system cancer and also twice the amount of breast cancer compared to the athletes, says Rose E. Frisch of the Harvard School of Public Health. The athletes were leaner in every age group from 20 to 80. Fat makes estrogen and it is known that excessive amounts increase risk of breast cancer or cancer of the uterus. Also studies show that, in general, exercise does not lower blood pressure. You will have to find something else for that.
Source: American Health Foundation, Washington Post Health Journal, Jan 14, 1992.

Information Brief

Health Advice

Common health recommendations include eating three to five servings each of vegetables and fruits every day and six or more servings of grain and three servings of milk, cheese or yogurt. Two or three servings of meat, poultry, fish, or eggs a day is about right with fats and oils used sparingly. And eat with gusto because the digestive system mirrors the mind. We don't process the food very well if we are angry or upset.

When it comes to vitamins and minerals, some new thinking has surfaced about the recommended daily allowance (RDA). For instance, immune system response can be improved by consuming 25 times more B_6 than the RDA. Also, T-cells return to the level of younger people with 15 milligrams of zinc daily. We are cautioned not to allow magnesium deficiency, since it plays a key role in the body's electrical activities that affect the heart beat and may also improve response to magnetotherapy. The experts say to be sure to take sufficient amounts, but don't overdose on beta-carotene and the vitamins C and E. Remember to avoid a buildup of vitamins D and especially vitamin A because they can become toxic. Take a minimum of 1,200 milligrams of calcium daily.

In addition to sound nutrition, we are told to limit ourselves to one alcoholic beverage a day if a woman and two a day for a man (a male can assimilate more because of greater stomach acids). Don't smoke. About 400,000 people a year die from diseases related to smoking.

Exercise several times a week for about 30 minutes or more even if it's limited to a good walk. And be sure to get in at least 20 minutes of strength training a week, regardless of age, repeated enough times so that the muscles feel nearly exhausted. Don't expect blood pressure to come down with just minor exercise. In any case, it might not come down at all. You'll have to work harder at that. Magnetotherapy has been shown to lower blood pressure in some cases.

Chapter 10

Peak Health from Natural Energy

Caring for Ailments That Appear Deceptive

Now that we have looked at some of the problems of the conventional health system and also the simplicity of keeping in good health, let us conclude by examining just four major ailments facing Americans that stymie most doctors, yet which we can do something about: pain, lack of sound sleep, chronic fatigue syndrome and premenstrual syndrome. Magnetotherapy fits these conditions rather well. Of the multiple of diseases and problems that exist, these cover a big piece of our health complaints. The prescribed methodology for these problems gives us an idea of what to do for most ailments, since the method of application is quite similar.

Pain

For pain, let us turn to Dr. Jay A. Goldstein's interpretation in his critical book, "Could Your Doctor Be Wrong?" He asks how is it possible for highly trained physicians not to know what to do. The answer is that relatively few doctors are trained in what the medical community calls the new specialty of pain treatment. Insurance companies do not like to pay for pain treatment if it is not connected to specific "cook book" disorders; it becomes expensive for the patient and not profitable for the doctor. About all most physicians will do is prescribe a pain-relieving drug that may have some short-term effect but may even be harmful over the long-term. Typical patients look for quick, easy cures, Goldstein says, while doctors succumb to desires for fast results even knowing serious pain can last months or years.

Fibromyalgia is a serious pain, Goldstein tells us, that involves 200-plus tender points where pain is felt on either side of the body or on the upper and lower parts of the body. These points are not strained or knotted muscles that result from overexertion or old tears in cartilage or other structures. If they were, the pain would disappear or be localized in a short time as the muscles heal. Trigger points or nodules and taut bands can cause a shortening of the muscles. They can be activated by trauma or mechanical stress and can cause gall bladder pain, non-ulcer dyspepsia (NUD), intestinal spasms, bladder pain, pseudoappendicitis, and menstrual cramps. Goldstein says tender points are also triggers that can shoot pain off to some other area of the body called referred pain (or myofascial pain). **

Dr. Goldstein recognizes causes and pain locations quite well, but his cures are mainly drug injections. For example, he recommends injections directly into the trigger points, treatment, he says, that not very long ago was either unheard of or regarded as quackery, yet today is common as physicians learn new techniques. Results can be amazing and instantaneous, relieving pain not only at the trigger point, he explains, but also at the distant referred pain site that may fall at the opposite side of the body. Providers need to be well versed in the location of trigger points in order to apply injections effectively; otherwise, the pain can be made worse if by error the physician treats tender points instead, or the pain may return if other associated factors such as poor posture or repetitive activities are not solved. Dr. Goldstein mentions only briefly alternative therapies such as acupuncture or proper exercise. Yet magnetotherapy can be applied to both trigger and tender points without fear of making a mistake by not knowing which point is which?

As ever, the standard establishment approach for pain is antidepressant and other drugs, such as Flexeril, Xanox, Motrin, Advil, Buspar, or Prozac. Drugs seem to be the expeditious, recommended therapy even when some drugs like Prozac have become very controversial as causing unacceptable side effects, even violence and wild behavior. Importantly, physicians need to be educated to the various alternative therapies in preference to the use of drugs, even those used directly at the pain site. More and more providers believe that the best treatment is one of the alternatives. This highlights the problem faced by medical injections,

---

*   The italicized text refers to more complex information.

which, after all, are a localized application of drugs that can spread to other parts of the body.

Using magnetotherapy, the physician would not need extensive training in acupuncture point location or in trigger or tender point identification. Even the lay person can safely apply a magnet on a painful area to relieve muscle tension or create a heat source, while increasing oxygen to the spot. What is unique about magnetotherapy is that one can apply magnets on various areas of the body, or sit or sleep on magnetic pads, that will treat many tense muscles in various known and unknown locations, such as distant and difficult referred pain sites simultaneously. Usually it is not merely one muscle that is at fault. Muscles may tense at a number of locations from a single problem source. Not even the best therapist can identify all pain sites, but overall application of magnetic fields will usually find them quickly and easily. Pain relief may come as rapidly as a few minutes or it may take days or weeks of magnetotherapy for more serious or prolonged ailments.

Of course, not all drugs are addictive or threatening and proper use can be justified when administered properly, especially when used in conjunction with alternatives that could take over as the treatment of choice after a period. **Countless Americans suffer needlessly from pain from wounds and many other causes, including the 23 million operations performed in the U.S. every year because doctors and nurses do not administer adequate pain killing medication or therapy, according to the newly created federal agency for Health Care Policy and Research. The agency has issued national guidelines for more aggressive treatment of pain that would speed recovery and reduce hospital stays.**

The conventional dose of pain killing drugs is less than half the amount needed for proper control, the Health Care Policy agency says, while the risk of addiction is small if used temporarily. Pain is a dangerous disease that can delay healing and accelerate cancer growth by suppressing the immune system and its "natural killer" cells. One of the key recommendations is that patients should become closely involved with doctors in pain control, including the use of several non-drug therapies such as breathing exercises and meditation, etc. But, not surprisingly, complete ignorance of the benefits of magnetotherapy is obvious or deliberately ignored by medical traditionalists. Since magnetotherapy has been approved by health departments around the world as an effective pain treatment, it appears some change is needed in the U.S. system. If pain is a dangerous disease, let's use the most effective and safest treatments.

Simply giving one or several muscle injections does not solve the problem over the long-term. This is why sleeping on a magnetic bed, or using magnets for 15 to 30 minutes daily as regular routine, is the best kind of preventative maintenance program. And you don't need a therapist standing over you. Once the physician has given the instruction and best course, the patient can continue therapy safely at home for a long time. Individuals must simply follow proper procedures, either given by the manufacturer of the magnetic product or a doctor or physical therapist, cautioning the correct use of the polarities and other factors. There is more than enough business to go around for all doctors.

Almost everybody agrees that the alternative therapies are safer than localized drug injections or internal drug use. The reason alternatives may not be recommended as standard treatment by the conventional medical community is because they take time, particularly true of massage or acupuncture or acupressure. On the other hand, a physician can just as easily prescribe a magnetic application, instructing his patient where, when and how to apply the treatment at home without the loss of either the doctor's or the patient's time. Instruction in magnetotherapy is rather simple, and doctors can actually see more patients with better results with this knowledge at hand. Millions of people are using magnetotherapy without ever having seen a doctor and many more are using it after having seen a doctor when they could not get results from conventional treatments.

Recall the case mentioned earlier of the husband who was in an auto accident twenty years ago and had suffered a broken neck and a crushed disk in his lower back. After three surgeries, he continued to suffer headaches, loss of hearing, and nausea from pain. After magnetotherapy and continual application, to this day he does not experience any headaches, doesn't snore, sleeps well, has more energy, and his hearing has largely returned. Numerous cases such as this are available for review.

Also, the case mentioned earlier of the woman from Florida who hurt her back in 1956. Doctors and chiropractors and massage therapists worked on her for years up to 1991. The recommended pharmaceutical supplements of minerals and vitamins did not cure her problem. Introduction to permanent magnets took the pain away within two days.

Her sciatic pain was also eliminated. All this occurred under the same lifestyle and the same foods. She now keeps fit with a magnetic maintenance program.

Persistent pain may be caused by some unusual or unsuspecting reason. It may be caused by post operative conditions or immobility from being on a sick bed too long or from having a leg or arm in a cast. If not diagnosed quickly, the ailment may become permanent like some we discussed where pain persisted for twenty years or more. When a cast is removed, for example, pain may become worse because of nearby nerve damage rather than from the original pain site, explains Dr. Goldstein. An unsuspecting physician, he says, may make matters worse by recommending another operation without realizing the new problem may have been caused by immobility from the first surgery. Magnetotherapy is not likely to make that mistake.

Pain whose location cannot be found is called chronic intractable benign pain or simply chronic pain syndrome. The doctor unfamiliar with trigger points (fibromyalgia) may say it's all in the head—the typical diagnosis for many unknown maladies. He might turn to cognitive-behavioral therapy as a possible solution; yet, it is best to explore all diagnostic methods, including all other alternatives. But remember that cognitive-behavior therapy and more likely, magnetotherapy may not be covered by insurance or may be covered at a lower rate.

Look briefly at the most common pain ailment—backache. It is the second most frequent complaint in the United States, after the common cold. Its medical costs and lost productivity are estimated at 60 to 100 billion dollars annually. Recently the world's most foremost experts on backaches came up with a revolutionary treatment, "For up to 90 percent of all back aches, the best treatment is no treatment at all," the doctors concluded at a 1992 conference in Washington, D.C. "We're used to immediate treatment and response in this country," said James Weinstein, a spinal surgeon from the University of Iowa, but "back pain has a natural course that does not require intervention . . . most back aches will get better by themselves over the course of a few weeks." Wisely they reported that extended bed rest may actually delay recovery because without normal motion that circulates blood to the spine, vital oxygen can be deprived.

Well there you have it—no solution. Yet millions of people are experiencing pain relief from back aches and other parts of the body by simply applying magnetic instruments or sleeping on magnetic beds which dramatically increase oxygen intake to the cells, as explained earlier.

Another serious pain problem is repetitive stress injury (cumulative trauma disorder). It has become so common that it now accounts for half of the 284,000 work place illnesses that occur each year, according to the Bureau of Labor Statistics. Complaints come from typists, computer operators, truck drivers, musicians, tailors, meat packers, journalists, and athletes who require intense muscle concentration.

Carpal Tunnel Syndrome (compression of the main nerve in the hand) probably accounts for 50 to 75 percent of all cases of repetitive stress disorder. Any of nine tendons to the hand can be injured, making them swell and fill with fluid, reports Dr. Goldstein. This places pressure on the median nerve, creating numb fingers and weakened hand muscles that can radiate pain up the arm. In older people, it may be related to diabetes, arthritis or an underactive thyroid gland, which various forms of stress can aggravate.

Treatment begins with rest. Doctors may prescribe splints to immobilize joints. Aspirin, ibuprofen, and diuretics can reduce swelling. Cortisone injections can sometimes help control inflammation but are only effective in a small number of cases and cannot be repeated more than twice because of harmful side effects, reports Goldstein. Ultrasound is a highly acceptable therapy that has been found effective because it heats tissues more deeply. On the other hand, magnetotherapy penetrates even more deeply into the body and the bone—as much as 17 inches or more. The power of one gauss can penetrate 30 inches if the magnet is the correct size and weight. Ultrasound is a sound wave entering the body in a higher and limited frequency of the full spectrum. Importantly, sufferers who continue a magnetic maintenance program on a daily basis will ameliorate further occurrence, keep muscles relaxed, and reduce symptoms over the long-term. If the body's energy levels are balanced at sufficiently higher levels, symptoms might recede altogether.

Some months ago, a neighbor of mine complained of severe backache attributed to her word-processing job which had not been materially relieved by many visits to the conventional doctor. I loaned her a simple 3"x5"x2" magnet which erased most of the pain in 30 minutes.

She tapes this 2,000 gauss, rather powerful, magnet to her back when going to work. One day while leaning against a metal pole on the Metro subway, she got stuck and missed her stop, but her back was a lot better! This from a $20 magnet that will last just about a lifetime. A heavy magnet such as this, which can penetrate through the entire body, is not usually necessary. Flat, flexible plastiform magnets may work as well. The deeper penetrating magnet is best used at home and interchangeably with other types of magnets to determine what best suits one's body condition, something you are more likely to find out from trial and error. Your doctor usually cannot spare the time for experimentation, or is not familiar with the appropriate routines, which is really part of the protocol that should be taught in medical school. So you end up taking care of your own life.

In an another similar Carpal Tunnel Syndrome case, I loaned my Magnet-X Corp. mattress—with its 309 negative oriented magnets—to a friend. Her pain was relieved within several days, after a night or two of mild stress necessary to throw off toxins. She wasn't sure whether it was all in her mind or the mattress. After a couple of weeks, I had to take back my only mattress. Her son stopped me on the street some time later and said his mother now knows the mattress works because the pain came back. When she places even smaller magnets on her back, the pain recedes. Anecdotal or not, this type of experience is repeated over and over again.

Sleep

Another area in which most physicians and therapists are undertrained is sleep disorder. In fact, little knowledge is available from anyone about why we sleep. Much can be done about snoring or sleep apnea (where one actually stops breathing and which can be fatal). Dreams are still a mystery. We do know sleep is closely related to our biological, circadian rhythms, allowing us to fall asleep and wake up about the same time daily.

Negative magnetic energy is in greater demand during wakeful periods than the brain and Earth can supply, therefore the need for sleep. Insufficient sleep causes stress and buildup of toxins which further interferes with proper sleep. Better sleep can usually come about by sleeping on a negative field magnetic bed. In this regard, an anti-stress level magnetic field has been documented by Dr. Philpott as producing the neurohormone melatonin by the pineal gland during periods of no sunlight. Deficiency of melatonin leads to physical and emotional disorders and development of infection and neoplasm.

Negative magnetism at the crown of the head and mid-sternum are excellent sleep inducers, as experienced by Philpott. In order to wake up more quickly and fully energized, circadian bright lights placed so that the light shines directly into the eyes for about 30 minutes (while eating breakfast or preparing for the day ahead) is recommended by many doctors as an additional therapy. If you have trouble waking up or feel overly drowsy in the morning, try the bright light routine. It is medically approved therapy and now fairly widely available.

Unfortunately, if you have a sleep problem, most doctors will simply prescribe sleeping pills. Just in the past week, I heard of another "miracle" sleeping pill that hit the market. Remember that insurance companies avoid paying for sleep problems. And health maintenance organizations usually do not have adequate facilities for testing or treating sleep disorders; yet, this is one of our most common ailments and another failure of a highly technological but misdirected health system. We sell billions of dollars of sleeping pills that do not cure insomnia and in many cases cause addiction. It is a terrible shame that millions of Americans must rely on a bottle of pills sitting next to the bed. It would be so much fairer if the drug manufacturers put their money into sleep research and real cures, while insurance companies stood up for solutions to these common problems.

Discussion of sleep disorders could easily fill a volume. Suffice it to say here that there are a variety of causes. Dr. Goldstein talks about transient insomnia which may be caused by jet lag, shift work, or stress. One may have to learn how to tune out problems of the day. Some have life-long insomnia from childhood, while others experience chronic fatigue syndrome, whereby a person is unable to sleep even if exhausted. Some have the problem of excessive sleepiness, sleep apnea, or "restless legs syndrome," recognized by the thrashing of arms and legs.

Snoring is a problem for many which Dr. Goldstein says may be cured by reduction in the increase of muscle tension in the tongue and throat muscles. The force of air down the windpipe causes overly relaxed muscles of the throat to vibrate because they are being pulled downward and closer together. The air and vibration produce the sound. Snoring occurs most often when one sleeps on his back because the tongue falls deeper into the throat. It occurs more in men than women and more in obese people and more with increases in age.

Sleep sufferers or snorers often turn to surgery or drugs. Halcion, as stated previously, is the world's most widely prescribed sleeping pill with over seven million Americans using it annually. Halcion is UpJohn Company's second best earner at 250 million dollars a year in ninety countries. The FDA approved its use in 1982, but the Dutch withdrew it in 1979 and Britain banned it in 1991, concluding that the risks outweigh the benefits. Dr. Anthony Kales, Head of Psychiatry at Penn State University Medical School stated, "This is a very dangerous drug. No other benzodiazetine has such a narrow margin of safety. The only justification for having it on the market is to insure the company's profitability. From a public health standpoint, there is no reason at all." The FDA is again reviewing it. Doctors are still prescribing it.

Why do we continue to insist that people need drugs to sleep? Fortunately, at least some habits are changing. Today thousands of people are sleeping on magnetic beds that improve sleep and even change peoples' lives. Many users report the need to sleep less hours yet with more comfort and arising more exhilarated. Since magnetic fields tend to oxygenate the tissues more effectively and reduce swollen tissue to open passages, snorers and sinus suffers report considerable improvement and, in some cases, complete recovery to a normal condition. It doesn't work on everybody, but it is effective for a high percentage of users. Some with excellent circulation and a high metabolism rate may not notice a remarkable difference at first. On the other hand, subtle changes over a period of time will normally take place to improve sleep and provide for a healthier, more vigorous body upon waking each day.

Dr. Dean Bonlie, who is researching the effects of magnetotherapy as reported earlier, has had unusual success in treating athletes. He says that increased molecular activity from the resonance of the brain's pulsed D.C. currents and resulting magnetic fields interacting with the geomagnetic field, supplemented by a strong negative magnetic field bed will 1) facilitate and enhance all chemical reactions in the body, 2) enhance cellular diffusion of gases, 3) and, conserve nutrients since the body has more energy to reconstitute enzymes, such as A.T.P. This enables the heart to accomplish its work with less effort. Some subjects report lower blood pressure, and all athletes have reported slower resting heart rates.

Bonlie has observed hundreds of clients who use magnetic beds who have demonstrated reduced stress and better sleep without side effects, except for the release of toxins. He is an advocate of using only the negative polarity, citing his own clinical research and case studies of the many beneficial effects of negative fields alone.

In athletes particularly, Bonlie says, one needs more than the irritant effects of a positive or bipolar application of magnetism. As soon as positive magnetic fields or intense heat or irritating medications are applied to the locale of pain, the brain responds with negative energy to counter this new irritant and relieve the original pain. But long-term healing cannot be obtained in this fashion. The safest course is from the use of negative magnetic fields only, he says. Pain is relieved and sound sleep more likely to result. And one may use the negative magnetic pads indefinitely, gaining a lifetime of good rest.

In Bonlie's own case, as stated earlier, he found he not only sleeps better by using a magnetic bed but also has experienced elimination of all symptoms from arthritis. No one can make a claim of cure for arthritis or degenerative joint reversal, but both Dr. H. L. Bansal and Dr. R. S. Bansal, of the Indian Institute of Magnetotherapy, claim extraordinary success in relief of pain and improved muscle motion on many patients with arthritis and diabetes. They also report that magnetotherapy cuts healing time as much as half or more for such injuries as sprains, strains, broken bones, and burns and cuts. Healing is also more effective, resulting in less scar tissue and better symmetry. By eliminating pain and stress, sleep improves naturally.

Chronic Fatigue Syndrome

Let us look at another culprit to our way of life, chronic fatigue syndrome (CFS). As we discussed in earlier chapters, it is a prime applicant for magnetotherapy, especially since the average doctor has no explanation for it and no cure. It affects millions of Americans and tens of millions worldwide. It is frequently misdiagnosed as a form of depression or senility, or more technically, dementia. As a consequence, doctors proceed to prescribe anti-depressants, while ignoring the real problem. If it is real dementia, a drug may help. Too often it is pseudodementia which may be diagnosed on a computerized Spect Scan that measures brain blood flow, explains Dr. Goldstein. In pseudodementia, reductions in blood flow will not occur in typical areas for Alzheimer's, as just one consideration, he points out.

The understanding of dementias, particularly in younger people can be greatly enhanced by the use of "functional brain imaging," the process which measures electrical, blood flow, metabolic and electromagnetic activity in the brain rather than simply taking a picture of it as MRI and CAT scans do. Dr. Goldstein informs us that evoked responses from visual, auditory, or bodily stimuli can affect the pathways of electrical and magnetic messages as they travel through the brain.*

CFS is considered a new disease by most doctors although it has been around for decades but not listed in the typical medical "cook book." Patients are sent back and forth among doctors without proper diagnosis. Dr. Goldstein wants us to know that it has some of the characteristics of flu-like symptoms and at one time it was called "Yuppie Flu" or "Raggety

---

* The italicized text refers to more complex information.

313

Ann Syndrome" because patients slumped from the lack of energy. Adults under the age of 45 seem most susceptible while the majority of the patients are women. It has been too often diagnosed as lyme disease, multiple sclerosis, hyperthyroidism, hepatitis, and lymphoma, among other conditions, Goldstein says.

Dr. Anthony L. Komaroff, Associate Professor of Medicine at Harvard and Chief of General Medicine at Brigham and Women's Hospital in Boston, believes CFS may be caused by the activation of dormant viruses and other infectious agents which cause some people's immune systems to malfunction. Remember that evidence exists that negative magnetic fields attack dormant viruses and infectious agents that harm our immune systems.

CFS is a psychoneuroimmunologic disorder (psychological, neurological, and immunological dysfunction), Dr. Goldstein says. Genetics, prior illness, environment, stress, age and gender may all be factors. It is not simply fatigue or all in the mind. **A check list of symptoms put out by the Centers for Disease Control include: fatigue, cognitive and nervous system disorders, psychological problems, recurrent flu-like illnesses, painful lymph nodes, severe nasal and other allergies, weight increase, muscle and joint aches, low grade fevers, night sweats, heart palpitations, severe premenstrual syndrome, herpes, recurrent urination, rashes, and hair loss. I.Q. scores can drop and one can have difficulty in driving an auto or reading street signs.** One must be careful not to confuse it with other diseases. It is difficult to find specialists in this disease, unless one turns to the alternative therapists.

Unfortunately, the conventional medical profession has found no cure for CFS. Some nutritional supplements may help but exercise may make it worse, according to Goldstein. He says tests can come back negative from your physician so you can become even more frustrated. Your doctor may try to explain it away as depression and have little time to spend on the real problem. Again, the typical cures recommended are a whole series of questionable drugs such as Nardil, Parnate, Tagnamet, and Prozac, among others. A patient is not supposed to over-exert himself or drink alcohol, deny the body sound sleep, or engage in any kind of stress related activities. Goldstein steps forward to say that psychotherapy, acupuncture, naturopathy, reflexology, and nutritional medicine may offer relief. Remember that magnetotherapy can override most of these alternatives.

It has been demonstrated that magnetotherapy is one of the medical alternatives for chronic fatigue syndrome, used extensively in Japan and half a dozen other countries. People from all over the world with CFS who have made regular use of magnetic beds or who have engaged in magnetic field maintenance programs, report improvements. Dr. Philpott's treatment is directed toward the pineal gland that is responsible for the production of melatonin. He secures a round neodymium magnet (negatively oriented) on the exact center of the crown of the head. Melatonin governs our biocycles, among other things, which are stress producing when disordered, affecting our emotional, mental and physical states. Surprisingly, some individuals have recovered in a few short nights, as observed clinically with procedures and results recorded by Philpott. Verification that these were actual CFS victims is difficult but they all had the signs. Whatever their reason for fatigue, lackadaisical attitude or minimum performance, magnetic treatment had a profound effect. Dr. Bonlie has treated seven cases of CFS successfully by using a strong negative magnetic bed plus other magnetic devices such as a necklace or bracelet during the day hours as well for the more difficult cases. He believes CFS is the result of the brain not being able to put out enough D.C. current due to a diminution of glial cells from age, lack of oxygen, or infection.

Premenstrual Syndrome

Our final consideration here is premenstrual syndrome (PMS), which has many of the same characteristics of chronic fatigue syndrome. Dr. Goldstein believes that CFS might even cause PMS. Virtually all women who have CFS also have severe PMS. The symptoms cause noticeable change in normal function of 40 percent of all women and severe alteration of lifestyle in two to ten percent.

Cures are illusive. Some women insist that natural progesterone helps, others observe no effect or even a worsening of the condition, according to Dr. Goldstein. Only one double-blind clinical study to support its use is available. In any case, progesterone may become addictive. Here again the conventional treatment is drug prescription and, in some cases, possibly nutritional supplements.

One theory for the cause of PMS is that women with it have lower blood levels of beta-endorphin after ovulation than women who do not have PMS. If this is the case, beta-endorphin would be low in the brain's hypothalamus, resulting in a form of narcotic withdrawal. *We already discussed the effect of electrical and magnetic fields that stimulate the concha of the ear that in controlled tests have resulted in drug addicts being cured of withdrawal symptoms. An increase of endorphin to the hypothalamus has been noted as one possible effect of this treatment. The results could very well be the same for PMS sufferers.* *

Significantly, providers of magnetotherapy report successful treatment of PMS cases with the use of magnetic beds or a nightly maintenance routine. Dean Bonlie states that numerous of his clients with PMS report complete removal of symptoms, cramps, depression and other signs. These happy people suggest other women try magnetic beds. Dr. Philpott suggests treatment on a regular basis to prevent development of symptoms—daily 30 to 60 minute applications between menstrual periods. During periods of discomfort, he recommends treatment of the ovaries with ceramic magnets or several plastiform magnets stacked together for greater gauss strength and penetration.

Indications are that we are dealing with similarly constricted body cells regardless of the malignancy or ailment, whether PMS, chronic fatigue syndrome, sepsis, cancer or some other infection. In each case, we need to get the cell back to a healthy state. We know that we can raise the energy and strength of normal cells, and recent evidence shows that even infectious cells can be restored. *The Memorial Sloan Kettering Cancer Center in New York City has developed a variety of drugs that have demonstrated that malignant cells can mature to resemble normal cells. John Laszlo of the American Cancer Society says, "We had always thought that when a cell moves in the direction of becoming a cancer cell it can never come back. But from these studies it's clear that at least some cancer cells can revert back to normal."* * At the very least, we can strengthen what is there.

Various studies have demonstrated that negative magnetic fields improve the health of human cells, drive out infectious growth, and convert

---

* The italicized text refers to more complex information.

cells to a normal alkalizing pH state. No one is bold enough to say that magnetic fields can cure cancer or sepsis or arthritis or any major disease, but successful human case histories exist for the elimination of symptoms for all of these by energizing the immune system to perform at a higher level. People may draw whatever conclusions they wish at this stage. Suffice it to say that more research and controlled, clinical studies are warranted and that they should proceed without delay.

Final Words

To discuss the gamut of diseases, their consequences and possible cures, would take volumes. This information simply touches on several major ailments that particularly lend themselves to magnetotherapy and that affect the majority of Americans and most people around the world. The principles of treatment are essentially the same for every ailment with variations primarily in the strength and polarity of the magnetic field and the duration of use. The two philosophies of which polarity to use should not complicate the treatment protocol. If one questions the polarity to be used, when in doubt always use the safest.

Prevailing experiments and case histories appear to show that negative fields are alkalizing and the positive fields acidic. Simple tests show the human blood sugar goes up with the positive fields and down with the negative. Epileptic seizures are excited with the positive fields and diminished with the negative. If the user applies the positive polarity or dual polarities for certain ailments because he believes treatment is quicker or more stimulating, he is advised to follow positive field treatment with negative field exposure for safety purposes, especially for long-term high gauss applications. The expert practitioners tell us that if the positive field has to be used at all, it can accomplish everything it needs to in minutes. Then it should be followed by 30 to 60 minutes, twice daily, of negative magnetic treatment to be on the safe side and to achieve a normal pH balance. Low gauss bipolar treatment is deemed safe.

The user should be sure to examine magnetic equipment closely. Some manufactures will not even inform you which polarity is which or what pole is facing your body. Some have no idea about the importance or the distinction and some don't care. To them, magnetism is magnetism and if people heal, that is enough. The long-term consequences of sleeping on positive magnetic fields can be harmful, stimulating cancer growth, infection and stress.

Japanese, as the biggest users of magnetotherapy (some 30 million devices), warn us that stress will occur after prolonged use of positive or dual polarities and that we should simply stop using the magnets for a period until the body readjusts or balances the fields. But meanwhile cell damage could occur from using the positive polarity.

The user should be careful to measure the polarity of devices by using a magnetometer or a simple compass, whose positive (south) polarized needle that points north will attract the negative (north) field of any other magnetic force or device, in addition to the Earth's north magnetic pole. In other words, the arrow head of a compass will point to the negative pole of a magnet. Some manufacturers have been taught to use the industrial rather than the scientific convention and are thoroughly mixed up which is north (negative) or south (positive). Take control of your own destiny. Don't rely on any one else. At least become a partner with the doctor and the supplier.

The body completely rebuilds itself every six months, except for brain tissue and certain connective tissue. This means that all of us have the opportunity to rejuvenate our health no matter how good or bad we feel now. Don't despair over a weak or ill system. Do something about it.

Magnetotherapy, under a daily maintenance program, can rid the body of toxic wastes, balance pH, and build more energy into the system, as the cells strengthen and receive more oxygen. Even with the use of the negative fields, as the acidic waste passes from the body, some people may feel stress and pain as they detoxify. This should not last more than a few days for most people. Understand it and bear with it. Sleep on the magnetic pad an hour or two the first few nights if you experience stress due to release of toxins, then gradually build up to a full night.

Some people have been known to get up in the middle of the night to walk off detoxification the first few nights. Yet after this initial period of detoxification, sleeping on a magnetic bed involves no work or stress. It feels good and is the easiest therapy, one which every person, regardless of energy or will can do and actually enjoy for a lifetime without being harassed about exercising or eating the right foods—things you are encouraged to do in any case.

The human system will improve and you will feel better. Heart rate and blood pressure can move to more normal counts. One may feel younger and livelier and live longer. Most aches and pains will disappear. Even serious illnesses can pass or at least be eased. There are too many successful cases not to believe this, while any placebo effect has proven secondary or minor. The thousands of cases, more nearly millions of self-induced alternative cures, never get into the medical literature. Perhaps a book should be written simply documenting 1000 or one million successful magnetotherapy histories. For some that may mean more than all the technical explanations.

Sampling of anecdotal cases has become necessary to show the range and depth of healing, otherwise no one would know what it is all about or its possibilities. More controlled tests are desired but that does not mean that we should discredit true case histories, unless there is evidence to the contrary. The people in these cases are willing to challenge the medical industry and the government, if necessary. This nation has more than enough research money to conduct all the studies necessary to verify every claim. We simply have to do it. Our priorities have been lobbied too much in the direction of chemicals and elaborate technologies. Let us begin to think more about the safety of people and prevention of disease.

The proper application of magnetotherapy has proven safe for humans. As to whether you should use it, no one can make that decision but you. Of course, for any serious ailment, see a medical professional, but if that fails, don't assume that to be the end. Try an inexpensive, simple magnet first to relieve a particular pain, then sleep on a magnetic pad and examine the course of your life. Perhaps there is no other way, for it may be a long time before the majority of the medical profession feels that magnetotherapy should be part of their sophisticated regimen of "cookbook" cures. No doubt many physicians will still look for standard, direct healing found in conventional medical books. Yet it may be time to change the book. Human spirit, and the desire to live on and live healthy will make the final judgment about this medicine.

Appendix I
Recommended Areas of Research for Magnetic Field Therapy,
by William H. Philpott, M.D.

1. Bronchitis, Bronchiectasis, Acute or Chronic Lung Infection
   Obtain adequate penetration, using the negative pole. During the day place stacked magnets on the back of the chest an hour at a time three times daily. Magnets should be placed on the left and right sides of the chest during day treatment as well. Night treatment can also include four 4"x6"x½" ceramic magnets one inch apart at the crown of the head.

2. Mitral Valve Prolapse
   Wear a 3"x12"x(1/8)" plastiform magnet over the heart during the day and/or night.

3. Negatively Magnetized Oxygen
   When breathing 100 percent oxygen, tape the negative pole of one or more ceramic mini-block magnets on the tubing to magnetize the oxygen.

4. All Types of Leukemias
   Use a magnetic bed of mini ceramic block magnets that provide a full field from the shoulders down. Alternative treatment is four ceramic magnets at the crown of the head. Also treat spleen, liver, rectal and chest areas with ceramic magnets several times daily for an hour each time.

5. Negative Magnetic Energy—Antibiotic Effect
   Electrolyzed normal saline and biological treatment with a negative magnetic field have been observed to have antibiotic value. Treat normal saline and cerebral spinal fluid and observe.

6. Magnetic Brain Treatment
   Observe for depression, anxiety, obsessions, compulsions, seizures occurring at night, schizophrenia, post-brain trauma, post-cerebral vascular accident, brain viral infections, cerebral arteriosclerosis, migraine headaches. Use a 4"x6"x½" ceramic magnet placed from the forehead to the occiput just above the ears. The magnet can be rotated from one side to the other.

7. Breast Cancer Prevention and Treatment
   Place ceramic magnet discs ¾"x(1/8)" of 850 gauss ¾" apart beneath the lining of the bra cup worn daily for preventive purposes. Use a ceramic mini-block 1¾"x¾" magnet of 3,950 gauss for treating cancer. Treat under the arms as well.

8. Post Central Nervous System Trauma
   It is observed that negative magnetic energy relieves cellular edema, oxygenates and oxidates, controls and normalizes neuronal excitation, governs healing, and resolves scar tissue. Positive magnetic energy excites neuronal functions

and is capable of reinstituting neuronal function inhibited by extension of disuse.

Apply negative magnetic energy to an area as large as the lesion being treated. In terms of the head, apply to both sides. Apply only negative polarity and as long as possible in the acute phase.

9. Hyperkinesis and Learning Disorders
These disorders are of common association and cause. Maladaptive reactions to certain food is a common cause related to IgG food allergies, non-immunologic hypersensitive food reactions, and food addictions. Avoidance period of three months from maladaptive foods followed by a four-day diversified rotation diet has a high level symptom relief value. Negative magnetic energy inhibits food maladaptive reactions. Sleep on a magnetic pad and treat by pre-meal exposure to liver, spleen, mid-chest and epigastric and temporal areas of the head and occipital area of the head.

10. Possible Ionization Damage Repair
Ionization is a disruption of an atom or molecule by strong electromagnetic energy causing ejection of electrons from the material ejected from the atom or molecules. It is postulated that a negative magnetic field can repair damage of cells.

11. Essential Hypertension
Essential hypertension encompasses 96% to 94% of hypertensive cases for which no specific identifiable illness exists; however, there is measurable evidence of abnormal organ functions such as hormonal, renal, and vascular systems. Environmental and various foods have been isolated as causes and treated by avoidance and a rotation diet. Further study of the impact of magnetic energy is recommended.

12. Leprosy
Leprosy is a worldwide disease with more than 20 million people affected. It is a chronic granulomatous systemic bacteria (mycobacterium lepral) infection in which skin and peripheral nerves are the most vulnerable. Negative magnetic energy gives evidence as a universal antibiotic and should be tested with controls as to its effect on this disease.

13. Osteomyelitis
This is caused by a bacterial infection of bone. A long duration of use of negative magnetic energy should be tested.

Appendix I (*cont'd*)
Recommended Areas of Research for Magnetic Field Therapy,
by William H. Philpott, M.D.

14. Glaucoma

Glaucoma is caused by pressure in the eyes due to improper drainage of fluid from the eyes. Cataracts are disordered carbohydrate metabolism ranging from hypoglycemia to frank diabetes mellitus and senility. A cause of cataracts is reduced oxygen to the eye lens. Evidence exists that negative magnetic fields oxygenate cells. Magnets placed next to the eye can pull fluid out.

15. Bone Spurs and Soft Tissue Bruises

Bone spurs occur after bruising heal tissue on the bone. Calcium deposits in the bruised area produce a spur. A negative magnetic field is known to dissolve calcium in soft tissue or in bone that is not part of the live tissue.

16. Insulin Dependent Diabetes Mellitus

Insulin dependent diabetes mellitus is caused by injury to pancreatic insulin producing beta cells. Viral infections such as mumps pan ceratitis has been considered a likely cause in some cases involving children. More recently, IgG cows milk allergy that initiates a pancreatic beta cell autoimmune reaction has been documented as a cause in a substantial number of cases. This causes cellular edema from evoked acidosis that produces insulin resistance. Edema can be caused by immune, non-immune, and addictive reactions.

An allergy survey should be conducted on the patient, food avoidance and rotation diet instituted, then treat with a negative magnetic field, and monitor. Although it has been demonstrated that adequate pretreatment with a negative magnetic field can block allergic, non-allergic and addictive reactions to foods, a four-day diversified rotation diet should also take place. This major disease of mankind is reversible, yet physicians aren't doing it. The clinical evidence is in (Philpott W.H. and Kalita D. **Victory over Diabetes: A BioEcologic Triumph**, Keats Publishing, New Canaan, Ct., 1983).

Dr. G.S., a researcher at the NIH whose daughter had diabetes, read the above book, called Philpott and said, "You are right." Other physicians would not believe that food allergy and addiction and maturity onset Type II diabetes mellitus have the same disordered chemistry until they visited the examination office and observed the blood sugar levels of patients over five days and reactions to single foods. Those who have observed have changed the way they practice.

Philpott is convinced that deterioration does not have to occur in the insulin dependent diabetic. He also states that we must learn that allergic and non-allergic maladaptive reactions and addictions allowed to function over a period of years leads to the final stage of diabetes mellitus, arteriosclerosis, amyotrophic lateral sclerosis, Alzheimer's disease, and likely several other degenerative diseases.

Appendix I *(cont'd)*
Recommended Areas of Research for Magnetic Field Therapy,
by William H. Philpott, M.D.

Alzheimer's cases were tested to have hyperammonemia, while none of senile cases showed this. Hyperammonemia is seen as diabetics, amyotrophic lateral sclerotics and Alzheimer's disease cases. An Alzheimer's case with treatment of the head in a negative magnetic field was observed to have a return of memory and orientation which lasted for four hours after removal of the negative magnetic field. The question arises whether the brain can heal, including the growth of new neurons.

Also atherosclerosis is speeded up in the diabetes mellitis disease and is always a part of the diabetic disease process. We have made a mistake, says Philpott, in diagnosing diabetes as a disease only in its late stage when the lasting blood sugar is higher than normal. For years prior to this, the same disease process is taking place.

Acute bouts of acidosis occurs in response to maladaptive foods, chemicals and addiction, the blood pH is sufficiently low during this period to cause cross-linking of amino acids that produce insoluble gels found in atherosclerosis deposited in arteries and gels in Alzheimers. The question arises, can these insoluble gels be reversed by raising the pH? There is clinical evidence in this respect. Treating atheromotous plaques has been resolved. Symptoms are relieved in a few minutes but plaque removal may take weeks or months.

Schizophrenic patients examined also had an assortment of chronic degenerative diseases, such as arthritis, lupus, multiple sclerosis, migraine headache, etc., including maturity onset type diabetes mellitus. Common denominators showed up between mental illness and associated physical degenerative diseases in patients. The role of pH and magnetic fields needs to be further explored.

17.   Rheumatic Diseases
Rheumatoid arthritis, bursitis, myositis, tendinitis and lupus have similar causes which are maladaptive reactions to foods, chemicals, inhalants, toxins and infections. Avoidance of the symptom evoking substances is primary, next is proper nutrition. Negative magnetic energy can relieve and even prevent inflammatory maladaptive reactions.

18.   Magnetic Water Floss and Negatively Magnetized Water for Tooth
        Scale and Gum Infection
Water is paramagnetic and the oxygen dissolved in water is paramagnetic. The negative field can inhibit bacterial and fungal growth. Water passing through magnetic flux produces an abundance of free electrons that prevent electrovalent bonding, therefore prevent or dissolve placque and calculus on the teeth as well as preventing bacterial colonization.

Appendix I (cont'd)
Recommended Areas of Research for Magnetic Field Therapy,
by William H. Philpott, M.D.

19.   Frontal and Maxillary Sinuses
Sinus infections may be viral, fungal or bacterial in origin or of mixed infections. Negative magnetic energy has been observed to be quite useful, increasing fluid flow in the sinus cavity and reducing inflammation.

20.   Obesity
Obsessive compulsiveness develops based on a learned artificial drive in response to withdrawal symptoms and symptom relief by eating the offending foods. Negative magnetic energy has been observed to be able to reduce food reactions and prevent food reactions by exposure to negative magnetic fields well ahead of consuming meals of otherwise symptom evoking foods.

21.   Osteoporosis
Bones repair under a negative magnetic field that pulls minerals into the area, including calcium. Sleeping on a magnetic bed will help pull minerals and calcium into the bones.

22.   Free Radical Induced Inflammation
Free radicals contain at least one unpaired electron. Free radicals are paramagnetic. "According to Quantum Mechanics, the spin of the odd electron of the free radical when placed in a magnetic field, may have two and only two orientations, one with and the other against the field." (New Encyclopedia Britannica, Vol.9, Micropaedia, 1986, pp.886-7.)
Free radicals evoke inflammation in biological tissues. Clinical observations show a rapid resolution of inflammation during exposure to a static negative magnetic field and an increase in inflammation from the positive magnetic field, while exposure to bipolar fields simultaneously at non-stressful gauss strength also reduces inflammation rapidly by attracting negative energy to the area.
Free radicals can be formed in a state of tissue hypoxia. Phagocytes produce free radical oxygen species to kill microorganism infections. The amino acid Taurine serves as an antioxidant to protect against the death of phagocytes after they kill bacteria.
The anabolic neurohormone, melatonin, has a control over free radical production. Melatonin controls oxidation-reduction, including antioxidant reduction by including a low c AMP-c GMP radio (Vacas, M., Sarmineuto, M., Cardinale, D., **Melatonin Increases c GMP and decreases c AMP levels in Rat Medical Basal Hypothalamus in Vitro**. *Brain Research*, 225:207-21 and Cutler, R., **Antioxidants, Aging, and Longevity**, in **Free Radicals in Biology**, Pryor, W. (ed.) *Academic Press*, Orlando.) An anti-stress magnetic field

evokes production of melatonin by the pineal gland (Semm, P., **Magnetic Sensitivity of Pineal Gland**, *Nature*, 1980, 228:206.)

A negative magnetic field controls free radical inflammation as it influences the paramagnetic free radicals and produces melatonin that prevents free radical production. Because the negative field increases tissue oxygenation and likely oxidation, the initiation of free radical formation is prevented since free radicals form in a tissue hypoxic state. (See review Fontenote, John M. and Levine, Stephen A., **Melatonin Deficiency: Its Role in Oncogenesis and Age-Related Pathology**, *Journal Orthomolecular Medicine*, 1st Qtr., 199 Vol.5 No.1 pp.22-4.)

23. Progressive Systemic Sclerosis
    This is a multi-system disorder characterized by inflammatory reaction of many organ systems as well as the skin. Commonly affected are the gastric intestinal tract, lungs, heart and kidneys. Cause is unknown but appears to have an autoimmune basis, as well as suspicions of viral infections and IgG food reactions. Cases have responded to magnetotherapy but controlled tests are wanting.

24. Dermatomyositis and Polymyositis
    Uncertain causes but suspicions much like the foregoing and treatment by magnetotherapy, rotation food diet, and nutritional supplements after proper assessment.

25. Laryngeal Polyps
    Likely develop from an irritation of the larynx, such as from tobacco smoking or similar cause. The viral infection is likely the cause of the polyp similar to skin warts and moles. Observations show that negative magnetic fields cause lesions to dry up and peel off, leaving normal skin. Treatment is usually from two to six weeks or more.

Appendix II
Nature of the Electron

Since the electron is such an important concept in the field of magnetotherapy, we should consider its being. Discovered in 1897, it is one of few elementary particles impervious to further subdivision. The positively charged nucleus in the center of the atom repels positively charged alpha particles but attracts or holds the negatively charged electrons, whose combined charge precisely balances the nucleus, within the sphere of the atom. This electronic sphere is 10,000 times larger than the nucleus and 2,000 times lighter. These concepts are simple and indisputable. The arrangement of the electrons is more in doubt, set in various waves, lengths and frequencies.

In quantum theory, the wave/particle duality of electrons lies at the heart of quantum mechanics. The higher the frequency, the higher the energy as formulated in Planck's law of 1918. All energy comes in discrete, irreducible bundles called quanta (when carried by light, called photon). The orbits of the electrons are not observable or measurable, while any attempt to examine an atom with a beam of light or other probe will disrupt the path of the electrons. The interior picture is a sealed book. However, the exclusions principle confirms that no two electrons can be in the same state of motion (same position and speed) at the same time, otherwise they would crash into each other.

The electron weighs 10^{-30} or nonillionth of a kilogram and the charge is so minute at 10^{19}, it would take 10 billion electrons to power a 100 watt light bulb for one second. Size is actually none at all, simply a mathematical point, yet an electron can be trapped between two negatively charged plates in a vacuum tube, called the Penning Trap, and photographed. The nucleus is 99.9 percent of the atom's weight, hovering like a BB in the center of the Superdome surrounded by empty space except for a few electrons. In this respect, the major constituent of the universe and the atom by far "is nothing, so shouldn't we be thinking about nothing," when we try to analyze the nature of this vacuum, asks Hans Christian Von Baeyer?

The oppositely charged antiparticle is the positron. Together with the electron, this particle carries no net electric charge. When converted into energy, their masses add up to the energy of the fluctuation that gave birth to them, such that the vacuum becomes momentarily polarized. The force is not caused by gravity or electricity but by the energized vacuum. The dream of medicine is to be able to pick off cells composed of noxious chemicals and radiation one at a time without harming the rest of the body. Magnetic fields possibly influence the polarization of the vacuum and its energy. Electrons may be added or their movement stimulated.

Source: Taming the Atom, Hans Christian Von Baeyer, 1992; author.

Appendix III
EcoMax™ *Technology for Ecology and Economy*

A fascinating product, several years in development and about to be marketed, is the EcoMax™ (Patented and Patents Pending in the U.S. and Overseas.) This product improves both fuel economy and emissions substantially on automobiles, trucks, buses, boats, and airplanes (that is, all combustion engines); and also reduces pollutants from lawn mowers, home and commercial heating systems, and other devices. Research and testing, for what could be a remarkable breakthrough, demonstrate that hydrogen carbon (HC), carbon monoxide (CO), and oxide of nitrogen (NOx) are reduced to a fraction of their normal output. On the other hand, CO_2 is substantially increased. A reading of 13 CO_2 or higher indicates complete or near complete burnout of HC and CO.

Scientifically, the EcoMax™ system functions by bipolar field magnetic generation which attracts appropriate fuel elements by using magnets of specific gauss strength and configuration to control the molecules of hydrogen carbons and oxygen. The most important activity taking place in any combustion engine, whether gasoline, diesel or propane, is the proper mixture of fuel (HC) and air (O). When magnets of the appropriate strength and placement polarize these two elements, a more complete mixture results and more efficient BTU combustion takes place; this process results in better fuel economy and performance. If this product functions as reported, this could be the most meaningful finding for both ecology and the economy; Al Gore ought to look at this one.

The magnetic system functions best when in place at least for 500 to 1,000 miles. With proper engine maintenance, magnetic system performance should last almost indefinitely. Results vary, of course, based on the condition of the engine. However, even for autos approaching or exceeding 100,000 miles of use, results have shown surprising readings. In a test of 15 autos, emissions were reduced substantially. A sample of three tests is shown below:

| Tested by: | Auto Make/ Odometer Reading | Test Emission Reading | | |
		HC (PPM)*	CO (%)	CO_2 (%)
Maryland Dept. of Transportation, Inspection Div. State Standards		*State Stds:* 0220	*State Stds:* 1.20	*State Stds:* 6.00
I Maryland Dept. of Transportation, Inspection Div.	1987 Chrysler Odometer 79,500	*After:* 0005	*After:* 0.00	*After:* 14.80
II Exxon Testing Station Rockville, MD	1984 Toyota Corolla Odometer 89,000	*Before:* 0170 *After:* 0007	*Before:* 1.08 *After:* 0.09	*Before:* 10.9 *After:* 14.50
III Tune-Up Center Gaithersburg, MD	1981 Datsun/Nissan Odometer 83,000	*Before:* 0160 *After:* **0005**	*Before:* 1.01 *After:* **0.09**	*Before:* 9.05 *After:* **13.50**
Now available for gas, diesel, propane, and alcohol fuel operated vehicles.	**Source:** Richard Z. Hricak NOVA Publishing Company 11607 Nebel Street, Rockville, MD 20852 301-231-8229			

* PPM equals parts per million.

Glossary

- **blastema**: mass of living substance capable of growth and differentiation

- **chelation**: forming coordinate bonds through two or more atoms important in enzyme deactivation. Bond energy is the amount of energy required to break a bond and produce neutral atoms. Coulomb's law—all bonds arise from the attraction of unlike charges. Binds to minerals to help them work normally or be eliminated by the body.

- **circadian rhythm**: the predominant biological cycle of all living things. In humans this pattern is approximately 24 hours and usually follows the lunar day. Biological cycles occur in almost all physical functions, including sleep, wakefulness, hormone levels, and numbers of white cells in the blood.

- **clinical**: dispassionate direct observation of the patient

- **collagen**: a protein that makes up most of the fibrous connective tissue that holds the body's parts together, such as in tendons, ligaments, and scar tissues. It also forms the basic structure of bone.

- **dedifferentiation**: reversion back to a more primitive state, or its original, embryonic, unspecialized form, often as preliminary to a major change

- **differentiation**: development from the one to the many; the simple to the complex; modification of body parts for performance of special functions; sum of processes whereby indifferent cells, tissues, and structures attain adult form and function

- **DNA**: the molecule in cells that contains genetic information

- **Earth's magnetic field**: .5 gauss having daily fluctuations of up to .1 gauss and ranging from .3 at the equator to .6 at the poles—based on geological measurement of magnetic particles in lake sediment as well as data from NASA's MAGSAT orbiter

- **electrolyte**: any chemical compound that when dissolved in water separates into charged atoms that permit the passage of electrical current through the solution

- **electromagnet**: a magnet consisting essentially of a soft-iron core wound with a current-carrying coil of insulated wire, in which the current produces the magnetization of the core

- **electromagnetic field**: the field of force associated with an accelerating electric charge, having both electric and magnetic components and containing a definite amount of electromagnetic energy

• **enzyme**: (Greek for fermentation) a catalyst to accelerate rates of reactions several orders of magnitude while experiencing no permanent chemical modification. It may not proceed in absence of temperature or pressure or in acidic pH.

• **free radical**: a molecule or atom that contains an unpaired electron but is neither positive or negative charged and is highly unstable or reactive. It is oxygen derived, fulfilling certain necessary physiological functions, but is also capable of great harm in excess or in the wrong place. (Free is often dropped because it can lead to confusion.)

• **gauss**: the unit of measurement used for measuring a magnetic field

• **gene**: portion of DNA molecule structured to produce to a specific effect in the cell

• **hertz**: (Hz) a unit of frequency equal to one cycle per second

• **in vitro**: experiment done in a dish on part of a living organism

• **in vivo**: experiment done on an intact, whole organism

• **magnet**: a body that attracts iron and certain other materials by virtue of a surrounding field of force produced by the motion of its atomic electrons and alignment of its atoms

• **magnetic field**: a condition in a region of space established by the presence of a magnet and characterized by the existence of a detectable magnetic force at every point in the region

• **magnetite**: a black mineral of iron oxide, which when magnetically polarized is called a lodestone, found in both man and animals

• **magnetometer**: instrument for comparing magnitude and direction of magnetic fields

• **magnetosphere**: is the complex structure of the magnetic field around the Earth, extending from about 400 to several thousand miles above the surface; it protects us from the solar-wind particles containing deadly ionizing radiation (such as x-rays) and other high energy radiation

• **neuron**: nerve cell

• **neutrino**: neutral and massless particle emitted during decay of other particles. Charge must be zero because it is undetected, yet discovered in order to meet the conservation laws of energy. Neutron possesses a magnetic moment, although the net charge is zero.

• **PEMF**: pulsed electromagnetic field

• **pH**: (potential for hydrogen) range of numbers expressing the relative acidity or alkalinity of a solution from 0 to 14. Neutrality is 7, above is alkaline and below acidic. pH provides a measure of the hydrogen ion concentration of a solution, such as in saliva or blood. For human blood the acceptable range is 7.5 to 7.6. Below this range indicates a health problem. For saliva the range is wider, a health problem is indicated below 7 or 6.5.

• **piezoelectric**: effect on a substance that changes mechanical stress into electrical energy, producing an electrical current when the substance is deformed by pressure or bending.

• **sciatic nerve**: main nerve in the leg that includes motor nerve fibers carrying impulses to the leg muscles and sensory nerve fibers carrying impulses to the brain.

• **sham**: having such poor quality as to be fake

• **undifferentiated**: unspecialized as referring to cells that are in a primitive or embryonic state

• **vector**: a carrier or a quantity possessing magnitude, direction, and sense (positivity or negativity), and commonly represented by a straight line resembling an arrow—length denotes magnitude, arrow denotes direction, position with respect to an axis denotes sense

Sources and References

Over 500 articles, books, reports, studies and scientific figures were reviewed. Only certain key sources are presented here. More than 100 interviews were also conducted.

Chapter 1

1. Davis, A.R. and Rawls, W., **Magnetism & Its Effects on the Living System**, *Acres USA*, Kansas City, MO, 1976
2. Becker, R.O. **Cross Currents**, *Jeremy P. Tarcher, Inc.*, Los Angeles, CA, 1990
3. Evans, John, **Mind, Body and Electromagnetism**, 1986
4. Philpott, William P., Choctaw, OK, interviews 1992-3
5. Barefoot, Robert R. and Reich, Carl J., M.D., **The Calcium Factor**
6. Dr. Dean Bonlie, MagnetiCo Inc., Calgary, Canada, D.D.S. interviews 1992-3
7. Robert Barefoot, interviews 1992-3
8. Robert O. Becker, interview June, 1993
9. Dr. John Zimmerman, Reno, Nevada, interviews, 1992-3
10. Office of Alternative Medicine, National Institutes of Health, Conferences and Reports, 1993
11. Bio-Electro-Magnetics Institute, Reno, Neveda, Journal Fall 1992, Spring 1993
12. Magnetic-X Corp. Calgary, Canada, documented case histories, 1992-3
13. MagnetiCo Inc., Calgary, Canada, documented case histories, 1992-3
14. *Journal of the National Medical Association*, September 1990
15. Gerber, Richard, **Vibrational Medicine**, *Bear & Co.*, 1968
16. Savitz, D.A. and Calle, E.E. (1987) Leukemia and Occupational exposure to electromagnetic fields: review of epidemiological surveys, J. Occup. Med 29:47-51.
17. Daniels, G.H. and Martin, J.B., Harrison's Principles of Internal Medicine, 11th Edition 1987, McGraw-Hill Book Company, pp.1701-5
18. Aharonov, Y and Bohm, D., **Significance of Electromagnetic Potentials in Quantum Theory**, *The Physical Review*, 115 485(1959)
19. New Encyclopedia Britannica, Vol.18, MACROPEDIA, 1986, pp.274-5

Chapter 2

1. Ring, John J., president American Medical Association, **An Alliance of Excellence**, Vital Speeches, April 1st, 1992
2. Dear, Julie, **Sharks and Cancer**, *Health Journal, Washington Post*, December 10th, 1991
3. **Chiropractors**, *Physician's Weekly, Whittle Communications Publications*, 1991
4. **Exercise Bench and Osteoarthritis**, *Health Journal, Washington Post*, December 10th, 1991
5. Becker, Robert O., M.D. and Selden, Gary **The Body Electric**, 1985
6. Philpott, William P., Dr. and Taplin, Sharon, **Biomagnetic Handbook**, Envirotech, Choctaw, OK, 1990
7. Pierrollos, John, **Core Energetics**, 1987
8. Gerber, Richard, **Vibrational Medicine**, *Bear & Co.*, 1968
9. **Int'l Conference on Medicine**, *Advances in Biomagnetism*, 1989
10. Evans, John, **Mind, Body and Electromagnetism**, 1986

11. Becker, R.O. **Cross Currents**, *Jeremy P. Tarcher, Inc.*, Los Angeles, CA, 1990
12. Davis, A.R. and Rawls, W., **The Magnetic Blueprint of Life**, *Acres USA*, Kansas City, MO, 1979
13. Davis, A.R. and Rawls, W., **The Magnetic Effect**, *Acres USA*, Kansas City, MO, 1975
14. Davis, A.R. and Rawls, W., **Magnetism & Its Effects on the Living System**, *Acres USA*, Kansas City, MO, 1976
15. Crease, Robert, **Biomagnetism**, State University of New York, Stony Brook, *Science*, Vol.245, September 8th, 1989
16. *U.S. News and World Report*, Vol.83 No.1, January 2nd, 1991
17. **Hunting for a Miracle**, *Health Magazine*, Feb-Mar, 1992
18. Semm, P., **Magnetic Sensitivity of Pineal Gland**, *Nature*, 228(1980): 206
19. Bradford, Robert W., Rodriquez, Rodrigo, Garcia, Jorge and Allen, Henry, **The Effect of Magnetic Poles on Accelerated Charge Neutralization of Malignant Tumors in Vivo**, *Robert W. Bradford Research Institute*, 1989
20. *BEMI Journal*, 1991
21. Cox, Allen, **Magnetic Field Reversals**, *Scientific American*, February 1967, pp.44-54
22. Gubbins, David and Bloxhan, Jeremy, **The Secular Variation of the Earth's Magnetic Field**, *Nature*, Vol.317, October 31st, 1985
23. Velikovsky, Immanuel, **Earth in Upheaval**, p.146

Chapter 3
1. Barnothy, M.F. **Biological Effects of Magnetic Fields**, *Plenum Press*, N.Y. Vol.1, 1964; Vol.2, 1969
2. Brodeur, Paul, **Currents of Death (Power Lines, Computer Terminals and the Attempt to Cover up Their Threat to Your Health**, N.Y., *Simon and Schuster*, 1989
3. Louis Slesin, editor, **Microwave News**, Grand Central Station, N.Y., N.Y.
4. Rosenblatt, Michael, **The Endogenous Opiate Peptides**, pp.378-82, **Harrison's Principles of Internal Medicine**, *McGraw-Hill Book Co.*, 1987
5. Fontenot, J. and Levihe, S.A., **Melatonin Deficiency: It's Role in oncogenesis and Age-Relative Pathology**, *Journal of Orthomolecular Medicine*, 1st quarter, 1990
6. Daniels, G.H. and Martin, J.B., **Harriso**n's Principles of Internal Medicine, *McGraw-Hill Book Co.*, pp.1701-5, 11th Edition, 1987
7. Harrison Salisbury, **The Uncertainty of Medicine**, *Bio-Electric-Magnetics Institute Journal*, Reno, NV, Fall, 1991
8. Dr. Boryl Payne, **The Body Magnetic** and **Getting Started in Magnetic Healing**, Boston University and Goddard College, 1989
9. Bansal, H.L., Dr., and Bansal, R.S., Dr., **Magnetic Cure for Common Diseases**, New Delhi; Bombay, India, 1983, 1990
10. Becker, Robert O., **The Body Electric**, 1985
11. Philpott, William P., Dr., **Biomagnetic Handbook**, 1990

12. Barefoot, Robert R. and Reich, Carl M., M.D., **The Calcium Factor: The Scientific Secret of Health and Youth**, 1992

13. **Biological Effects of Power Frequency Electric and Magnetic Fields**, Carnagie Mellon University, Pittsburg, PA, 1989, grant from Department of Energy, Public Policy Section

14. **Evaluation of the Potential Carcinogenicity of Electromagnetic Fields**, July 1991, Environmental Protection Agency (EPA)

15. **Electric Field Exposure**, *Microwave News*, May/June 1990

16. Herbert, Lawrence F., **Colorado Public Utilities Commission Report**, *Bio-Electric-Magnetics Institute Newsletter*, 1990-1991

17. Narayan, P.V. Sarker, M.D., **Bioelectric Effects**, *Bioelectromagnetics and Biomedicine Journal of the Madvar Institute of Magnetobiology*, India, Dec. 1988

18. **The Surgeon General's Report on Nutrition and Health**, *US Dept. of Health and Human Services, Public Health Service,* 1988, No. 88-50210

19. Fisher, Michael, Editor, **Guide to Clinical Preventive Services**, An assessment of Effectiveness of 169 Interventions, *Report of the U.S. Preventive Services Task Force*, 1989

20. **Healthy People**, *Health Promotion and Disease Prevention Objectives*, U.S. Dept. of Health and Human Services, Public Health Service 91-50213, Sept. 1990

21. Hacmac, Edward A., **An Overview of Biomagnetic Therapeutics**, D.C., Jan 1991.

22. Trapper, Arthur, et al., **Evolving Perspective on the Exposure Risks from Magnetic Fields**, *Journal of the National Medical Association*, September 1990, 82:9

23. Philpott, William P., M.D., interviews 1991-1993

24. Adey, W.R., **Tissue Interactions with Non-Ionizing Electromagnetic Fields**, *Physical Review* 61:435-514

25. Chinbrera, A.; Nicolini, C., and Schwan, H.P., Editors, **Interaction Between Electromagnetic Fields and Cells**, Plenum, New York, 1985

26. Wilson, B.W.,; Steven, R.G.; and Anderson, L.E., Editors, **Extremely Low Frequency Electromagnetic Fields: The Question of Cancer**, *Battelle Press,* Columbus, Ohio, 1990

27. London, S.J. and Thomas, D.C., et al., **Exposure to Residential Electric and Magnetic Fields and Risk to Childhood Leukemia**, *American Journal Epidemial*, 1991, 134:923-37

28. Stachly, M.A., **Applications of Time-Varying Magnetic Fields in Medicine**, *Critical Review Biomedical Engineering*, 1990, 18:89-124

29. Blackman, C.F. and Benanem S.G., et al., **Effects of ELF (1-120 Hz) and Modulated (50 Hz) RF Fields on the Efflux of Calcium Ions from Brain Tissue in Vitro**, *Bioelectromagnetics*, 6:1-11

30. Lednev, V.V., **Possible Mechanism for the Influence of Weak Magnetic Fields on Biological Systems**, *Bioelectromagnetics*, 1991, 12:71-5

31. **Evaluation of the Potential Carcinogenicity of Electromagnetic Fields**, *EPA*, 1990, #600/6-90/005B

32. Morgan, M,C.; Florig, H.K.; Nair, I.; Hester, G.L., **Controlling Exposure to Transmission Line Electromagnetic Fields: a Regulatory Approach That is Compatible with the Available Science**, *Public Utilities Fortnightly*, March 17, 1988:49-58

Chapter 4

1. Bansal, H.L., Dr, **Magnetic Cure for Common Diseases**, 1983; 1990
2. Lightwood, R. **The Remedial Electromagnetic Field**, *Journal Biomedicine*, England, September, 1989, Vol.11
3. Kristiansen, Thomas, M.D., **Ultrasound Therapy**, *Preventive Medicine*, Aug. 1991
4. Sharrard, W.J.; Sutcliffe, M.G.; Robson, M.J.; and Macachern, A.G., **Treatment of Fibrous Non-Union Fractures by Pulsing Electromagnetic Stimulation**, *Journal of Bone Joint Surgery*, Br., 1982, 64(2):189-93
5. Basset, Andrew, Dr., **Protocol for Electromagnetic Therapy**, Columbia University Orthopaedic Hospital, Presbyterian Medical Center, NYC
6. Begliani, L.V.; Rosenwasser, M.P.; Cavilo, N.; Schink, M.M.; and Basset, C.R., **Pulsing Electromagnetic Fields**, *Journal of Bone Joint Surgery*, 1983, April 64(4):480-5
7. Marcer, M.; Musatti, G.; and Bassett, C.A., **Ununited Fractures**, *Clinical Orthopaedics*, 1984 Nov(190):260-5
8. Bassett, Andrew L., M.D.; ScD; Mitchell, Sharon N., RN; and Gaston, Sawnie R., M.D., **Ununited Fractures and Failed Arthrodeses**, *JAMA* 1982, 247:623-8
9. Bassett, C.A.; Schink-Ascani, M.; and Lewis, S.M., **Steinberg Ratings of Femial Head Osteonecrosis**, *Clinical Orthopaedics*, 1989, September (246):172-85
10. Bender, A.; Par, G.; Hazleman, B.; and Fitton-Jackson, S., **Persistent Rotator Cuff Tendinitis**, *Lancet*, 1984, March 31, 1(8379):695-8
11. Brighton, C.T. and Pollack, S.R., **Treatment of Recalcitrant Non-Union**, *Journal of Bone Surgery*, 1985, April 67(4):577-85
12. Simmons, J.W., **Treatment of Failed Posterior Lumbar**, *Clinical Orthopaedics*, 1985, March (193):127-32
13. Hargreaves, Ann and Lander, Janice, **Use of Transcutaneous Electrical Nerve Stimulation**, May/June 1989
14. Frymoyer, John W., Cats-Baril, William L., **Estimated Direct Cost of Back Pain**, 1990
15. Brighton, Carl T., M.D., **Electrically Induced Osteogenesis**, symposium sponsored by Dept. of Orthopaedic Surgery, Univ. of Pennsylvania, Phil, PA, 1989
16. Connolly, John F., M.D., **Analysis of Consecutive Fractures**, Chairman, Dept. of Orthopaedic Surgery and Rehabilitation, Univ. of Nebraska Medical Center and Chief of Orthopaedic Surgery, Omaha Veteran's Administration Hospital
17. Foley-Nolan, Darrah, M.D., **Treatment of Neck Pain**, Mater Misericordia Hospital, Dublin Ireland, Dept. of Rheumatology and Rehabilitation
18. Windmill, Ian M., Dr., Ph.D, **Facial Nerve Stimulation with Magnetic Fields**, Division of Communicative Disorders, Univ. of Louisville, Kentucky

19. Le Claire, Richard, M.D., Vourgouess, Jean, M.D., **Periarthritis of the Shoulder**, February 1989, Tenth Int'l Conference of Physical Medicine and Rehabilitation, Toronto, Canada

20. Stewart, David and Judith, **Destablization of an Abnormal Physiological Balanced Situation, Chronic Musculoskeletal Pain**, Dept. of Biological Research, Medi-Electronics Research and Development Corp., Loretto, Ontario, Canada, 1989

21. Lud, G.V. and Demeckiy, A.M., Professor, **Use of Permanent Magnetic Fields in Reconstructive Surgery of the Main Artery**, Head of Dept. of Surgery, Vitebsk Medical Institute Vitebsk, USSR, 1990, Acta Chirurgiae Plasticaes

22. Wunch-Bender, F., **The Influence of Static Magnetic Fields on Skin Temperature and Blood Flow in Man**, Dept. of Radiology, Univ. of Kiel Medical School, Federal Republic of Germany, 1984

23. **Emerging Electro-Magnetic Medicine**, Conferences sponsored by FDA at Tulsa University, Tulsa, OK, 1989

24. O'Connor, M.E. and Bentall, N.Y., **Electromagnetic Congress Proceedings**, *Springer-Verlay*, 1990, May:25-8

25. **PEMF for Persistent Neck Pain**, Double-Blind, Placebo Controlled Study of 20 patients, Orthopedics 1990, April, 13(4):445-51

26. **Pulsed Magnetic Fields, Observations, in 353 Patients Suffering from Chronic Pain**, *Minerva, Anestesial*, 1989 July-Aug., 55(7-8): 295-9

27. **The Conservative Treatment of Osteonecrosis of the Femoral Head**, *Clinical Orthopaedics*, 1989, Dec, (249):209-18

28. Taylor, Keith, et al., **Effect of a Single 30 Minute Treatment of High Voltage Pulsed Current on Edema Formation in Frog Hind Limbs**, *Physical Therapy*, Jan, 1992.Vol.72, No.1, p.63

29. Matanoski, O., et al., **Leukemia in Telephone Lineman**, Dept. of Epidemiology, Johns Hopkins Univ., Baltimore, MD., Bio-Electromagnetic Society Annual Meeting, June 23-7, 1991

30. Bassen, Howard, et al., **Reduction of Electric and Magnetic Field Emissions from Electric Blankets**, Center for Devices and Radiological Health, FDA, Rockville, MD, BEMS Annual Meeting, June 1991

31. Phella, A. A., et al., **On the Sensitivity of Cells and Tissues to Electro-Magnetic Fields**, Bioelectrochemistry Laboratory, Dept. of Orthopaedics, Mount Sinai School of Medicine, N.Y., N.Y. and Dept. of Biophysical and Electronic Engineering, Univ. of Genoa, Italy, BEMS Annual Meeting, June 1991

32. Maret, G. and Kiepenheuer, J., **Bioeffects of Steady Magnetic Fields**, Les Houches, France, 1986; 02NLM; OT 34 B6124

33. Isakov, J.F.; Geraskin, U.I.; and Rudokov, S.S., et al., **A New Method of Surgical Treatment of Funnel Chest with Help of Permanent Magnets**, *Chir. Pediatr*, 21/5.361, 1980

34. Batken, Stanley and Tabisah, F.L., **Effects of Alternating Magnetic Fields (12 gauss) of Transplanted Neuroblastoma**, *Res. Comm. in Chem. Path. and Pharm.*, 16/2, 351, 1977

35. Migushima, Y.; Akaoka, I.; and Nishida, Y., **Effects of Magnetic Field on Inflammation**, *Experientia*, 31/12/1411, 1975

Chapter 5

1. Zimmerman, John, Ph.D., Bio-Electric-Magnetics Institute, Reno, NV, interviews 1991-1993
2. Park, Harold, M.D., Vancouver, Washington, interviews Apr. 1992 - Aug. 1993
3. Sun, Camin, Professor @ Beijing Institute of Technology; Stanish, W.D.; and Kozey, J.W., **Test of Therapeutic Electro Membrane**, Orthopaedic and Sport Medicine Clinic, Nova Scotia, Canada, 1990
4. Zablotsky, Ted J., M.D., **The Application of Permanent Magnets in Musculoskeletal Injuries**, Oct. 1989
5. Randall, B.F.; Imig, C.J.; Hines, H.M., **Effects of Some Physical Therapies on Blood Flow**, Arch Phys. Med., 1952, 33:73
6. Gubbins, David and Bloxhan, Jeremy, *Scientific American*, December 1981, pp.71-5
7. Kolm, Henry H. and Freeman, Arthur J., **Intense Magnetic Field**, *Scientific American*, April 1965, pp.66-9
8. Lefebyer, M.; Wiesendanger, M.; Cherlin, D., Blackinton, D.; and Mehta S., **Modulation of Lymphocyte Function in Low Frequency Electric and Magnetic Environments**, *FASEB journal*, Abstract # 2433
9. Terry, H.J., **The Electromagnetic Measurement of Blood Flow During Arterial Surgery**, *Biomed Engineering*, 1970, 7:466-72
10. Broeringmeyer, R. and M., **Energy Training Manual**, *BioHealth Enterprises*, Murray Hill, KY
11. Payne, Buryl, **Getting Started in Magnetic Healing**, Psychophysics Labs, 214 Matt Ave, Santa Cruz, CA, 1988
12. Barnathy, Madeleine F., **Biological Effects of Magnetic Fields**, Vol.I & II, *Plenum Press*, NY & England, 1974
13. Maret, G. and Kiepenhener, J., Editors, **Bio Effects of Steady Magnetic Fields**, O2 NLM, Qt 34, 1986
14. Trappier, Arthur, et al., **Evolving Perspectives on the exposure Risks from Magnetic Fields**, Sept 1990
15. Nakaemo, Kyoichi, **Magnetic Field Deficiency Syndrome and Magnetic Treatment**, *Japanese Medical Journal*, 2745, Dec 4, 1976
16. Philpott, William P., Critical Review of Holger Hannemann's Book, **Magnetic Therapy—Balancing Your Bodies Energy Flow for Self Healing**, *Sterling Publishing Co.*, N.Y., N.Y., 1992
17. Philpott, William P., **Comparisons of Theoretic Formulations, Diagnostic Techniques and Therapy Techniques Between Richard Broeringmeyer and William P. Philpott, Application of Biomagnetics**, 1992
18. Philpott, William P., **A Critical Review and Evaluation of Currently Practiced Magnetic Therapy**, *Philpott Medical Services*, Choctaw, OK, April 1991

Chapter 6
1. Bansal, H.L., M.D., **Magnetic Cure**, 1983, 1990
2. Philpott, William P., **Biomagnetic Handbook**, 1990, reference papers 1991
3. Chokrovertz, Sudhansu, Editor; 49 Authors, **Magnetic Stimulation in Clinical Neurophysiology**, Boston, Butterworths, 1990, ISBN 0-409-90151-2, LC 89-804
4. **Biomagnetism Discipline Opening New Windows on the Workings of the Brain, Heart, and Other Organs**, *Research News*, September 1989, Int'l Conference on Biomagnetism, New York University (Aug 14-18, 1989)
5. Kenko, Nippon; Kenkyukai (KK), Zoshin; and Miyazaki, Akihiro, Professor, **Magnetic Pad Efficacy Test Results**, Kagoshima Univ., 1990-1
6. **Magnetic Water Conditioners**, *U.S. Dept. of Energy*, 1986 study
7. Busch, Kenneth, M.D. Baylor University, January 1992
8. Collins, Denver, State Industries, January 1992
9. **Field Tests of Descaling**, *New Scientist magazine*, City University of London, June 1992

Chapter 7
1. Heimlich, Jean, **What Your Doctor Won't Tell You**
2. **Causes of Cancer**, *Health Journal, Washington Post*, January 14, 1992
3. Heney, Daniel Q., **Breast Cancer and X-rays**, December 26, 1991
4. Becker, Robert O., **The Body Electric**, 1985
5. Sugarman, Carol, **American Dietetic Association Nutrition Survey**, *Health Journal, Washington Post*, December 17, 1991
6. Baghurst, Peter, **Breast Cancer and Fiber**, *Australia Commonwealth Scientific and Industrial Research Organization*
7. **Cholesterol Levels**, *JAMA*, October 1991
8. Barefoot, Robert R. and Riech, Carl M., M.D., **The Calcium Factor**, 1992
9. Hersey Harry, **New Answers to Old Questions**, 1989
10. Philpott, William P. M.D., **Magnetic Handbook**
11. **Osteoporosis Research, Education and Health Promotion**, *U.S. Dept. of Health and Human Services*, Public Health Service, NIH, September 1991
12. **Pioneering Cancer Electrotherapy**, *Medical Tribune*, 1987
13. **Alcohol Detoxification Case Study**, Magnetico Inc., Calgary, Alberta, Canada, February 12, 1992
14. **Case Histories of Symptom Relief and Longer-Term Rehabilitation**, *Nikken Providers and Personal Users*, Taped Interviews and Follow-up, January 1991-March 1992
15. **Case Histories and Evaluation**, *Magnetic X Corp*, Calgary, Alberta, Canada, November 1991-April 1992
16. Jenkins, Richard Dean, **The Healing Power of Magnets**, *Alternative Medicine*, February 1992
17. Santivani, M.T., **The Art of Magnetic Healing**, *B. Jain Publishers*, New Delhi, 1986

18. Holzapfel, E.; Crepan, P.; and Philppe, C., **Magnet Therapy**, *Thorson's Publishing Group*, 1986
19. Horowitz, N. and Stavish, S., **Pioneering Cancer Electrotherapy**, *Medical Tribune*, 1987
20. **Unconventional Cancer Treatments**, *Office of Technology Assessment*, 1989-90
21. Philpott, William H., **Brain Allergies**, 1980
22. Patterson, Margaret A., **Effects of Neuro-Electric Therapy in Drug Addiction**, Bulletin on Narcotics, London, England, Vol.XXVIII, No.4, October-December 1976
23. Wen, H.L. and Cheung, S.Y.C., **Treatment of Drug Addiction by Acupuncture and Electrical Stimulation**, *Asian Journal of Medicine*, 1973, 9:138-41
24. Sainsbury, M.J., **Acupuncture in Heroin Withdrawal**, *Medical Journal of Australia*, 1974, 2:102-5

Chapter 8
1. Breggen, Peter R., **Toxic Psychiatry**
2. Jenkins, Richard Dean, **Healing Power of Magnets**, *Fitness Magazine*, February 1992
3. Myozaki, Akikero, **Magnetic Pad Efficacy Test Results**, Kugoshima University School of Medicine, Japan
4. Park, Harry, Interview October, 1992
5. Tyler, Paul, **EMR and the Brain; A Brief Literature Review**, FDA Conference, 1990
6. Patterson, Margaret A., M.D., **Bulletin on Narcotics**, October-December 1976, Vol.XXVIII, No.4

Chapter 9
1. Cohn, Victor, **Cost Control Programs**, *Health Journal, Washington Post*, February 25, 1992
2. Wolfe, Sidney M., *Washington Post*, January 19, 1992
3. Ferguson, Tom, M.D., **Patient, Heal Thyself**, *Futurist*, January-February 1992
4. **American Health Foundation: Benefits of Exercise**, *Health Journal, Washington Post*, January 14, 1992
5. Chokroverty, Suahansu, et al., **Magnetic Stimulation in Clinical Neurophysiology**, Boston Butterworths, 1990, ISBN 0-409-90151-2, LC 89-804
6. Tassinari, C.A., **Epileptic**, *Neurology*, July 1990, 40(7):1132-3
7. Delpizzo, Vincent and Keam, Donall, **Carcinogenic Potential**, Australian Radiation Laboratory, February 1989, ARL/T Ro82 OJ NLU: Qt 34 C265
8. *Washington Post*, May 6, 1993, p.A17
9. *Health Journal, Washington Post*, May 11, 1993, p.8
10. Rosenbaum, Maj-Britt, M.D., **Doctor, Doctor**, *Mademoiselle*, February 1993, p.96
11. Hallett, Mark, M.D. and Cohen, Leonard, M.D., **A New Method for Stimulation of Nerve and Brain**, *Journal of American Medical Association*, Vol.262:4, July 28, 1989

12. *Health Journal, Washington Post*, October 1991, March 6, 1992; February 25, 1992; January 14, 1992; December 24, 1992
13. Becker, Robert O., M.D., **The Body Electric**, 1985
14. *Havard Health Letter*, August 1991
15. Gazette, Gaithersburg and Hackman, Fyllis, December 1991
16. **Pathways** (Winter 1991-2)
17. Redfearn, J.W.T. and Lippold, O.C.J., **A Preliminary Account of the Clinical Effects of Polarizing the Brain in Certain Psychiatric Disorders**, *British Journal of Psychiatry*, 1964, Vol.110, p.773
18. Lippold, O.C.J. and Redfearn, J.W.T., **Mental Changes Resulting from the Passage of Small Direct Currents through the Human Brain**, *British Journal of Psychiatry*, 1964, Vol.110, p.76

Chapter 10

1. Goldstein, J.A., M.D., **Could Your Doctor be Wrong?**, 1989
2. Weil, Andrew, M.D., **Natural Health, Natural Medicine**, 1990
3. Fontenot, J.N., and Levine, S.A., **Melatonin Deficiency: Its Role in Oncogenesis and Age-Related Pathology**, *Journal of Orthomolecular Medicine*, December 1, 1991, Vol.5 No.1
4. Daniels, O.H. and Martin, J.B., **Growth Hormone, Harrison's Principles of Internal Medicine**, 11th Edition, 1987, pp.1701-5
5. Semm, P., **Magnetic Sensitivity of Pineal Gland**, Nature, 1980, 228:206
6. Weide, Zhory, **The Effects of Growth of Hela Cells Due to Strong Exposure to Constant Magnetic Fields**, Life Science Lab., Shenzhen University, Shenzhen, China, BEMS Annual Meeting, June 1991
7. Erman, Milton, et al., **Low-Energy Emission Therapy Treatment for Insomnia**, Division of Sleep Disorders, Scripps Clinic and Research Foundation, La Jolla, CA, BEMS Annual Meeting, June 1991
8. Kato, Masamichi, et al., **Effects of 50 Hertz Rotating Magnetic Fields on Melatonin Secretion of RAT**, Dept. of Physiology, Hokkaido Univ., School of Medicine, Criepi, Japan, BEMS, June 1991

INDEX

For information on where to obtain additional copies of this book or background knowledge on the sources, or for other questions, please write or call:

 NOVA Publishing Company
11607 Nebel Street
Rockville, MD 20852

Phone: 1-800-637-0067 or 301-231-8229
Fax: 301-816-0816

ISBN 0-9639560-1-9